STATISTICS IN THE PHARMACEUTICAL INDUSTRY

THIRD EDITION

Biostatistics: A Series of References and Textbooks

Series Editor
Shein-Chung Chow
Duke University School of Medicine
Department of Biostatistics and Bioinformatics
Durham, NC, USA

1. *Design and Analysis of Animal Studies in Pharmaceutical Development,* Shein-Chung Chow and Jen-pei Liu
2. *Basic Statistics and Pharmaceutical Statistical Applications,* James E. De Muth
3. *Design and Analysis of Bioavailability and Bioequivalence Studies, Second Edition, Revised and Expanded,* Shein-Chung Chow and Jen-pei Liu
4. *Meta-Analysis in Medicine and Health Policy,* Dalene K. Stangl and Donald A. Berry
5. *Generalized Linear Models: A Bayesian Perspective,* Dipak K. Dey, Sujit K. Ghosh, and Bani K. Mallick
6. *Difference Equations with Public Health Applications,* Lemuel A. Moyé and Asha Seth Kapadia
7. *Medical Biostatistics,* Abhaya Indrayan and Sanjeev B. Sarmukaddam
8. *Statistical Methods for Clinical Trials,* Mark X. Norleans
9. *Causal Analysis in Biomedicine and Epidemiology: Based on Minimal Sufficient Causation,* Mikel Aickin
10. *Statistics in Drug Research: Methodologies and Recent Developments,* Shein-Chung Chow and Jun Shao
11. *Sample Size Calculations in Clinical Research,* Shein-Chung Chow, Jun Shao, and Hansheng Wang
12. *Applied Statistical Design for the Researcher,* Daryl S. Paulson
13. *Advances in Clinical Trial Biostatistics,* Nancy L. Geller
14. *Statistics in the Pharmaceutical Industry, 3rd Edition,* Ralph Buncher and Jia-Yeong Tsay
15. *DNA Microarrays and Related Genomics Techniques: Design, Analysis, and Interpretation of Experiments,* David B. Allsion, Grier P. Page, T. Mark Beasley, and Jode W. Edwards

STATISTICS IN THE PHARMACEUTICAL INDUSTRY

THIRD EDITION

EDITED BY

C. RALPH BUNCHER
University of Cincinnati Medical Center
Cincinnati, OH, U.S.A.

JIA-YEONG TSAY
Organon Pharmaceuticals U.S.A., Inc.
Roseland, NJ

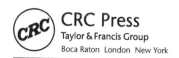

CRC Press
Taylor & Francis Group
Boca Raton London New York

CRC Press is an imprint of the
Taylor & Francis Group, an **informa** business
A CHAPMAN & HALL BOOK

First published 2006 by Chapman & Hall

Published 2019 CRC Press
Taylor & Francis Group
6000 Broken Sound Parkway NW, Suite 300
Boca Raton, FL 33487-2742

First issued in paperback 2022

ISBN 13: 978-1-03-247787-9 (pbk)
ISBN 13: 978-0-8247-5469-3 (hbk)

DOI: 10.1201/9781315275888

Library of Congress Card Number 2005043985

Library of Congress Cataloging-in-Publication Data

Statistics in the pharmaceutical industry / [edited by] C. Ralph Buncher, Jia-Yeong Tsay.-- 3rd ed.
    p. cm. -- (Biostatics ; 14)
  ISBN 0-8247-5469-7 (alk. paper)
  1. Pharmacy--Statistical methods. 2. Pharmaceutical industry--Statistical methods. 3. Drugs--Testing. I. Buncher, C. Ralph (Charles Ralph), 1938- II. Tsay, Jia-Yeong, 1944- III. Biostatistics
(New York, N.Y.)
RS57.S8 2005   2005043985

Visit the Taylor & Francis Web site at
http://www.taylorandfrancis.com

and the CRC Press Web site at
http://www.crcpress.com

To Maxine and Tung-Ying

Series Introduction

The primary objectives of the Biostatistics Book Series are to provide useful reference books for researchers and scientists in academia, industry, and government, and also to offer textbooks for undergraduate or graduate courses in the area of biostatistics. This book series will provide comprehensive and unified presentations of statistical designs and analyses of important applications in biostatistics, such as those in biopharmaceuticals. A well-balanced summary will be given of current and recently developed statistical methods and interpretations for both statisticians and researchers or scientists with minimal statistical knowledge who are engaged in the field of applied biostatistics. The series is committed to providing easy-to-understand, state-of-the-art references and textbooks. In each volume, statistical concepts and methodologies will be illustrated through real world examples.

As indicated by the authors of this volume, there is a rapid change in pharmaceutical research and development since the publication of the second edition of this book. New concepts and advanced technologies have enabled more flexible and efficient pharmaceutical research and development in the past decade. These new concepts and advanced technologies include the use of adaptive (or flexible) design in early phase of clinical research and development, the determination of non-inferiority margin in non-inferiority trials for proving superiority over placebo, and the establishment of a predictive clinical model using genomic data for personalized medicine. Similar to previous editions, this volume provides a well-balanced summarization of statistical designs and analyses that are commonly encountered in pharmaceutical research and development. It covers important topics in pharmaceutical research and development such as clinical trial designs, interim analysis and adaptive design in clinical trials, post-marking studies and adverse drug experiences, statistical challenges in pharmacogenomics, and global harmonization of drug development. As a result, it can serve as not only a textbook for a course in biopharmaceutical statistics at senior level of undergraduate or graduate level but also as a useful reference book for pharmaceutical scientists and researchers in the health related area. In addition, this volume also provides pharmaceutical scientists and researchers an innovative way of thinking for evaluation of the effectiveness and safety of an investigational new drug or therapy. It would be beneficial to biostatisticians and pharmaceutical scientists and researchers who are engaged in the areas of pharmaceutical research and development.

Shein-Chung Chow

Preface to the Third Edition

Wow — and we thought that the decade from the first to the second edition was one of rapid change. The changes in the pharmaceutical industry in the last decade, from the second to this third edition, have been even more enormous. For example, the industry and all of its thinking have become global so that planning from the very beginning of a new drug to its marketing are done on an international basis. The regulatory authorities have made great strides in harmonization so that there are fewer small and time consuming differences from one country to another. Computer power has permitted an increased level of statistical sophistication in analyses and in improved communication over the internet and intranet. Now one designs clinical trials that are adaptive and thus provide flexibility and also raise interesting new statistical issues of validity. Proving superiority over placebo is becoming less important and trials that show equivalence with (or superiority to) a known effective medication are thus more common and important.

This book then tries to convey the excitement of the pharmaceutical industry to an audience including those who work there on the industry side or the regulatory authorities who review the work of the industry and wish to learn about a different area, to those who may work there in the future and wish to learn more about the industry before making that decision, and to those who just wish to understand more about the role of statistics in this research and these companies. These chapters are written by those on the front lines in the industry and at the regulatory agencies. The views of those who originate the statistics and those who then evaluate the analysis are both here. While their roles may give these statisticians different viewpoints, their goals are the same: see that studies are designed to prove safety and efficacy and good manufacturing and find new medications that are marketable while weeding out the chemical candidates that have some defect. The answers vary with different classes of drugs and this variety is also illustrated in this volume.

We the editors express our thanks to the authors of these chapters who have recorded their knowledge and experience to make it easier for others to achieve the same level with fewer hurdles. The sophistication of the authors' thinking has been a blessing to the editors.

C. Ralph Buncher
Jia-Yeong Tsay

Preface to the Second Edition

This volume started out as a simple revision which was to become the second edition of our book *Statistics in the Pharmaceutical Industry*. Then the appreciation of the enormous changes in the industry in recent years emerged.

In a decade of rapid change in this field, have come, in large numbers, the new initials of PCs (personal computers), CANDAs (computer-assisted new drug applications), CROs (contract research organizations), AIDS (acquired immunodeficiency syndrome), as well as biotechnology, biomonitoring, pharmacoepidemiology, molecular biology, meta-analysis, designer drugs, international planning, work stations, and so forth. Diseases for which there was no pharmaceutical therapy are now routinely treated, and the expectation is that new genetic and molecular knowledge will make possible treatment for virtually all diseases.

The result is that this book not only was completely revised by updating every chapter from the first edition, but also was expanded by adding many chapters to cover new areas that were still in their infancy during the development of the first edition. We believe that reading this book will enlighten readers—be they students in statistics, faculty members, statisticians, OS nonstatisticians—about the pharmaceutical industry and the many roles played by the biostatistician within that industry. Even those readers with background in the industry may find interesting ideas in the words of others whose experience may differ from their own.

We wish to thank the authors of these chapters who used their practical knowledge to make this revision possible. They have many years of experience in the pharmaceutical industry, whether working for government or industry or both. Their efforts will enable the reader to speed the process of building experience and understanding.

We thank the many people at Marcel Dekker, Inc., who have worked on this book and helped bring it to fruition. We also thank Brenda Riggins in the Division of Biostatistics at the University of Cincinnati for her special efforts which facilitated this volume.

C. Ralph Buncher
Jia-Yeong Tsay

Preface to the First Edition

This book is the culmination of many years of difficult work by numerous people. The idea of a book devoted to the lessons learned by those working in the pharmaceutical field had its genesis in 1973. After an initial flare of interest, the idea lay dormant for three or four years. Then the current group was assembled to bring the thought to fruition. Even this final stage has taken a number of years for all of the usual reasons associated with busy persons trying to put together a volume while also having the rest of their duties undiminished. We are proud that this book fulfills most of our dreams.

AUDIENCE FOR THIS BOOK

For whom is this book written? The editors and authors have discussed this question extensively, especially since this is the first book that we know of devoted to applied statistics in the pharmaceutical industry. We agreed to keep in mind four audiences in particular as the chapters were written.

The principal audience for this book is the graduate student in statistics or biostatistics. We believe that these students can use this volume to find out much more than is currently available about opportunities in the pharmaceutical industry, which is one of the major employers of biostatisticians. It is hoped that some academic institutions will choose to use this volume as a textbook in a seminar type of course, perhaps held jointly with students in pharmacology, pharmacy, or research methods. Secondly, the book has been sprinkled with topics that the authors believe would be good thesis subjects for those who are looking for work which will be of use and interest to others. Finally, we believe that this book provides much general information on applied statistics which will help enlarge the perspective of the student training for a career in the field of statistics, whether that field is on the applied side or in the theoretical world. Many new employees in the pharmaceutical industry also fit into this category.

A second audience for this book consists of the statistics faculty members who have had little or no acquaintance with the pharmaceutical industry. We believe that these statisticians, who have a wider perspective and a greater depth of experience than the students, will be able to sort out which problems in the industry are similar to problems that they are already working on and which problems are relatively unique to the industry. We all agree that there are many valuable contributions that academic statisticians could make toward solving problems facing the pharmaceutical industry. We hope that this book will help provide a greater bridge between industry and academia.

A third audience for this book consists of other persons interested in the pharmaceutical industry who are not statisticians. Many of the chapters in this book can be read and understood by those with no statistical training or only minimal training in statistics. We are thinking of those working in clinical fields, pharmacology, chemistry, quality control, company management, legal departments, and data managers. Each of these persons can find a wealth of experience summarized and presented. These lessons are explained in the hope that other professionals will not have to relearn problems and pitfalls that exist for almost every drug and almost every company. Clearly, members of regulatory agencies and persons wishing to know more about the inner workings of the pharmaceutical industry also fit into this category.

Finally, we believe that the pharmaceutical industry currently documents its statistical and other evidence better than any other segment of our society. As more and more comparable problems—for example, concerns with the value and safety of nontherapeutic chemicals and other environmental agents—become greater concerns for industry and regulatory agencies, we foresee that parts of industry and government other than the pharmaceutical industry and the Food and Drug Administration will be doing the same extensive work and documentation that has been pioneered in the pharmaceutical industry. We think that those other industrial/governmental interfaces will profit by learning the lessons of the pharmaceutical industry and applying them in their own spheres as appropriate.

READING THIS BOOK

Chapter 1 describes the development of a chemical into a new drug for those unfamiliar with the process or with the vocabulary of the industry. The other chapters are in chronological order with respect to drug development.

This book has been written with the idea that many if not most readers will read only a few chapters. We recommend that those unfamiliar with the industry read the introductory chapter and then a few of current interest. It is hoped that after learning some of the material, the reader will find additional chapters to be of interest and will pick up the volume again to gain additional insight and perspective.

This book has been designed to show many of the problems and solutions of the statistical portion of the biopharmaceutical industry. The principal emphasis throughout is on the problems that occur and the solutions that are used in practice rather than in theory. The chapters in this book are written with the personal experiences of the authors in the pharmaceutical industry in mind. Thus the book manifests a diversity in subject matter as well as style and attitude toward statistical problems.

An attempt has been made to explain the problems discussed in each chapter before describing some of the solutions. As in most areas of human endeavor, it is easy to miss some of the subtleties of the problem if one has never been exposed to it. Thus the book does require some sophistication in understanding the problems of finding out the truth about a drug, forming impressions of the truth when only part of the data is at hand, convincing others that your understanding of the situation is the correct one, and documenting the material so that an outside reviewer (even one who may be a doubter) can be convinced that a pharmaceutical product is sufficiently safe and efficacious or, in other words, sufficiently well understood to be suitable for marketing.

We thank the authors of these chapters for their cooperation and help during this project. Special thanks go to Charlie Dunnett for key suggestions in this process. Two other persons not mentioned elsewhere were essential to the successful completion of this project. They are Hannah Aron and Elaine Sirkoski who are Staff Assistants in the Division of Biostatistics and Epidemiology at the University of Cincinnati. They did much of the organizing and communicating and all of the typing of this final copy. We thank Hannah and Elaine for a superior job well done.

C. Ralph Buncher
Jia-Yeong Tsay

Contributors

Mirza W. Ali
Otsuka Maryland Research
  Institute, Inc.
Rockville, Maryland

Ronald J. Bosch
Department of Biostatistics
Harvard School of Public Health
Boston, Massachusetts

C. Ralph Buncher
University of Cincinnati College
  of Medicine
Cincinnati, Ohio

Chi-wan Chen
Center for Drug Evaluation and
  Research
Food and Drug Administration
Rockville, Maryland

T. Timothy Chen
National Cancer Institute
National Institutes of Health
Bethesda, Maryland

Wen Jen Chen
Center for Drug Evaluation and
  Research
Food and Drug Administration
Rockville, Maryland

Yusong Chen
Biostatistics/QDS
Wilmington, Delaware

George Y. H. Chi
Clinical Biostatistics/Hematology
  and Oncology
Johnson and Johnson
  Pharmaceutical Research
  & Development, L.L.C.
Raritan, New Jersey

John Constant
Global Product Development
  Services
PRA International
Vancouver, BC, Canada

Satya D. Dubey
Office of Biostatistics (HFD-700)
Food and Drug Administration
Rockville, Maryland

Charles W. Dunnett
Department of Epidemiology
  and Biostatistics
McMaster University
Hamilton, ON, Canada

Peter H. van Ewijk
Clinical Trial Operations
N.V. Organon, The Netherlands

Roger E. Flora
Global Product Development
  Service
PRA International
Richmond, Virginia

Charles H. Goldsmith
Department of Epidemiology and
    Biostatistics
McMaster Universtiy
Hamilton, ON, Canada

Paul S. Horn
Department of Mathematics
University of Cincinnati
Cincinnati, Ohio

Bernhard Huitfeldt
AstraZeneca R&D
Global Clinical Science
Sweden

Irving K. Hwang
School of Public Health,
    UMDNJ
Irving Consulting Group
Pluckemin, New Jersey

Roswitha E. Kelly
Division of Biometrics
    1 (HFD-710)
Food and Drug Administration
Rockville, Maryland

K. K. Gordon Lan
Adventis Pharmaceuticals
Bridgewater, New Jersey

Daphne T. Lin
Center for Drug Evaluation and
    Research
Food and Drug Administration
Rockville, Maryland

Karl K. Lin
Center for Drug Evaluation and
    Research
Food and Drug Administration
Rockville, Maryland

Qing Liu
Statistical Science
Johnson and Johnson Pharmaceutical
    Research and Development
Titusville, New Jersey

Cynthia G. McCormick
Food and Drug Administration
Bethesda, Maryland

Mamoru Narukawa
First International Organization
    Division
Economic Affairs Bureau
Ministry of Foreign Affairs
Tokyo, Japan

Robert T. O'Neill
Office of Biostatistics
Rockville, Maryland

Amadeo J. Pesce
Department of Pathology
University of Cincinnati
Cincinnati, Ohio

Gordon Pledger
Statistical Science
Johnson and Johnson Pharmaceutical
    Research and Development
Titusville, New Jersey

C. Frank Shen
Exploratory Development, Global
    Biostatistics and Programming
Bristol-Myers Squibb Co.
Princeton, New Jersey

Weichung Joe Shih
Division of Biometrics
University of Medicine and Dentistry
    of New Jersey
New Brunswick, New Jersey

Ted M. Smith
Auxilium Pharmaceuticals
Norristown, Pennsylvania

Masahiro Takeuchi
Division of Biostatistics
Kitasato University
   Graduate School
Tokyo, Japan

Jia-Yeong Tsay
Clinical Trial Operations
Organon Pharmaceuticals
   USA Inc.
Roseland, New Jersey

Yi Tsong
Center for Drug Evaluation and
   Research
Food and Drug Administration
Rockville, Maryland

Lianng Yuh
Antigenics
Lexington, Massachusetts

Kim E. Zerba
Statistical Genetics and Biomarkers
Clinical Discovery Biostatistics and
   Data Management
Bristol-Myers Squibb Co.
Princeton, New Jersey

Table of Contents

1 Introduction to the Evolution of Pharmaceutical Products

C. Ralph Buncher and Jia-Yeong Tsay

CONTENTS

I. INTRODUCTION

There are many amazing statistics about the pharmaceutical industry. A United States government agency has announced that almost half of the people in the country used a prescribed pharmaceutical product in the last month.[1] On an age-specific basis, this usage includes one quarter of children, more than 60% of middle aged adults and more than 80% of older adults. One in six people used three or more drugs including almost half of those aged 65 and over. This is an amazing testimony to the accomplishments of the scientists working in this industry and producing effective and valuable medications over the last half century — although some doubters would give much of the credit to improved marketing.

These achievements do not come without great expenditure. DiMasi et al.[2] report that the "estimated average out-of-pocket cost per new drug is US $403 million" although total costs may be twice as high. Clearly this is an industry that requires tremendous resources of both money and people.

In addition to the tremendous productivity of the industry, there has also been a tremendous amount of structural change. Perhaps the largest change of the last decade or so is the emphasis on globalization instead of the more traditional country by country approach. One of the major improvements is that the regulatory authorities of various countries, and particularly the United States (U.S.), European Union (E.U.), and Japan, have worked to bring their rules into line with each other so that more of the research and development data can be applied to fulfill requirements in multiple countries. This streamlining of the system should make global drug development more efficient and less costly.

One of the most profound effects on international drug development from globalization is the establishment of various International Conference on Harmonization (ICH) guidelines. Through these ICH guidelines the E.U., U.S., and Japanese regulatory authorities will use similar rules and regulations with much of the common data for the new drug application for marketing in these regions. ICH-M4[3] provides guidance for the Common Technical Documents (CTD) that may be submitted to E.U., U.S., and Japanese regions for submitting marketing applications. The CTD consists of five modules. Module 1 is region specific and for regional administration information. Modules 2 to 5 are technical parts and intended to be common for the three regions.

Also there is more offshore outsourcing such as more pharmaceutical companies having their data entry or data management done in India or China. This trend seems to be gradually becoming the norm for major pharmaceutical companies. The results of offshore outsourcing show that it provides reduced cycle times, error rates, and costs. More recently some companies have expanded their offshore outsourcing into biostatistical operations as indicated by Mehra[4] who presents some success stories on offshore outsourcing in data management and biostatistics.

Part of the globalization effort has involved restructuring of companies. Companies have merged and purchased each other at a rapid rate. For example, most of the companies represented by the authors of the first edition of this book are no longer distinct entities. These mergers offer the positive benefit of each company learning the best practices of the other with the usual overtones of power struggles and defending of one's "turf". The result seems to be a continued vibrant industry that will continue to produce more valuable drugs to treat and cure the ills to which the human body is subject.

Another important change is the standard to prove efficacy. In times past, one used a placebo as the basic concurrent control; subject to the usual concerns for ethical treatment, i.e., one did not stop a patient from taking a physiologically important medication. In the current world, the number of physiologically important medications has grown to such an extent that those planning clinical trials now must frequently, if not usually, design trials to compare the new medication with a standard active drug. According to McGinn[5] an article in the revised Declaration of Helsinki states that "an experimental treatment should always be compared against the best available treatment. Only when there is no such treatment available anywhere in the world can a new drug be compared against a placebo." This transition has led to trials that emphasize proving noninferiority or equivalence to an active medication rather than superiority over a placebo. Statisticians trained in alpha and beta errors of hypothesis testing immediately realize that proving noninferiority or equivalence is statistically a very different package. For further details, readers are referred to Chapter 12.

One of the products of this type of methodological research is a greater emphasis on adaptive clinical trials (see Chapters 13 and 14). The old concept of doing a study while everyone is in a completely blindfold condition has given way to the Data and Safety Monitoring Committees. These committees have the role of deciding in the middle of the study whether the study should continue or be stopped early. The standard situations for stopping early, even if they are not common occurrences, are: efficacy has already been proven, side effects are too severe in one group, or the results are so far from the desired outcome that the goal will not be achieved in the time remaining.

One obvious conclusion from these statements is that the statistical analysis is now more complicated and complex than in past times. Ubiquitous statistical software has enabled more complex analyses to become routine. More is expected from the analysis than in past times. Subgroups need to be studied and various alternatives considered before the analysis is considered complete. This is particularly so in the large global trial, which may be sufficient to provide required evidence of efficacy by a single trial for the new drug application (NDA), if adequate subgroups can be proved to be statistically significant.[6] The ultimate goal is finding identifiable subgroups in the data set that can have different standards of treatment set for them. Thus, for one example, if one can identify those who metabolize the drug slowly, they can be given smaller doses than the standard and those who metabolize rapidly can be given larger doses. While these attempts at Pharmacogenomics and "Individualized Drug Therapy" are ongoing and "more than 800 pharmacogenetics/genomics reviews" have been published, no one should underestimate the problems in making this a part of routine medicine.[7]

A number of statistical tools that were once novel have become mainstream and are used routinely, as appropriate. These include generalized estimating equations, several varieties of multivariate analysis, and mixed models. We should also note that this sophisticated analysis of data, especially the efficacy data, is an excellent example of the increased productivity that the hardware and software enable. (By the way, do you know that the originator of the term "software" was the late and great statistician John Tukey?)

Knowledge is the seed from which new drug preparations are grown. Molecular studies in biology are blossoming forth at such exceptional speed that new knowledge is created daily. The enterprising and astute are capable of using this new knowledge as a springboard towards new pharmaceutical products. The new products mean better health for the public and possible prosperity for the company that develops the product.

Thus the key decision points are: (i) whether we the sponsors are convinced that we should test this new molecular entity in humans based on results from animal and laboratory studies only, (ii) whether we the sponsors are convinced that the drug works and is safe in humans, (iii) whether we the sponsors now have sufficient information to convince the Food and Drug Administration (FDA) and regulatory authorities in other countries and the medical community that this medication as we now manufacture is safe and effective, and (iv) whether the FDA and other regulatory authorities will approve the drug for marketing.

II. MOLECULAR BIOLOGY

In the last decade, the ability to understand the role of individual chemicals, which can cause or prevent disease, has increased faster than at any time in human history. Much of this knowledge has been generated through studies of the genetic material, the proteins created from genes, and the role played by each. Collectively, this work is called "Molecular Biology" and involves proteins through concepts such as proteomics. Those who work in molecular biology are converting these theoretical concepts into realities and statisticians are measuring the progress.

Most statisticians working in the industry get to learn and be proficient in some of the biologic and medical terminology even if they have never learned it during their prior education. One can read statements such as "until recently, it was common practice for a pharmaceutical company to market a chiral drug as the racemate".[8] In this case one needs to know that if there are four different chemical groups attached to a carbon atom, then two mirror-image forms called enantiomers or optical isomers are possible. These are chiral drugs. Generally, Nature creates just one of them but human manufacturing creates both in equal numbers which is a "racemic" mixture. Usually only one form is of therapeutic value but both can cause side effects. If the manufacturing process is able to produce only the form that is therapeutic, then the incidence of side effects will be reduced.

This explosion in molecular biology is one of the great changes in the last decade in the pharmaceutical industry that we have identified. Another by-product of molecular biology is the proliferation of smaller companies consisting of only a small number of researchers who are experts in a niche area of medicine and chemistry. Through molecular biologic techniques, these researchers can produce a new candidate drug. With the help of other companies, they can develop this candidate into a new drug, or they can sell or out-license the medication to another, usually larger, company that will undertake the approval process. Alternatively, the company may be purchased by a larger company because of the value of the new drug candidate.

Another major change in the last decade is the use of computing equipment. The new machines, and the wondrous software also now available, give the statistician instant ability to explore data sets, to represent the data graphically, to calculate results, do an influence analysis, and to do other complex analyses. As a result the level of sophistication in statistical analysis is much higher because of the ability to do more extensive analysis and because of the desire to see those alternatives. Thus one can present alternative analyses with difficult patients both in and out to see if there are any qualitative differences, one can differentially weight the observations, one can see what happens if you omit an investigator from a combined analysis, and one can do formal or informal meta-analysis of the results. Concepts such as data mining and bioinformatics have become part of the vocabulary of statisticians in this industry.

Many potential problems arise because a statistician in the pharmaceutical industry produces data that are to be evaluated by other statisticians, particularly those at the FDA. Anyone who has ever tried to review a major work of another statistical analyst realizes that there are important points to be resolved. The first major point concerns the ability to follow a complex analysis, because most statistical work is only reported in a skeletal outline. One needs to be able to follow exactly which patients were included in the analysis. Were all data points used, or were some outliers rejected, presumably for valid reasons?

Moreover, the ability to store and retrieve alternative analyses makes the system effective. These abilities have led in turn to the desire to transmit all of this information intact from the sponsor's statisticians to those of the FDA. Statisticians at the FDA usually want to pursue their own alternatives in analyzing a data set rather than just checking the analysis of others. This sequence of events can be facilitated by the electronic format of the NDA submission. We note that electronic storage devices change about once a decade and that two decades later it may be impossible to read the files that have been stored for future reference. Thus every group must consider every five to ten years whether data that was previously stored must be stored again on a newer electronic storage device.

Another trend in the last decade is the ability to monitor drug levels and the effects of medications in various body fluids and tissues. More and more, physicians are able to take into account the characteristics of individual patients and thus to tailor doses to just the right level for each. The sources of variation in optimal dose can be genetic differences, such as different varieties of the same enzyme, or different physical characteristics, such as differences in body weight. While statisticians find the variance to be informative, physicians find that variation is mostly a problem in optimal therapy. By tailoring doses of medication, the physicians improve their ability to treat but at times make the statistician's job a little more challenging. These abilities to make informative extra measurements and the resulting explosion of data to be analyzed also make the statistician's job more interesting.

The final trend in the last decade is seen to be the changes in the structure of the industry. The pharmaceutical industry no longer is focused within individual countries but rather it has become an international marketplace with efficacy and safety research focused on the world market. Much of Europe is now one unit rather than many separate countries. Thus, the old information problem was how do we best get safety and efficacy information in this one country;

now the question is more like the following: in which country should we do each piece of research to optimize our opportunities to do research, our costs, the information we obtain, and the information necessary to convince the authorities in many lands to let us market the medication. Optimizing the research has also resulted in restructuring within the companies. Thus companies that used to do all of the work themselves will now frequently, if not always, use outside contractors to carry out some or all of the research and statistical functions that used to be internal. A whole new sub-industry has grown up of Contract Research Organizations which include, among other capabilities, all of the statistical functions necessary in clinical trial research. Chapter 18 contains more information on this subject.

III. ISSUES IN DRUG DEVELOPMENT

This first chapter attempts to accomplish three tasks. The first is to outline briefly the steps involved in the pharmaceutical industry from creation of a new molecular compound in the laboratory until, for some tiny fraction of those compounds, a new drug is available on the market. Bouckenooghe[9] estimates that "out of 10,000 molecules discovered, synthesized, and screened, only about 50 are found to have potential as a drug and progress to preclinical *in vitro* and animal testing. Further, only 10 make it to Phase I and just three make it to Phase II, leading hopefully to one product that can get licensed as a human medicine." This brief description is primarily to allow those unfamiliar with the process to have a better idea of the many interrelated steps involved in this long and frequently unsuccessful effort. Second, the outline will emphasize the role of the statistician in each of these phases, because that is a purpose of this volume. Finally, the chapters in this book will be introduced at the point that the description of the development of a new drug relates to that chapter.

There are three main issues in drug development: safety, efficacy, and manufacturing. Safety must first be proven in cell based and whole animal research before a drug is permitted to be used in humans. Then the safety must again be proven in humans to justify long-term clinical rather than experimental use of a drug. Finally, after the drug has been approved for marketing, investigators will search for rare side effects of a drug in those patients who have used the drug. Efficacy must be proven in clinical testing of a drug for the medical purpose intended in typical groups of patients. Prior to this time, a chemical has been selected because it has been found to be "active" in some subhuman biologic screen or because of considerations in molecular biology or chemical structural analysis. After success in screening, this chemical has been sufficiently tested in animals so that one can infer that the drug is likely to be clinically useful in humans. Finally, a drug must be manufactured. What was once a newly active chemical created by molecular biologists or chemists in a laboratory must be produced in a pilot plant operation and then later manufactured in large batches with careful quality control so that each individual dose of the medication will exhibit the high standards of safety and efficacy expected.

Obviously, these developments are not made independently of each other. A drug that does not dissolve as intended may show restricted efficacy, for example, relief of pain for only two hours rather than the intended eight hours. Reformulation of the medication might serve to improve the efficacy. Drug side effects may disappear if the medication is given at mealtime or at bedtime and as a result enhance efficacy. A drug that has been found to be highly efficacious and easy to manufacture may turn out on lifetime toxicity testing to cause malignant tumors in rats, thus abruptly ending a research program.

Currently one thinks of a typical duration of time from creation of the chemical structure in the laboratory until a drug is marketed to be on the order of 7 to 12 years. Safety, efficacy, and marketing are each studied for a majority of that period; however, proving safety requires the most time. On the time scale, the lifetime of a drug may be divided into: preclinical time, the period from creation of the chemical to its first use in humans; clinical studies, during which time the drug is being tested in humans; and finally post-approval, during which time the drug is being sold commercially.

In the preclinical stage, one must learn about the characteristics of the drug to such an extent that it makes good sense to the sponsor (pharmaceutical company) and to the Federal FDA to try this drug in human beings. In order to reach this stage, the sponsor must be reasonably sure of the drug as shown in various tests of cell preparations and short-term animal toxicity testing in at least two species. Also, the sponsor will want to know that there is a reasonable indication that the drug will have the desired positive effect as predicted by tests in animal species and known molecular configurations.

Finally, the sponsor will have to be able to manufacture test lots of the proposed medication so questions of dosage form and amount and procedure for the preparation must be resolved. Typically, these experimental quantities of the drug will be made in a pilot plant operation or in special laboratories that make sufficient quantities of the drug for experimental purposes. As a by-product of this research, the sponsor will have studied the metabolism of the drug in animals to know whether it accumulates in the tissues or whether it is excreted rapidly. Likewise, questions about the active form of the drug, whether it is the parent compound or some metabolite of it, will have been tentatively answered. Doses that have been proven effective in animals will be extrapolated to the likely therapeutic human dose and then to a fraction of that dose to provide a margin of safety for initial testing.

All of this material is carefully written up by the sponsor and submitted to the U.S. Food and Drug Administration or regulatory authority in another country to ask for an exemption so that the chemical may be tested in humans as an Investigational New Drug (IND). This submission is usually called submission for an IND. Regulations allow the FDA 30 days in which to deny the IND or to ask additional questions that were not adequately answered in the submission.

The clinical trials before drug approval are divided into three categories: Phase I, Phase II, and Phase III. Phase I studies are the earliest studies in humans, involving perhaps 20 to 80 subjects in total. Usually these persons are healthy volunteers. Questions to be answered concern the short-term toxicity of the drug in clinical pharmacology studies that provide data concerning absorption, distribution, metabolism, and excretion (ADME) of the drug and which establish the safe dosage range for the drug as well as likely side effects; occasionally some inferences regarding effectiveness may be made. These studies are characterized statistically by few subjects who are carefully observed but multiple measurements per patient.

Phase II studies involve perhaps 100 to 300 patients with the disease of interest who are studied in carefully supervised controlled clinical trials. These studies show the drug's fundamental effectiveness in restricted circumstances. As a by-product, one usually obtains dose–response curves in humans for effectiveness and side effects. Common adverse effects can be detected during Phase II. Tests for the serum level or other level of the medication may be incorporated into the research, especially if there is sizeable genetic variation in metabolism of the medication.

Phase III trials involve proving efficacy in typical patients. During this phase, various levels of the severity of the disease are studied and patients using various concomitant medications provide information on a more clinical and less experimental usage. The total number of persons studied in this phase rarely exceeds 3500 patients and frequently is much smaller, usually 1000 to 3000.[10]

During this phase, efficacy is proven conclusively, and safety, with the exception of rare adverse events, is also demonstrated. A sponsor must notify the FDA of any serious adverse events, which implies close monitoring of the data as well as statistical tests of various results from clinical evaluation of safety. The monitoring of the studies may be done by the sponsor or by a Contract Research Organization (see Chapter 18), and some of this work could be outsourced to workers in another country.

All of the data on the three clinical phases with respect to human research is submitted electronically as part of the NDA. Details can be seen in the FDA Guidance[11] on the electronic submission of NDAs. The NDA will contain results of the animal pharmacological and toxicological studies as well as the human pharmacology studies and the "adequate and well-controled" clinical studies demonstrating the drug's efficacy and side effects. Data from long-term animal toxicity testing — for example, lifetime studies in rats lasting about two years — are included in this submission. All of the manufacturing information must also be contained in the submission indicating all of the ingredients that go into the drug and whether the ingredients are active or inactive, included for the purposes of taste, color, physical characteristics of the tablet, or packaging, as in the case of a capsule.

The total submission that could easily be equivalent to 500 to 1000 volumes, each one up to 2 in. thick in the old day of paper submission now can be loaded to only one DLT Tape of pocket size. The period of preparing an NDA by the sponsor, reviewing the NDA by the FDA, and then reaching a resolution about points for which there is insufficient information for the FDA reviewer to sign off on that part of the submission often involves several years. By law, the FDA is to respond to a submission in 60 days to determine if the NDA is complete and fileable. In recent years the FDA has made this complex review process more rapid, i.e., a ten month review timeline for a standard submission. A separate fast track has been added for those drugs that are especially innovative or of use in life threatening diseases for which few or no alternatives are available. For this type of priority NDAs have a six month review timeline. An important part of the submission and of the final NDA approval is the precise labeling to be used with the drug. In the labeling, the many thousands of pages of research and development are compressed into a few dozen paragraphs, which summarize the research with the drug.

After the drug has been approved by the FDA, the sponsor is permitted to manufacture and sell it. During this postmarketing period, usually called Phase IV, a number of other questions may be answered. These questions concern relative efficacy of the new drug compared with others for the same or similar purpose. Also likely to be answered is the question of the effects of prolonged use of the medication and whether any rare side effects can be discovered. In some instances, approval is made contingent on doing particular Phase IV studies. For further discussion on Phase IV postmarketing studies, see Chapter 17.

IV. PRECLINICAL TESTING

Frequently, the effect of drugs can be investigated by using a molecular preparation, a cell preparation, or an animal or portion of an animal as a test system with the characteristic that increasing doses will produce increasing effects. A particular concern is whether the drug will cause cancer in its use. Drs. Lin and Ali report in Chapter 2 on how the FDA reviews animal toxicity data on the carcinogenic potential of a new medication. The more general measurement of the effects of medication on an animal is termed bioassay. Bioassays are particularly good ways of telling how potent a new drug is relative to a standard drug or treatment. Finney[12] provides a detailed discussion on statistical methods in bioassay, although logistic regression has supplanted some older methods. Bioassay procedures are particularly important in the preclinical phase of drug development, but also have great importance in further animal and human testing during the clinical phases of research and in quality control.

A vital area in pharmaceutical research is the area of animal pathology and toxicology. Procedures have been formalized in response to rules and regulations about "good laboratory practices." One part of the good laboratory practices refers to the recording and analysis of toxicity data. In addition, there is activity on optimal experimental designs to be used in the practical world of toxicity testing. In that world, animals die for causes unrelated to the experiment, particular samples are sometimes lost through technical error, and practical matters of cost limit the size of experiments. Thus, what is needed are experimental designs that are at once powerful (in the statistical sense of being able to observe a difference if it is truly there) and robust (in the statistical sense that if assumptions, such as a particular variable being normally distributed, are not met, the analysis is still valid; and in the laboratory sense that loss of a few test animals or samples should not invalidate the experiment).

V. TOXICITY TESTING

There are numerous methods for testing toxicity of potential drugs. The first major factor is whether the test is to be of acute or chronic exposure. If of acute exposure, then one can administer a single dose to an animal and find out whether there are any apparent toxic effects. Actually, several different doses are administered. Alternatively, a small number of doses may be given and tested for toxicity. In chronic toxicity tests, the drug is given on a continuous basis, perhaps over the lifetime of the test animal. Numerous unsolved problems are involved with this procedure. If one is simply trying to determine the effects on a test animal, the above procedure is reasonable as it stands, though limited by the problems of sampling error, size of experiment, and so forth. If, however, one is interested in using a test animal as a surrogate for a human, then it is implicit that the test animal handle the drug biochemically and pharmacologically in a manner similar to the human, if not identical. Thus, a test animal that metabolizes a drug in a different manner than does the human, is not likely to be a valid surrogate.

There are many statistical and practical problems in these tests. Short-term acute experiments can be done during the preclinical testing phase. Lifetime experiments, on the other hand, require at least two years of observation in rats, a frequently used test animal; and then perhaps another year for finishing the experiment, preparing the numerous slides, reading and evaluating the slides, and producing a statistical analysis of the resulting data. Thus, a chronic rat study can require a duration of the order of three years. Practicality suggests that such studies should be done only after one is reasonably sure that the drug is going to be used in humans. Statistical problems involve mortality and sampling. It would be reasonable to schedule a certain number of animals to begin a study and then to sacrifice a fixed randomly selected proportion at each of several checkpoints in the study. Unfortunately, some animals may die from "natural" causes or there may be laboratory problems assumed to be unrelated to the drug or exposure. Thus, any statistical design must be robust with respect to these anticipated untoward effects.

Questions about optimal number of animals are also of great importance. Since we would all prefer to expose as few animals as practical to these studies and animal experiments for toxicity are extremely expensive, they should be done in the most efficient manner possible. The statistician can save pharmaceutical companies a great deal of resources (animals, employee time, space, and money) with an optimally designed experiment; of course statistically, concern for sensitivity always dictates as large an experiment as possible.

VI. CLINICAL TESTING

After drugs have been tested extensively in experimental animals and the FDA has issued an IND exemption, the drug can be tested for the first time in Phase I human trials. Choosing the proper doses to use in humans is an interesting statistical problem. One can assume that on a fixed number of milligrams of drug per kilogram of body weight, the effects of the drug are constant. For anticancer drugs this is frequently amended to use the unit of milligrams of drug per square meter of body-surface area of the animal. In these or other projections (frequently extrapolations, because the experimental animals are much smaller than the humans about to be tested) there is ample room for more statistical work to predict what dose in humans will have the same effect as a dose shown to have been effective in an experimental animal. Differences in metabolic processes, in disease processes, in species-specific modifying factors, in genetic characteristics, in diet and nutrition, and other factors are such that some of the experimental data in animals may be totally inappropriate to use in such a projection. Obviously, portions of this problem are beyond the role of the statistician; however, the statistical problem involves making estimates of an effective dose in humans that is not unduly affected by meaningless data points from a particular animal species.

Finally, the eventful day arrives and the drug is used for the first time in humans in a Phase I trial. Initial doses are chosen to be especially safe and usually include placebo controls. The experimental program in humans usually reproduces the results found in animals. First, acute single-dose studies, then short-term studies of more than one dose, and finally studies of several different doses on a longer-term basis are done. The goal of the initial studies is to find out about the toxicity of the drug in humans. What side effects, if any, are found in persons taking what is thought to be a large dose of the drug? What are the characteristics of these side effects? In order to be as certain as possible about any adverse effects, each volunteer or patient is given an extensive physical examination before taking the drug and then again after taking the drug, and for longer-term experiments at various intervals while taking the drug. These examinations include liver function tests, kidney tests, blood chemistry, urine chemistry, eye testing, and various other studies designed to provide more data about the organ systems that might be adversely affected by the drug. An extensive battery of laboratory tests is usually included in these initial clinical pharmacology studies. Most of these tests will not be necessary in later studies when more is known about the clinical pharmacology of the drug.

The statistical characteristic of these initial studies is that they include a large number of observations on a small number of persons. Thus, the ability to be inclusive in characterizing the effect of the drug on the handful of persons who have taken it is quite good, based on repeated measures/correlated observations in the study persons. On the other hand, the small number of such subjects in these early trials means that inferences about the next persons to take the drug are subject to large prediction errors.

Drs. Dubey, Chi, and Kelly discuss the role of the FDA statisticians in the review of IND and efficacy and safety evaluation of new drug applications in Chapter 3. That chapter includes the operating rules for these drug trials based on published federal rules, regulations, and guidelines. Moreover, the results of the studies must be of a quality to convince the FDA statisticians; therefore, it is necessary to understand the criteria used in making these evaluations. Drs. Buncher and Tsay sketch a number of the important points that should be considered in Chapter 4 on clinical trial designs. This area of statistical work involves many statisticians in the pharmaceutical industry. Accordingly, a number of other chapters are devoted to various aspects of clinical trials.

Patients who are studied in a clinical trial are supposed to be representative of those persons who will later take the drug. Studies at the University of Rochester School of Medicine and Dentistry have made apparent how much selectivity is involved concerning the patients who actually take part in modern regulated pharmaceutical research. Writings from Drs. Weintraub and Calimlim in Chapter 5 describe the selection of both inpatients and outpatients participating in clinical trials.

Each different class of drugs involves special problems with respect to carrying out clinical trials. For example, antibiotics generally involve short-term trials, while drugs for the cardiovascular system involve tests over months and even years. Trials with geriatric patients differ from those with persons in the middle of life. A major area of research is pharmaceutical preparations to be used to control or cure cancer. Dr. Chen discusses statistical aspects of these cancer trials in Chapter 6 and Dr. Shih provides further discussion on more recent statistical issues and development of these trials in Chapter 7. Another field of interest is hormone replacement therapy (HRT) for men who suffer testosterone deficiency. Dr. Smith explains this therapeutic area of male HRT trials in Chapter 8. Dr. McCormick follows with a discussion of clinical trials of analgesic drugs in Chapter 9.

HIV/AIDS is a difficult area for medical research. No cure has been found, although progress in developing treatments has been made. In Chapter 10, Drs. Bosch and Buncher discuss statistical issues in HIV/AIDS research.

VII. PLACEBO EFFECTS AND OTHER TOPICS

In order to know the effects of a drug, one must separate the pharmacological effects from the medical aura effects. The accepted way to do this is to compare the active drug with a pharmacologically inert substance. The substance is designated a placebo from the Latin for "I shall please." The placebo is well known to be a good analgesic; it cures or reduces headaches, backaches, postoperative pain, etc. Side effects from placebo therapy are even more extensive than the list of conditions that are aided by the placebo. Headaches, nausea, vomiting, dizziness, and so forth have all been caused by the administration of placebos. The placebo effect is discussed in Chapter 11 by Dr. Buncher. When a placebo is considered inappropriate as a control in a trial for ethical or other reasons, a positive treatment is usually used for a noninferiority or equivalence trial. In this case the objective is to show the test drug is no worse than or equally good as the active treatment in efficacy. Dr. Hwang presents an interesting discussion on this topic in Chapter 12.

Studies used to be completed first and then were subject to statistical analysis. Many prefer to know how the study results are proceeding even as the study is ongoing for ethical, financial, and scientific reasons. An area in statistics on these interim analyses and relevant adaptive designs has developed. Drs. Liu and Pledger in Chapter 13, and Drs. Hwang and Lan in Chapter 14 have extensive discussion on interim analysis and adaptive design. Dr. O'Neill provides the regulatory view of these methods in Chapter 15. Genomics advanced rapidly in the last decade. Its application in pharmaceutical development has shown its importance. In Chapter 16 Drs. Zerba and Shen discuss statistical challenges in pharmacogenomics. There are also many studies of medications that start after the NDA has been granted. Drs. Buncher and Tsay discuss these Phase IV postmarketing studies in Chapter 17. A group of companies known collectively as Contract Research Organizations have grown up to provide statistical and clinical trial management services for the sponsors of medications. Drs. Flora and Constant discuss the role of these organizations in drug development in Chapter 18.

VIII. GLOBAL DRUG DEVELOPMENT

Globalization is an industrial trend. The pharmaceutical industry is no exception. The high cost and long duration to develop a new drug present a compelling pressure to the pharmaceutical companies to seek alternatives with lower cost and shorter time in the drug development process. For a global pharmaceutical company, simultaneous clinical development in different parts of the world is a common practice now. Harmonization in the relevant processes is a key to success. Drs. van Ewijk, Huitfeldt, and Tsay discuss a clinical statistical perspective in global harmonization of drug development in Chapter 19. In the global drug development, the sponsor hopes to use much of the same clinical data collected in different countries to submit new drug applications in different countries of the world. However, many countries require clinical data from their local country. If no clinical trials were done in that country, some bridging studies may be required in order to convince the country's authority that extrapolation of foreign clinical data to their population is valid. Narukawa-san and Professor Takeuchi discuss bridging strategies for global drug development in Chapter 20.

IX. MANUFACTURING

Everyone is familiar with the concept of thousands of tiny capsules or tablets being carefully produced by a pharmaceutical manufacturer. Obviously, with a little reflection we realize that this sort of production requires a tremendous amount of development before it becomes a reality. The chemical that has been tested in animals and found to be active must be given to humans. If the chemical is to be given in tablet form, the tablet must dissolve, typically in the stomach of the person taking the medication. The tablet must not break up into chunks in some people and dissolve neatly in other people. Therefore, other ingredients must be added to the tablet to give it proper disintegration and dissolution characteristics to hold the tablet together before it is taken, to be less affected by temperature and humidity, and to yield various other favorable properties. This is a part of the field of drug formulation.

Another part of the formulation process involves the human reaction rather than physical reactions. For example, what does the tablet taste like? Perhaps a sweetener must be added to avoid a bitter taste. Perhaps something must be added to prevent the tablet from feeling chalky. Other ingredients will be added to change the color of the tablet. In the case of capsules, a gelatin will be used with the addition of food coloring to give the capsule a particular identifying color or set of colors.

After the initial formulation work is completed, the drug is tested in humans in the original Phase I and Phase II studies. During these early studies some problem with the formulation may be discovered. Meanwhile, pilot plant preparation of the drug is being worked on. At later stages full-scale manufacture of the drug will be planned and accomplished. Required changes in the drug at any of these stages will require a restart of many of the formulation steps. Checking procedures and other steps preparatory to a formal quality control program must also be worked out. The statistician is often involved at the time of bioavailability studies when various pharmacokinetic parameters are studied. Drs. Yuh and Chen cover these issues in Chapter 21.

The statistician works with other employees in the quality control field to be certain that the drug is manufactured to the best standards possible. This field is usually called "Current Good Manufacturing Practices (cGMP) in Manufacturing, Processing, Packing, or Holding the Drugs" and is described in the FDA cGMP Guidance (see http://www.fda.gov/cder/guidance/index.htm).[13] Another practically important and statistically interesting question concerns the stability of a drug. For how long after the drug is manufactured can it be considered clinically adequate? These time periods are typically measured in years. Dr. Tsong and his collaborators at the FDA discuss stability testing of pharmaceutical preparations in Chapter 22.

X. OTHER ISSUES

A classical statistical problem is that of multiple comparisons that must be considered when there are more than two treatment groups in the experiment or more than two measurements on each subject simultaneously. If a drug may have one of four activities and we wish to claim only one of them, then we must take account of the fact when setting a "0.05 level" of Type I error that there are four random chances that the drug will be shown to be effective rather than just one. In a similar manner, if there are ten chemicals competing to become a drug, the possibility that at least one of them will be better than the placebo by chance is certainly enhanced by the fact that it is one of ten. Again, the probability levels must be properly adjusted. Drs. Dunnett and Goldsmith discuss this problem and some of the solutions in Chapter 23 on when and how to do multiple comparisons.

Finally, there are many clinical tests that may have an accepted range of normal values. Some tests are new enough that the "normal range" is not clearly established. All statisticians understand that "normal" means everything from Gaussian to typical to acceptable depending on the context. Those subjects whose measurements are outside of acceptable values may be considered potentially unhealthy or to have a side effect of the medication. Thus statisticians sometimes have to define these normal ranges (also called reference ranges or reference intervals) or to validate the intervals established by others. Drs. Horn and Pesce discuss in Chapter 24 various methods of creating these reference intervals.

We hope that the readers will have many stimulating thoughts and lessons in reading these chapters by statisticians and others who are well experienced in the pharmaceutical industry.

REFERENCES

1. National Center for Health Statistics, Health, United States, 2004 with Chartbook on Trends in the Health of Americans with special feature on Drugs, Hyattsville, 2004 (http://www.cdc.gov/nchs/hus.htm).
2. DiMasi, J.A., Hansen, R.W., and Grabowski, H.G., The price of innovation: new estimates of drug development costs, *J. Health Econ.*, 22, 151–185, 2003.
3. ICH-M4 Guideline, Organization of the Common Technical Document for the Registration of Pharmaceuticals for Human Use, 2000 (see http://www.ich.org or http://www.fda.gov/cder/guidance/index.htm).
4. Mehra, M., Building an offshore biometrics center: a case study, presented at *DIA 40th Annual Meeting*, June 17, 2004.
5. McGinn, P.R., World Medical Association adopts new research standard that puts patient first: a revised Declaration of Helsinki reiterates that the well-being of the patient outweighs advancement of clinical research, even in the poorest of countries. AMNews correspondent, December 18, 2000 (http://www.ama-assn.org/amednews/2000/12/18/prsa1218.htm).
6. FDA Guidance for Industry, Providing Clinical Evidence of Effectiveness for Human Drugs and Biological Products, May 1998 (http://www.fda.gov/cder/guidance/index.htm).
7. Nebert, D.W., Jorge-Nebert, L., and Vesell, E.S., Pharmacogenomics and "individualized drug therapy" — high expectations and disappointing achievements, *Am. J. Pharmacogenomics*, 3, 361–370, 2003.

8. Nugent, W.A., RajanBabu, T.V., and Burk, M.J., Beyond nature's chiral pool: enantioselective catalysis in industry, *Science*, 259, 479–483, 1993.

9. Bouckenooghe, A., Achieving regulatory success in phases IIIb and IV, *Appl. Clin. Trial.*, 13(8), 34 2004.

10. Glossary of clinical research terminology, *Appl. Clin. Trial.* Vol. 11, No. 12, p. 30, December 2002.

11. FDA Guidance for Industry, Providing Regulatory Submissions in Electronic Format-NDAs, January 1999 (http://www.fda.gov/cder/guidance/index.htm).

12. Finney, D.J., *Statistical Methods in Biological Assay*, 3rd Ed., Hafner, New York, 1978.

13. Food and Drug Administration Regulations, Current good manufacturing practices for finished pharmaceuticals. Code of Federal Regulations, Title 21, Part 211, 2004.

2 Statistical Review and Evaluation of Animal Carcinogenicity Studies of Pharmaceuticals

Karl K. Lin and Mirza W. Ali

CONTENTS

I. INTRODUCTION

The risk assessment of a new drug exposure in humans usually begins with an assessment of risk of the drug in animals. It is required by law that the sponsor of a new drug conducts nonclinical studies in animals to assess the pharmacological actions, the toxicological effects, and the pharmacokinetic properties of the drug in relation to its proposed therapeutic indications or clinical uses. Studies in animals, designed for assessment of toxicological effects of the drug, include acute, subacute, subchronic, and chronic toxicity studies, tumorigenicity, reproduction, and pharmacokinetic studies.

The Divisions of Biometrics, Center for Drug Evaluation and Research (CDER), Food and Drug Administration (FDA) are responsible for statistical reviews of results of long-term (or chronic) animal carcinogenicity experiments submitted by drug sponsors to FDA as parts of their investigational new drug (IND) or new drug application (NDA) submissions. Long-term animal carcinogenicity studies usually are conducted on sexes of mice and rats for the majority of the normal lifespan of those animals. The primary purpose of these studies is to determine the oncogenic potential of the new drug. There are different ways to use the results of long-term animal carcinogenicity studies in determination of oncogenic potential of chemical compounds. The first way is to use the results merely for screening of unsafe chemical compounds. The second way is to do risk assessments of chemicals in humans, which involves extrapolations of results from animals to humans, and from high to low doses. The third way is to verify scientific hypotheses about the mechanisms of carcinogenesis.

Statisticians in CDER are not involved in extrapolating animal carcinogenicity study findings beyond the ranges of doses studied or to species other than those studied, nor are they involved in investigation of mechanisms of carcinogenesis. Accordingly, statisticians in the CDER develop a quantitative assessment of the risk of a drug for each species and sex of rodent, and the reviewing pharmacologists and medical officers apply their knowledge of mammalian similarities and interspecies differences to extrapolate qualitatively from rodent to human beings.[1]

The statistical interest in detecting oncogenic potential of a new drug, is to test if there are statistically significant positive dose–response relationships in tumor incidence rates induced by the new drug. The phrase "positive dose–response relationship" in this chapter refers to the increasing linear component of the effect of treatment, but not necessarily to a strictly increasing tumor rate as dose increases. However, the review and evaluation of the results of long-term animal carcinogenicity experiments studying the oncogenic potential of a new drug is a complex process. The final interpretation of the study results involves issues that require statistical as well as nonstatistical biomedical judgments. The statistical issues, in carrying out an animal carcinogenicity experiment, include the validity of design of the experiment, the appropriateness of methods of statistical analysis of experimental data, adjustment for the effect of multiple tests, and the use of comparable historical data in the final interpretation of the results.

There is a vast amount of statistical literatures on these issues. The techniques or methods of analysis, and decision rules adopted by FDA statisticians in their reviews are based on current literature, inputs derived out of consultations with outside experts, our research, and best scientific judgments, although it is recognized that some of the issues are still without consensus of opinion among experts in evaluation of animal carcinogenicity studies. The majority of the methods of analysis and interpretation, described in this book chapter, are based on those included in the draft FDA Guidance for Industry: Statistical Aspects of the Design, Analysis, and Interpretation of Chronic Rodent Carcinogenicity Studies of Pharmaceuticals,[2] and an article on carcinogenicity studies of pharmaceuticals by the first author.[3]

Besides reviewing the reports submitted by sponsors, statisticians in the CDER also need tumor data on computer readable media from drug sponsors to perform additional statistical analyses, which they believe are appropriate and necessary to evaluate the analyses and conclusions contained in the reports. The Agency has issued guidelines for formats and specifications for submission of animal carcinogenicity study data.[4] To expedite the statistical review, sponsors are urged to submit the tumor data on computer readable media using the Agency's recommended formats and specifications along with their original, initial submissions of the hardcopy NDA or IND.

The purpose of this chapter is to provide some guidance in the design of animal carcinogenicity experiments, method of statistical analysis of tumor data, interpretation of study results, presentation of data and results in reports, and submission of tumor data to FDA statistical reviewers that drug sponsors can follow in their preparations for the nonclinical parts of IND and NDA submissions. A discussion on the validity of the design of experiment is given in Section II. This is followed by an extensive discussion on methods of statistical analysis in Section III. In Section IV, a discussion on how the results should be interpreted is given. A brief discussion on carcinogenicity studies using transgenic mice is given in Section V. Discussions on data presentation and submission are given in Section VI. Finally, some concluding remarks are given in Section VII.

II. VALIDITY OF THE DESIGN

In evaluation of the validity of experimental designs, statistical reviewers check if randomization methods are used in allocating animals to treatment groups, to avoid possible biases caused by animal selections, and if a sufficient number of animals are used in an experiment to ensure reasonable power in the statistical tests used. It has been recommended that, in a standard four-treatment-group experiment, each dose group and concurrent control group should contain at least 50 animals of each sex. If interim sacrifices are planned, the initial number should be increased by the number of animals scheduled for the interim sacrifices.

In general, based on the results of sponsors' single dose, short-term sub-chronic toxicity studies, FDA statisticians, reviewing pharmacologists, medical officers, and CDER Carcinogenicity Assessment Committee (CAC) members will evaluate the appropriateness of the doses used in animal carcinogenicity experiments. However, in negative studies (i.e., studies in which no significant positive dose–response relationships or drug related increases in tumor incidence rates were detected) the statistical reviewers working with other FDA scientists will perform an additional evaluation on the validity of the designs of experiment, to see if there are sufficient animals living long enough to get an adequate exposure to the chemical and to be at risk of forming late-developing tumors. Also of concern is whether the doses used are high enough and close enough to the maximum tolerated dose (MTD) to present a reasonable tumor challenge to the tested animals.[5]

The adequacy of the number of animals surviving, the length of exposure, and the appropriate dose strength depend on species and strains of animals employed, routes of administration, and other factors (see the discussion in Haseman[6]). A general rule is that a 50% survival rate in any group between weeks 80 and 90 of a two-year study will be considered as a sufficient number and an adequate exposure. However, the percentage can be lower or higher if the number of animals used in each treatment or sex group is larger or smaller than 50, so that there will be between 20 and 30 animals still alive during these weeks. In consultations with reviewing pharmacologists and medical officers, FDA statistical reviewers often followed the criteria proposed in Chu et al.[7] in their evaluation to see if the high dose used is close to the MTD and presents a reasonable tumor challenge to the animals. Based on results of 200 National Cancer Institute carcinogen bioassays, these investigators considered a high dose to be close to the MTD if: (a) there was a detectable weight loss of up to 10% in the dosed group relative to the controls, (b) the animals exhibited clinical signs or severe histopathologic toxic effects that could be attributed to the chemical in the dosed animals, (c) there was a slightly increased mortality in the dosed animals compared with the controls.

The appropriateness of the high dose is always addressed in the CDER/CAC meetings during the final determinations of the oncogenic potential of new drugs under review at the FDA. It is an important, controversial, and complicated issue in the evaluation of validity of designs of animal experiments. Information about body weight gain, mortality, and clinical signs and histopathologic toxic effects still are used to resolve the issue. Other information, such as pharmacokinetic and metabolic data, is also often needed in evaluation of dose selection.

The International Conference on Harmonization (ICH) guidance entitled *S1C Dose Selection for Carcinogenicity Studies of Pharmaceuticals*[8] is an internationally accepted guidance for dose selection for carcinogenicity studies, and sponsors are advised to consult this document. The guidance allows for approaches to high dose selection based on toxicity endpoints, pharmaco-kinetic endpoints (multiple of maximum human exposure), pharmacodynamic endpoints, and maximal feasible dose.

III. METHODS OF STATISTICAL ANALYSIS

A. TEST OF INTERCURRENT MORTALITY DATA

Intercurrent mortality refers to all deaths not related to the development of the particular type or class of tumors that are being studied for evidence of carcinogenicity. Like human beings, older rodents have a many times higher probability of developing or dying from tumors than those of younger ages. Therefore, it is essential to identify and adjust the possible differences in intercurrent mortality (or longevity) among treatment groups to eliminate or reduce biases caused by the differences. It is pointed out that "the effects of differences in longevity on numbers of tumor-bearing animals can be very substantial, and so, whether or not they appear to be, they should routinely be corrected for when presenting experimental results."[5,9] The following examples demonstrate the above important point.

Example 1.[9] Consider an experiment consisting of one control group and one treated group of 100 mice each. A very toxic but not tumorigenic new drug was administered to the animals in the diet for two years. Assume that the spontaneous incidental tumor rates for both groups are 30% at 15 months and 80% at 18 months of age and that the mortality rates at 15 months for the control and the treated groups are 20% and 60%, respectively, because of the toxicity of the drug. The results of the experiment are summarized in Table 2.1. If one looks only at the overall tumor incidence rates of the control and the treated groups (70% and 50%, respectively) without considering the significantly higher early deaths in the treated group caused by the toxicity of the drug, one will conclude erroneously that there is a significant ($p = 0.002$, one-tailed) negative dose–response relationship in this tumor type (i.e., the new drug prevents tumor occurrences). The one-tailed p-value is 0.5 when the survival-adjusted prevalence method is used.[9]

TABLE 2.1
Data for Example 1

	Control			Treated		
	T	*D*	%	*T*	*D*	%
15 Months	6	20	30	18	60	30
18 Months	64	80	80	32	40	80
Total	70	100	70	50	100	50

T = incidental tumors found at necropsy, D = deaths.

Example 2.[10] Assume that the design used in this experiment is the same as the one used in the experiment of Example 1. However, we assume that the treated group has a much higher early mortality than the control (20% vs. 90%) before 15 months, and that the drug in this example induces an incidental tumor that does not cause the animal's death, either directly or indirectly. Also assume that the incidental tumor prevalence rates for the control and treated groups are 5% and 20%, respectively, before 15 months of age, and 30% and 70%, respectively, after 15 months of age. The results of this experiment are summarized in Table 2.2. Note that the age-specific tumor incidence rates are significantly higher in the treated group than those in the control group. The survival-adjusted prevalence method yielded a one-tailed p-value of 0.003; this shows a clear tumorigenic effect of the new drug. However, the overall tumor incidence rates are 25% for the two groups. Without considering the significantly higher early mortality in the treated group, one would conclude that the positive dose–response relationship is not significant.

Before analyzing the tumor data, the intercurrent mortality data are routinely tested first by FDA statisticians to see if the survival distributions of the treatment groups are significantly different or if there exist significant dose–response relationships. Cox's Test,[10–12] the generalized Wilcoxon or Kruskal–Wallis test,[12–14] and the Tarone trend tests[9,15,16] are routinely used to test for the heterogeneity in survival distributions and significant dose–response relationship (trend) in mortality.

There is an issue on the use of the results from tests of intercurrent mortality data in the determination whether a survival-adjusted method should be used in the analyses of tumor data. If we treat the test for heterogeneity in survival distributions or dose–response relationship in mortality as a preliminary test of significance,[17] then a level of significance larger than 0.05 should be used. A very large level of significance used in the preliminary test means that survival-adjusted methods should always be used in the subsequent analyses of the tumor data.

TABLE 2.2
Data for Example 2

	Control			Treated		
	T	*D*	%	*T*	*D*	%
Before 15 Months	1	20	5	18	90	20
After 15 Months	24	80	30	7	10	70
Total	25	100	25	25	100	25

T = incidental tumors found at necropsy, D = deaths.

B. CONTEXTS OF OBSERVATION OF TUMOR TYPES

The choice of a survival-adjusted method to analyze tumor data depends on the role that a tumor plays in causing the animal's death. Tumors can be classified as "fatal," "mortality-independent (or observable)," and "incidental" according to the contexts of observation described in Peto et al.[9] Tumors that kill the animal either directly or indirectly are said to have been observed in a fatal context. Tumors that are not directly or indirectly responsible for the animal's death, but are merely observed at the autopsy of the animal after it has died of some unrelated causes, are said to have been observed in an incidental context. Tumors, such as skin tumors, whose times of criterion attainment (i.e., detection of the tumor at a standard point of their development) other than the times or causes of death, are the primary interest of analyses and these are said to have been observed in a mortality-independent (or observable) context. To apply a survival-adjusted method correctly, it is essential that the context of observation of a tumor be determined as accurately as possible.

Different statistical techniques have been proposed for analyzing data of tumors observed in different contexts of observation. For example, the death-rate, onset-rate, and prevalence methods are recommended for analyzing data of tumors observed in fatal, mortality-independent, and incidental contexts of observation, respectively.[9] Peto et al. also demonstrate the possible biases resulting from misclassifications of incidental tumors as fatal tumors, or fatal tumors as incidental tumors.

C. STATISTICAL ANALYSES OF INCIDENTAL TUMORS

The prevalence method described by Peto et al.[9] is routinely used by FDA statisticians in testing for a positive dose–response relationship in prevalence rates of incidental tumors. Briefly, this method focuses on the age-specific tumor prevalence rates to correct for intercurrent mortality differences among treatment groups in the test for positive dose–response relationships in incidental tumors. The experimental period is partitioned into a set of intervals plus interim sacrifices (if any) and terminal sacrifices. The incidental tumors are then stratified by those intervals of survival times. The selection of the partition of the experiment period does not matter very much as long as the intervals "are not so short that the prevalence of incidental tumors in the autopsies they contain is not stable, nor yet so large that the real prevalence in the first half of one interval could differ markedly from the real prevalence in the second half."[9]

In each time interval and for each group, the observed number of animals with a particular tumor type found in necropsies, is compared with number of animals that died in the time interval and expected to have the tumor type found in the necropsies under the null hypothesis so that there is no dose–response relationship. Finally, the differences between the observed and the expected numbers of animals found with the tumor type after their deaths are combined across all time intervals to yield an overall test statistic using the method described in Mantel.[18]

The following derivation of the Peto prevalence test statistic uses the notations in Table 2.3. Let the experimental period be partitioned into the following M intervals $I_1, I_2, ..., I_M$. As mentioned before, interim sacrifices (if any) and terminal sacrifices should be treated as separate intervals.

The number of autopsied animals expected to have the particular incidental tumor in group i and interval k under the null hypothesis that there is no treatment effect is

$$E_{ik} = O_{.k} P_{ik}.$$

The covariance of $(O_{ik} - E_{ik})$ and $(O_{jk} - E_{jk})$ is

$$V_{ijk} = P_{ik}(\delta_{ij} - P_{jk})$$

where

$$\delta_{ij} = \begin{array}{ll} 1 & \text{if } i = j \\ 0 & \text{otherwise} \end{array}$$

Define

$$O_i = \Sigma_k O_{ik}$$
$$E_i = \Sigma_k E_{ik}$$

TABLE 2.3
Notation Used in the Derivation of Peto Prevalence Test Statistic

		Interval									
		I_1		I_2		...	I_k		...	I_M	
Group	Dose	R_1		R_2		...	R_k		...	R_M	
0	D_0	O_{01}	P_{01}	O_{02}	P_{02}	...	O_{0k}	P_{0k}	...	O_{0M}	P_{0M}
1	D_1	O_{11}	P_{11}	O_{12}	P_{12}	...	O_{1k}	P_{1k}	...	O_{1M}	P_{1M}
$\vdots$	$\vdots$	$\vdots$	$\vdots$	$\vdots$	$\vdots$	...	$\vdots$	$\vdots$	...	$\vdots$	$\vdots$
i	D_i	O_{i1}	P_{i1}	O_{i2}	P_{i2}	...	O_{ik}	P_{ik}	...	O_{iM}	P_{iM}
$\vdots$	$\vdots$	$\vdots$	$\vdots$	$\vdots$	$\vdots$		$\vdots$	$\vdots$	$\vdots$	$\vdots$	$\vdots$
r	D_r	O_{r1}	P_{r1}	O_{r2}	P_{r2}	...	O_{rk}	P_{rk}	...	O_{rM}	P_{rM}
Sum		$O_{.1}$	$P_{.1}$	$O_{.2}$	$P_{.2}$	...	$O_{.k}$	$P_{.k}$	...	$O_{.M}$	$P_{.M}$

R_k: number of animals that have not died of the tumor type of interest but come to autopsy in the time interval k, P_{ik}: proportion of R_k in group i, O_{ik}: observed number of autopsied animals in group I and interval k found to have the incidental tumor type, $O_{.k} = \Sigma_i O_{ik}$.

and

$$V_{ij} = \Sigma_k V_{ijk}$$

The test statistic T for the positive linear trend in the incidental tumor rate is defined as

$$T = \Sigma_i D_i (O_i - E_i)$$

with estimated variance

$$V(T) = \Sigma_i \Sigma_j D_i D_j V_{ij}$$

Under the null hypothesis of equal prevalence rate among the treatment groups, the statistic

$$Z = T/V(T)^{1/2}$$

is approximately distributed as standard normal.

As mentioned above, to use the prevalence method, the experimental period has to be partitioned into a set of intervals plus interim (if any) and terminal sacrifices.

The following partitions (in weeks) are used most often by FDA statisticians in two-year studies: (a) zero to 50, 51 to 80, 81 to 104, interim sacrifice (if any) and terminal sacrifice, (b) zero to 52, 53 to 78, 79 to 92, 93 to 104, interim sacrifice (if any), and terminal sacrifice (proposed by National Toxicology Program), or (c) Partition determined by the "ad hoc runs" procedure described in Peto et al.[9]

This method uses a normal approximation in the test for a positive dose–response relationship in tumor prevalence rates. The accuracy of the normal approximation depends on: the numbers of tumor-bearing animals in each group, in each interval, the number of intervals used in the partition, and the mortality patterns. However, it is known that under regularity conditions, the approximation will not be stable and reliable when the numbers of tumor occurrences across treatment groups are small. In this situation, an exact permutation trend test based on an extension of the hypergeometric distribution (discussed in Section III.F) is used to test the positive dose–response relationship in tumor prevalence rates.

Although Peto et al.[9] proposed general guidelines for partitioning the experimental period into intervals in the prevalence method, there is no unique way to do the partition. Test results could be different when different sets of intervals are used. Dinse and Haseman[19] applied ten different sets of intervals to the same tumor data set and got ten different p-values ranging from 0.001 to 0.261. Because of the lack of a unique way to partition the experimental period, some regression-type methods have been proposed as alternatives for analyzing incidental tumor data from animal carcinogenicity experiments. The logistic regression method[19–22] and Cochran–Armitage trend test methods[23,24] are two of those proposed alternatives. The main advantage of the regression type methods is that these adjust for the differences in intercurrent mortality by including the survival time as a continuous regression variable. This makes it unnecessary to partition the experimental period into intervals. Another advantage of these methods is that the other variables having effects on the prevalence rates, such as body weight and cage location, can also be incorporated into the model as covariates.

The logistic regression model is defined as

$$E(Y_i) = \frac{e^{a+bD_i}}{1 + e^{a+bD_i}}$$

without adjustment for intercurrent mortality differences, and as

$$E(Y_i) = \frac{e^{a+bD_i+F(t_i)}}{1 + e^{a+bD_i+F(t_i)}}$$

with adjustment for intercurrent mortality differences, where $E(Y_i)$, D_i, and t_i are the expected value of Y_i, the dose level, and survival time, respectively, of animal i and

$$F(t) = c_0 + c_1 t_i + c_2 t_i^2 + \cdots + c_p t_i^p$$

The following statistic

$$Z = \frac{\hat{b}}{\hat{V}(\hat{b})^{1/2}}$$

which is approximately distributed as a standard normal, is used to test the positive dose–response relationship in a specific incidental tumor. The term $\hat{V}(\hat{b})$ in the above equation is the variance of the estimated regression coefficient $\hat{b}$.

However, there is another issue in using the logistic regression method. The functional form of $F(t_i)$ has to be specified in the logistic regression model to indicate the effect of survival time on tumor prevalence rate. Like partitioning the experimental period into intervals in the Peto prevalence method, there is no unique way of determining the functional form and different functional forms of $F(t_i)$ can yield different results.

Armitage[23] applies the one-way analysis of variance model to the dependent variable Y, individual animal tumor status (i.e., $Y = 1$ if an animal developed the tumor of interest and $Y = 0$ otherwise) using the dose variable as the grouping variable to obtain the sum of square components of various sources of variation as shown in Table 2.4.

However, because the dependent variable Y assumes only values of zero and one, the test procedure for the linear contrast in regular analysis of variance has to be modified. Armitage suggested the use of the following alternative statistic

$$\chi_0^2 = \frac{S_1}{(S_1 + S_2 + S_3)/T}$$

which is distributed approximately with one degree of freedom under the null hypothesis of no positive dose–response relationship. The above analysis of

TABLE 2.4
Analysis of Variance Table

Source of Variation	D.F.	Sum of Squares
Treatment	r	$S_1 + S_2$
Linear	1	S_1
Departure from linearity	$r - 1$	S_2
Error	$T - r - 1$	S_3
Total	$T - 1$	$S_1 + S_2 + S_3$

T is the total number of animals used in the study. There are $r + 1$ treatment groups including the control.

---

variance approach to the trend test is equivalent to the test of significant positive slope of the regression equation of Y and X. Here the score variable X can take the values $X_1 = -r/2, X_2 = -(r - 2)/2, ..., X_r = r/2$, or any set of $r + 1$ equally spaced numbers for the case of $r + 1$ groups. If the fitted regression equation is expressed as

$$Y_i = \hat{a} + \hat{b}X_i$$

then the test statistic

$$Z = \frac{\hat{b}}{\hat{V}(\hat{b})^{1/2}}$$

which is distributed approximately as a standard normal is used to test the positive dose–response relationship.

The Cochran–Armitage regression methods are survival-unadjusted. The results from the unadjusted methods are reasonably unbiased if the intercurrent mortalities among the treatment groups are not significantly different. For experiments experiencing significant differences in intercurrent mortality, the Cochran–Armitage trend test procedures can be modified to adjust for the effect of the survival differences. Two different modifications can be made. The first is to use the survival time as a covariate and perform the analysis of covariance; the second is to include the linear term or quadratic term or both in the regression analysis as other independent variables in addition to the score variable X.

The computations in the modified Cochran–Armitage regression method are much simpler than those in the logistic regression method. However, it does not satisfy the condition of constant variance in regression analysis. The modified Cochran–Armitage regression method also has a shortcoming similar to the logistic regression method, i.e., there is no unique way to determine the functional relationship between survival time and tumor incidence.

Lin[25] conducted an empirical study using tumor data from three experiments to compare the Peto prevalence method with the logistic regression and the modified Cochran–Armitage regression type test procedures, with the following results. The p-values from the logistic regression methods assuming the effect of survival time on tumor incidence rate was linear and linear and quadratic forms were similar in the three studies used. However, this is not true in the case of the modified Cochran–Armitage regression method. The p-values from the model including only a linear term of survival time were in general appreciably larger than those from the model including the linear and quadratic terms.

The p-values from the Cochran–Armitage method using linear survival time as a covariate or as an independent regression variable were close to those from the logistic regression method also adjusted by the linear term of survival time, although those were somewhat larger. There was no clear pattern in p-values from these two test procedures when the linear and the quadratic terms of survival time are included.

The p-values from the Peto prevalence method were in general smaller than those from the Cochran–Armitage regression method adjusted by the linear term of survival time. There was no clear pattern in p-values between the two methods when the quadratic term of survival time was added to the Cochran–Armitage method. There was no clear pattern in p-values when the Peto prevalence method was compared with the logistic regression method.

The p-values from the unadjusted logistic and the unadjusted Cochran–Armitage test procedures were virtually identical, and were not very different from the p-values from the Peto prevalence method in the study in which there is no significant difference in mortality.

Finally, in terms of decision making, the Peto prevalence, the adjusted logistic regression, and the adjusted Cochran–Armitage regression methods reached consistent conclusions (either all methods reject or accept, at a given level of significance, the null hypothesis of no positive dose–response relationship in the tumors tested in the three studies).

Before the issues related to the functional form of the effect of survival time on tumor incidence rate and the power and the conservativeness of the logistic regression and the modified Cochran–Armitage regression test procedures are fully studied, FDA statisticians will continue to recommend the Peto prevalence method in analyzing incidental tumor data from animal experiments.

D. STATISTICAL ANALYSES OF FATAL TUMORS

In their reviews and analyses of animal carcinogenicity study data, FDA statisticians routinely use the death-rate method described in Peto et al.[9] to test the positive dose–response relationship in tumors observed in a fatal context.

The notations of Section III.C with some modifications will be used in this section to derive the test statistic of the death-rate method. Now let $t_1 < t_2 < \cdots < t_M$ be the time points when one or more animals died. Use these time points to replace the intervals adopted in the prevalence method. The notations in Table 2.3 are redefined as follows:

R_k = The number of animals of all groups just before t_k.

P_{ik} = The proportion of R_k in group i (the same as in the prevalence method).

O_{ik} = Observed number of animals in group i just before t_k found to have the fatal tumor.

$$O_{.k} = \sum_i O_{ik} O_{ik}$$

As in the prevalence method, the test statistic T for the positive dose–response relationship in the fatal tumor is defined as:

$$T = \sum_i D_i(O_i - E_i)$$

with estimated variance

$$\hat{V}(T) = \sum_i \sum_j D_i D_j V_{ij}$$

where D_i, O_i, E_i, and V_{ij} are defined similarly as in Section III-C. Under the null hypothesis of equal death rates among the treatment groups, the statistic

$$Z = \frac{T}{\hat{V}(T)^{1/2}}$$

is distributed approximately as a standard normal.

E. STATISTICAL ANALYSES OF TUMORS OBSERVED IN INCIDENTAL AND FATAL CONTEXTS

When a tumor was observed in a fatal context for a set of animals and in an incidental context for the remaining animals in an experiment, data should be analyzed separately by the prevalence and death-rate methods. Results from different methods can then be combined to yield an overall result. The combined overall result can be obtained by simply adding together either the separate observed and expected frequencies and variances, or the separate T statistics and their variances.

F. EXACT ANALYSIS

As mentioned in the previous sections, the prevalence and death-rate methods use a normal approximation in the test for positive dose–response relationship (trend) in tumor rates. The adequacy of the normal approximation may depend on factors, viz., the number of tumor-bearing animals, scores assigned to the treatment groups, number of intervals used in partitioning the study period, etc. It is particularly true that when the number of tumor-bearing animals is "small," the normal approximation is unreliable and tends mostly to underestimate the exact p-values.[26] Under this situation, the use of an exact permutation trend test is suggested[10,27] to test for dose–response relationship in tumor rates. The exact trend test is a generalization of the Fisher exact test to sequences of $2(r+1)$ tables.

1. The Exact Method

The exact method is derived by conditioning on the row and column marginal totals of each of the $2(r+1)$ tables, formed from the partitioned data set of Table 2.3. Consider the kth interval I_k (in Table 2.3) and write it as in Table 2.5. Now let the column totals $C_{0k}, C_{lk}, ..., C_{rk}$, and the row totals $O_{\cdot k}$ and $A_{\cdot K}$ be fixed. Define

$$P_{jk} = \frac{C_{jk}}{R_k}$$

Then the quantities $E_{ik} = O_{\cdot k}P_{ik}$, $V_{ijk} = P_{ik}(\delta_{ij} - P_{jk})$, and $V(t)$ as defined in Section III.C are all known constants.

Now let z be the observed value of Z. Then (under conditioning on the column and row marginal totals in each table) the observed significance level or

$$p\text{-value} = P(Z \geq z) = P\left[\frac{\sum D_i(O_i - E_i)}{\sqrt{V(T)}} \geq z\right] = P\left[\sum D_i O_i \geq y\right]$$

$$= P\left(\sum_i D_i \sum_k O_{ik} \geq y\right) = P\left(\sum_k \sum_i D_i O_{ik} \geq y\right) = P\left(\sum Y_k \geq y\right)$$

$$= P(Y \geq y)$$

where $Y = \sum Y_k = \sum_i D_i O_{ik}$ and $y = \sum y_k$, the observed value of Y.

We compute this p-value $[P(Y >= y)]$ from the exact permutational distribution of Y. Given the observed row and column marginal totals in

---

TABLE 2.5
The Data in the kth Time Interval I_k is Written as a $2(r+1)$ Table

Group		1	...	i	...	r	
Dose	D_0	D_1	...	D_i	...	D_r	Total
Number with tumor	O_{0k}	O_{1k}	...	O_{ik}	...	O_{rk}	$O_{\cdot k}$
Number without tumor	A_{0k}	A_{1k}	...	A_{ik}	...	A_{rk}	$A_{\cdot k}$
Total	C_{0k}	C_{1k}	...	C_{ik}	...	C_{rk}	R_k

a $2(r+1)$ table, generate all possible tables having the same marginal totals. Let S_k $(k = 1, 2, ..., K)$ be the set of all such tables generated from the kth observed table. Form a set of K tables taking one from each S_k. Assuming independence between the K tables, the above expression for the p-value can now be written as

$$p\text{-value} = \sum [P(Y_1 = y_1)...P(Y_K = y_K)]$$

where $y_k = \sum_i D_i O_{ik}$ $(k = 1, 2, ..., K)$, the sum is over all sets of K tables such that $(y_1 + y_2 + \cdots + y_k) \geq y$, the observed value of Y, and $P(Y_k = y_k)$ is the conditional probability given the marginal totals in the kth table,

$$P(Y_k = y_k) = \frac{\binom{C_{0k}}{O_{0k}}\binom{C_{1k}}{O_{1k}}...\binom{C_{rk}}{O_{rk}}}{\binom{R_k}{O_{\cdot k}}}$$

Example. Consider an experiment with three treatment groups (control, low, and high) with dose levels $D_0 = 0$, $D_1 = 1$, and $D_2 = 2$, respectively. Suppose the study period is partitioned into the intervals zero to 50, 51 to 80, 81 to 104 weeks, and the terminal sacrifice week. Consider a tumor type (classified as incidental) with the data shown in Table 2.6.

Since all the observed tumor counts (i.e., O's) in the first two time intervals are zeros, the data for these intervals will not contribute anything to the test

---

TABLE 2.6
Tumor Count Table

Time Interval (Weeks)		Dose Levels 0	1	2	Total
0–50	O	0	0	0	0
	C	1	3	3	7
51–80	O	0	0	0	0
	C	4	5	7	16
81–104	O	0	0	2	2
	C	10	12	15	37
Terminal sacrifice	O	0	1	0	1
	C	35	30	25	90

O = observed tumor count, C = number of animals necropsied.

TABLE 2.7
All Possible Configurations of $o_{.1}$ and the Corresponding Hypergeometric Probabilities

Configurations			y_1	$P(Y_1 = y_1)$
0	0	2	4	.15766
0	2	0	2	.09910
2	0	0	0	.06757
0	1	1	3	.27027
1	0	1	2	.22523
1	1	0	1	.18018

statistic and we may neglect these intervals. The observed tables formed from the last two intervals are as follows:

	Observed Table 1					Observed Table 2			
Dose	**0**	**1**	**2**	**Total**	**Dose**	**0**	**1**	**2**	**Total**
O	0	0	2	$2 = o_{.1}$	O	0	1	0	$1 = o_{.2}$
A	10	12	13	$35 = a_{.1}$	A	35	29	25	$89 = a_{.2}$
C	10	12	15	$37 = R_1$	C	35	30	25	$90 = R_2$

We will now generate all possible tables from Observed Table 1. Since the marginal totals are fixed, we may generate these tables by distributing the total tumor frequency $o_{.1}$ ($= 2$) among the three dose groups. Thus each table will correspond to a configuration of this distribution of $o_{.1}$. The configurations, the values of y_1, and the $P(Y_1 = y_1)$ are shown in Table 2.7.

To illustrate the computation of y_1 and $P(Y_1 = y_1)$ consider the last row. Here $y_1 = (D_0 \times 1) + (D_1 \times 1) + (D_2 \times 0) = (0 \times 1) + (1 \times 1) + (2 \times 0) = 1$, and

$$P(Y_1 = 1) = \frac{\binom{10}{1}\binom{12}{1}\binom{15}{0}}{\binom{37}{2}} = \frac{10 \times 12 \times 2}{37 \times 36} = .18018$$

The configurations and probabilities obtained from Observed Table 2 are given in Table 2.8.

Note that the first configuration $(0, 0, 2)$ in Table 2.7 corresponds to the Observed Table 1 with a value of $y_1 = (0 \times 0) + (1 \times 0) + (2 \times 2) = 4$ and a probability of .15766, and the second configuration $(0, 1, 0)$ in Table 2.8 corresponds to the Observed Table 2 with a value of $y_2 = (0 \times 0) + (1 \times 1) + (0 \times 0) = 1$ and a probability of .33333. Thus the observed value of

TABLE 2.8
All Possible Configurations of $o_{.2}$ and the Corresponding Hypergeometric Probabilities

Configurations			y_1	$P(Y_1 = y_1)$
0	0	1	2	.27778
0	1	0	1	.33333
1	0	0	0	.38889

$y = y_1 + y_2 = 4 + 1 = 5$. Now the exact

p-value (right-tailed) $= P(Y = Y_1 + Y_2 \geq 5)$
$$= P(Y_1 = 4, Y_2 = 1) + P(Y_1 = 4, Y_2 = 2) + P(Y_1 = 3, Y_2 = 2)$$
$$= (.15766 \times .33333) + (.15766 \times .27778) + (.27027 \times .27778)$$
$$= .17142$$

For the purpose of comparison it may be noted that the normal approximated p-value for the data set in the above example is .0927.

2. Comparison of Exact and Approximate Methods

As mentioned before, the use of exact p-values has been suggested when the number of tumor-bearing animals is small. However, the magnitude of this "smallness" is not known. Mantel[28] suggested the use of the exact procedure whenever the total number of tumor-bearing animals is five or less. However, a simulation study by Ali[26] showed that in a four-group experiment with 50 animals in each, the normal approximated p-value may severely underestimate the exact p-value even when the total number of tumor-bearing animals is as large as ten. In Ali's simulation, survival data for the four groups were generated under the proportional hazard assumption with a baseline Weibull model for the control group, and the tumor-bearing animals were distributed in one or more of the four survival time intervals: zero to 50, 51 to 80, 81 to 104, and over 104 weeks (i.e., the terminal sacrifice week).

FDA reviewers routinely apply the exact trend test whenever the total number of animals bearing the tumor type of interest across treatment groups is 12 or less.

An inherent feature of the exact method (as described above) is that p-values are computed from (conditional) null distribution which is discrete. Depending on the extent of this discreetness, the exact method will result in a conservative test in the sense that its actual significance level will, usually, be smaller than the nominal level. The extent of this conservativeness may play an important role in determining the experimentwise Type I error rate (also referred to as the false-positive rate) when performing multiple tests to significance in an experiment designed to test an "overall experimentwise" hypothesis. Under such circumstances, it is useful to gain knowledge of the actual significance levels of the individual tests.

The scenario just described fits an animal carcinogenicity study. In a typical animal carcinogenicity study, four parallel experiments (two species each with two sexes) are run. In each experiment, a combination of 20 or more organ or tissue types with several lesion types are tested for positive linear trend in tumor rates across the treatment groups. Thus the number of tests performed per experiment could be as high as 60 or more. Because, for many tumor types, the incidence is a relatively rare event, it is usually the case that each of a large class of (relatively rare) tumor types will be observed in only a few animals. Hence the number of exact trend tests performed will also be large. Thus the experimentwise false-positive rates will depend heavily on the actual significance levels of the individual exact tests. In addition to the issue of false-positive rates, the question of false-negative rates also arises in a parallel context.

Some knowledge about the Type I and Type II error rates of an exact trend test compared with approximate tests can be found in the results of a simulation study by Ali.[26,29] In this study, the actual significance levels and power of the exact trend test was compared with three approximate tests for the special case of a small number of tumor-bearing animals. Data for the simulation were generated under various Weibull models for survival time, and time to tumor, and tests were computed using four different score sets for the treatment groups. For details on the results of this study the reader is referred to the paper by Ali.[26] Here we will state only the main results comparing the exact test and its normal approximation version.

The actual attained significance levels (as estimated by 10,000 simulated experiments) were compared with the nominal 5% and 1% levels. Five Weibull models each with three score sets resulted in 15 cases to consider. The average number of tumor-bearing animals among these 15 cases ranged from 2.5 to 7.9. The attained significance levels of the exact test ranged from .82% to 1.7% when the nominal level was 5%, and from .08% to .32% when it was 1%. Hence it is clear that the exact test was always very conservative in rejecting the null hypothesis of "no trend" when the tumor prevalence rates across treatment groups were equal. On the other hand, the significance levels attained by the normal approximated test ranged from 3.01% to 8.36% corresponding to a nominal level of 5%, and from .31% to 2.09% when the nominal level was 1%. It is seen that the normal approximation was very unstable in the sense that the significance levels fluctuated above and below the nominal level.

Ali[26] also performed power comparisons between the two tests. The power was computed under various Weibull alternatives for tumor prevalence functions. The average number of tumor-bearing animals ranged from 4.4 to 9.5. The power of the exact test corresponding to a 5% nominal level ranged from 2.14% to 15.09%, and between .35% and 4.46% when the nominal level was 1%. Thus, in the case of very low total tumor rates, it is almost impossible for the exact test to detect increasing tumor prevalence across the treatment groups. In the case of the normal approximation test, the power ranged from 6.2% to 33% at the 5% nominal level, and between 1% and 12.8% when the nominal level was 1%. Hence, although the normal approximation improved the power, it was not high enough to make a real difference.

G. STATISTICAL ANALYSIS OF DATA WITHOUT INFORMATION ABOUT CAUSE OF DEATH

The widely used prevalence method, the death-rate method, and the onset rate methods for analyzing incidental, fatal, and mortality independent tumors, respectively, and described in previous sections, rely on good cause-of-death information. There are situations in which sponsors have not included tumor lethality and cause-of-death information in their statistical analyses and electronic data sets. Under those situations, statistical reviewers in CDER either treated all tumors as incidental or relied on cause-of-death assessments by the reviewing pharmacologists and toxicologists in the Center. There are consequences in misclassifying tumors as lethal or not in survival-adjusted statistical tests. The prevalence method will reject the null hypothesis of no positive trend less frequently than it should as the lethality of a tumor increases.[9,30] This will increase the probability of failing to detect true carcinogens.

The Bailer–Portier poly-3, and poly-6 (in general poly-k) tests[30,31] have been proposed for testing linear trends in tumor rates. These tests are basically modifications of the survival unadjusted Cochran–Armitage test[23,32] for linear trend in tumor rate. If the entire study period is considered as one interval, the data for a particular tumor type will be in the form of Table 2.9. The notations in Table 2.9 to be used to explain these tests are the same as those in Table 2.3 except that the kth interval now is the entire study period. The second subscript, k, for the kth interval was dropped from the notations.

The Cochran–Armitage test statistic for linear trend in tumor rate is defined as[23]:

$$\chi_{CA}^2 = \frac{R\{R\sum O_i D_i - O\sum C_i D_i\}^2}{O(R-O)\{R\sum C_i D_i^2 - (\sum C_i D_i)^2\}} \quad \text{or} \quad = \frac{\{\sum D_i(O_i - E_i)\}}{\sum E_i D_i^2 (\sum E_i D_i)^2 / O}$$

where $O = \sum O_i$, $A = \sum A_i$, $R = \sum C_i$, $E_i = OC_i / R$.

TABLE 2.9
The Data Using the Entire Study Period as an Interval

Group	0	1	...	i	...	r	
Dose	D_0	D_1	...	D_i	...	D_r	Total
# w. tumor	O_0	O_1	...	O_i	...	O_r	O
# w/o tumor	A_0	A_1	...	A_i	...	A_r	A
Total	C_0	C_1	...	C_i	...	C_r	R

The test statistic χ^2_{CA} is distributed approximately as χ^2 on one degree of freedom.

The Cochran–Armitage linear trend test is based on a binomial assumption that all animals in the same treatment group have the same risk of developing the tumor over the duration of the study. However, as noted previously, the animal's risk of developing the tumor increases as study time increases. The assumption is thus no longer valid if some animals die earlier than others. It has been shown that as long as the mortality patterns are similar across treatment groups, the Cochran–Armitage test is still valid, although it may be slightly less efficient than a survival-adjusted test.[30] However, if the mortality patterns are different across treatment groups, the Cochran–Armitage test can give very misleading results.

The Bailer–Portier poly-3 test adjusts for differences in mortality among treatment groups by modifying the number of animals at risk in the denominators in the calculations of overall tumor rates in the Cochran–Armitage test to reflect "less-than-whole-animal contributions for decreased survival."[31] The modification is made by defining a new number of animals at risk for each treatment group. The number of animals at risk for the ith treatment group C_i^* is defined as

$$C_i^* = \sum W_{ij}$$

where W_{ij} is the weight for the jth animal in the ith treatment group, and the sum is over all animals in the group.

Bailer and Portier[31] proposed the weight W_{ij} as follows:

$W_{ij} = 1$ to animals dying with the tumor, and
$W_{ij} = (t_{ij}/t_{\text{sacr}})^3$ to animals dying without the tumor

where t_{ij} is the time of death of the jth animal in the ith treatment group, and t_{sacr} is the time of terminal sacrifice.

The power of three used in the weighting is from the observation that tumor incidence can be modeled as a polynomial of order of three of age. Similarly the poly-6 test (or the general poly-k test) assigns the weight $W_{ij} = (t_{ij}/t_{\text{sacr}})^6$ (or $W_{ij} = (t_{ij}/t_{\text{sacr}})^k$) to animals dying without the tumor when the tumor incidence is close to a polynomial of order six (or order k).

The class of Bailer–Portier poly-k tests are carried out by replacing the C_i's by the new number of animals at risk C_i^*'s in the calculation of the above Cochran–Armitage test statistic.

The class of Bailer–Portier poly-k tests adjust differences in survival, do not need the information about cause of death, and call for only a (the terminal) sacrifice. Results of simulation studies by Bailer and Portier,[31] and Dinse[30] show that the tests performed very well under many conditions simulated. They are also relatively robust to (not affected greatly by) tumor lethality.

Bieler and Williams[33] pointed out that, since animal survival time is generally not a fixed quantity, the numerators and denominators of the adjusted quantal response estimates.

$$p_i^* = O_i / C_i^*$$

are both subject to random variation.

Bieler and Williams[33] proposed a test called the ratio trend test (also called Bieler–Williams poly-3 test), which is another modification to the Cochran–Armitage linear trend test. The ratio trend test employs the adjusted quantal response rates calculated in Bailer and Portier[31] and the delta method[34] in the estimation of the variance of the adjusted quantal response rates $p_i^* = O_i / C_i^*$.

The computational formula for Bieler–Williams ratio trend (modified C–A) test statistic is given as follows:

$$\chi_{BW}^2 = \frac{\sum m_i p_i^* D_i - (\sum m_i D_i)(\sum m_i p_i^*) / \sum m_i}{\{c[\sum m_i D_i^2 - (\sum m_i D_i)^2 / \sum m_i]\}^{1/2}}$$

where

$$c = \sum\sum (r_{ij} - r_{i.})2 / [R - (r+1)]$$

$$m_i = (C_I^*)^2 / C_i$$

$$r_{ij} = y_{ij} - p^* w_{ij}$$

$$r_i = \sum r_{ij} / C_i$$

y_{ij} = tumor response indicator (zero = absent at death, one = present at death) for the jth animal in the ith group.

Bieler and Williams[33] showed that the Bailer–Portier poly-3 trend test is anticonservative when tumor incidence rates are low and treatment toxicity is high. Their study also showed that for tumors with low background rates, the ratio trend test (Bieler–Williams poly-3 test) yielded actual Type I errors close to the nominal levels used and was observed to be less sensitive than the Bailer–Portier poly-3 trend test to misspecification of the shape of tumor incidence function and the magnitude of treatment toxicity.

The ratio trend test (Bieler–William poly-3 test), like the Bailer–Portier poly-3 test, adjusts differences in survival, does not need the information about cause of death, and results only in a (the terminal) sacrifice. Results of simulation studies[33,35] show that the tests performed well under many simulated conditions. It is also shown to be relatively robust to (not affected greatly by) tumor lethality, misspecification of the shape of tumor incidence function, and the magnitude of treatment toxicity. The ratio trend test (Bieler–William poly-3 test) should be used to replace the asymptotic tests that depend on the information of tumor lethality and cause of death when the information is unavailable.

H. COMBINED ANALYSIS OF TUMOR TYPES OBSERVED IN FATAL AND INCIDENTAL CONTEXTS BY EXACT PERMUTATION TEST

When a tumor type is observed in a fatal context in some animals and incidental context in other animals, and the total number of animals bearing the tumor type is not small, the appropriate method is to compute a pooled Z-statistic as described in Section III.E. However, when the total number of tumor-bearing animals is "small," e.g., less than ten, the normal approximation may not be adequate, and the p-value derived from a Z-test will not be reliable. One may be tempted to use the exact method described in the previous section using all tables formed for incidental tumors and fatal tumors. But as several authors have noted[36–38] this method is incorrect. A fundamental flaw in this approach is that the tables formed for fatal tumors are not conditionally independent as in case of incidental tumors. This is because animals can contribute to the total number-at-risk in more than one table. Heimann and Neuhaus have developed an exact permutation test that corrects this problem, but it assumes that the intercurrent mortality (i.e., the censoring distributions) among the dose groups is equal. In the case of unequal censoring the computing intensive test may yield worse results than the asymptotic test.[38] An alternative is to use the exact permutation trend test proposed by Mancuso et al.[37] for the combined analysis of incidental and fatal tumors. The test is an exact permutational version of the poly-3 test proposed by Bailer and Portier[31] and described in the previous section. The number of tumor-bearing animals over the entire experiment period can be exhibited as in Table 2.9.

The derivation of the exact poly-3 test is facilitated by first describing an exact permutation version of the Cochran–Armitage (CA) test. (Refer to the previous section for a description of the CA test.) An exact permutation version of the CA test can now be based on the permutation distribution of the test statistic $Y = \sum D_i O_i$, given the fixed row and columns marginal totals. In particular, the p-value $= P[Y \geq y|$ the row and column marginal totals], where y is the value of Y computed from the observed table. Let s be the number of tables that can be generated from all possible permutations of the cell counts given the fixed marginal totals such that the value of $Y \geq y$. Then the probability of observing a kth such table is given by

$$P_k = \frac{\binom{C_0}{O_{0k}}\binom{C_1}{O_{1k}}\cdots\binom{C_r}{O_{rk}}}{\binom{R}{O}}, \qquad k = 1, 2, \ldots, s.$$

The p-value then equals $\sum P_k$. In the above formulation it is assumed that all R animals were exposed to equal duration of risk, i.e., for the entire experiment period.

The survival-adjusted exact permutation trend test is based on the weighting scheme of the poly-3 test described in the previous section. In particular, let $[C_i^*]$ be the largest integer that does not exceed C_i^*. The adjusted exact test results are obtained by replacing C_i with $[C_i^*]$ and R with $R^* = \sum[C_i^*]$ in the computation of P_k and thereby the p-value as $\sum P_k$.

IV. INTERPRETATION OF STUDY RESULTS

Interpreting results of carcinogenicity experiments in an overall evaluation of the carcinogenic potential of a new drug is a complex process. Because of inherent limitations — such as small number of animals used, low tumor incidence rates, and biological variation — a carcinogenic drug may not be detected (i.e., a false negative error is committed). Also because of a large number of statistical tests performed on the data (usually two species, two sexes, 20 to 30 tissues examined, and four dose levels), there is a great potential that statistically significant positive dose–response relationships in some tumor types are purely caused by chance of random variation alone (i.e., a false positive error is committed). Controlling these two types of error is the central element in the interpretation of study results and involves statistical and nonstatistical biological judgments.[5] Therefore, it is important that an overall evaluation of the carcinogenic potential of a drug should be made based on the knowledge of statistical significance of positive dose–response relationships, historical control data,[5] and information of biological relevance.

The controls of the two types of error are also directly related to tests of statistical significance used. In the context of a question whether one should test for heterogeneity or positive dose–response relationship (trend) with respect to dose, Peto et al.[9] make the following recommendation: "If two or more dose levels are studied, statistical tests for positive trend with respect to the actual dose-levels tested will usually be more sensitive than the standard alternative statistical methods with respect to any real carcinogenic effects that may exist. In other words, when there is a fairly consistent positive trend in the experimental results, the p-value yielded by a test for heterogeneity will tend to be less impressive than the p-value yielded by a test for trend" (pp. 338, 339).

In general, FDA statistical reviewers follow this recommendation and test for a positive dose–response relationship in tumor incidence rates in their reviews.

Based on biological information, the overall false positive error in animal carcinogenicity studies, caused by the effect of multiple tests of statistical significance, can be controlled by reducing the number of variables evaluated. This can be achieved by combining certain tumor types. McConnell et al.[39] proposed the following guidelines for combining tumors: (a) tumors of the same histomorphogenic type with substantial evidence of progression from benign to malignant stage; (b) tumors, such as hyperplasia and benign tumors, in which criteria for differentiating then become unclear; (c) tumors in other organs or tissues but of the same histomorphogenic type; and (d) tumors of different morphologic classifications but with comparable histomorphogenesis.

These are statistical methods and use a Bonferroni type of adjustment for the effect of multiple comparisons.[28,40,41] This group of methods takes into consideration the fact that all tests performed on data pertaining to different tumors at the same or different sites are not independent, and significant results are not possible in some of the tests. The above modifications to the Bonferroni adjustment reduce the number of multiple tests performed and thus increase the power of the tests.

Tarone[41] proposed a modification of the Bonferroni method for discrete data. Since the statistical tests (trend or pairwise comparison tests) are based on discrete null distributions of the test statistics, Tarone's *modified Bonferroni method* is particularly suitable for correcting the effect of multiple tests in tumor data analysis. Tarone's modification method is conditional on the marginal totals of (two by two) or (two by c) tables. Using Tarone's notation the method is described here.

Suppose there are I sites (i.e., tissue and tumor combinations) for which a significance test can be performed. Let α_i be the minimum achievable significance level at site i, where $i = 1,2,...,I$. The minimum achievable significance level is the minimum of the observed p-values under all possible permutations of the animals of the given sex in the given experiment. For each integer k, let $m(k) =$ number of the I sites for which $\alpha_i < \alpha$, where α is the nominal significance level. Let K be the smallest value of k such that $m(k)/k \leq 1$, and let R_k denote the set of indices satisfying $K\alpha_i < \alpha$. A statistical test at site i will be considered to yield a significant result only if i is contained in R_k and $P_i < \alpha/K$, where P_i is the observed p-value for site i. Note that K is the modified Bonferroni correction factor. It can be readily seen that the overall false positive error rate (i.e., the probability of rejecting the null hypothesis, say, of no trend at any site) is bounded by α.

Tarone has suggested a further refinement of the modification method by considering the fact that, in most cases, the total probability in the rejection regions (as defined above) of the $m(k)$ tests will be less than α. Under this situation, it may be possible to expand one or more of the $m(k)$ rejections, or even outside the set R_k by adding points until the overall false positive error rate does not exceed α.

In the same spirit, Fears et al.[42] showed that in animal carcinogenicity studies, the issue of multiple tests is a problem only for the tumor types with high incidence rates. Since the majority of the tumor types in animal studies of human drugs have very low incidence rates and the final determination of the oncogenic potential of a new drug is based on results of statistical tests as well as relevant biologic and pathological information, it is argued[42-44] that the false error rates in animal carcinogenicity studies are not as large as some people previously thought.[45] Haseman[44] showed that if a comparison of tumor rates in high dose vs. control groups is carried out at the 0.01 level for all commonly occurring tumors and at the 0.05 level for all rare tumors, then the overall false positive error rate associated with this approach in NCI/NTP carcinogenicity studies appears to be no more than 7% to 8%.

Farrar and Crump[46,47] proposed an alternative method to adjust for the effect of multiple tests, and the effect of dependencies that may exist between tumors on the overall false positive error. In the proposed method, simple functions of p-values from conventional tests applied to each individual tumor (approximation or exact permutation, pairwise comparisons or trend tests) are evaluated for statistical significance using a Monte-Carlo procedure that treats individual animals as units of variation. The functions of p-values of individual pairwise and trend tests can be the minimum p-value or the product of a fixed number, K, of the smallest p-values. For material that causes tumors at only a single site, the minimum p-value may be a meaningful summary statistic, and the test based on this statistic may also be more powerful. However, for less specific carcinogens, the product of the K smallest p-values, which combines information from K sites, may be more appropriate.

As mentioned above, the statistical significance of a chosen function of the p-values used as the test statistic is then evaluated using a Monte-Carlo randomization (permutation) procedure. Animals are randomly assigned to treatment groups with the number of animals assigned to each treatment group being preserved. The test statistic is recomputed for each reassignment. The proportion of the statistics that are at least as extreme as the observed minimum p-value (or the product of the K smallest p-values) computed from the original data is used as the estimated overall false positive error.

A method related to the Farrar–Crump method but independently developed by Heyse and Rom[48] deals exclusively with the use of the minimum of the p-values from all exact permutation trend tests and random permutations in the adjustment for the effect of multiple statistical tests. In this method, the overall false positive error is estimated by the following formula (using the authors' notation):

$$P_{[1]}^* = 1 - \prod_{j=1}^{r}(1 - P_{(i)}^*) = P_{[1]}^* - P_{(i)}^* P_{(j)}^* + \cdots + (-1)^{n+1} P_{(i)}^* P_{(j)}^* \cdots P_{(r)}^*$$

where

$P_{[1]}^* =$ estimated overall false positive error.

$P_{(i)}^* = Pr(S_{(i)} \geq S_{(i)}^*) =$ the largest p-value that is attainable (with given number of tumors at site i) and is smaller than or equal to P_1.

$S(i) =$ A random variable assuming score of measuring trend from the exact permutation trend test.

$S_{(i)}^* =$ The observed value of $S_{(i)}$ that satisfies the definition of $P_{(i)}^*$ above.

P_1 = Minimum of the p-values from the exact permutation trend tests on individual sites and tumors.

n = The number of $P^*_{(i)}$ components in each term of $P^*_{[i]}$.

$$P^*_{(i)}P^*_{(j)}...P^*_{(r)} = Pr(S_{(i)} \geq S^*_{(i)} \text{ and...and } S_{(t)} \geq S^*_{(r)})$$

The above probabilities of joint events are calculated from multivariate randomization distributions of trend measure scores, $S_{(i)}s$.

r = the number of site/lesion combinations tested.

The above formula considers possible dependencies between sites and tumors. However, the authors showed empirically that "the independence assumption may prove to be a biologically reasonable approximation for the data of this sort."

Westfall and Young[49] proposed another method for controlling the experimentwise false error rate. In this method, all p-values are adjusted for the multiplicity of testing using vector-based bootstrap resampling method. In the test for positive dose–response relationship in tumor incidence rates using the survival-unadjusted Cochran–Armitage linear trend test,[23,24] the p-values can be adjusted for the effect of multiple tests by the above method as follows:

1. Assume the observed data are $x_{11},...,x_{1n_1},...,x_{g1},...,x_{gn_g}$, where each x_{ij} is a $kx1$ vector, and g is the number of treatment groups.
2. Compute the k unadjusted p-values, pv_k, for all lesion or site combinations using the Cochran–Armitage trend test.
3. Generate a prespecified number (with desired accuracy), say, 10,000, of replicate samples of the observed data $x_{11},...,x_{1n_1},...,x_{g1},...,x_{1n_g}$, with bootstrap resampling. Let $x^*_{11},...,x^*_{1n_1},...,x^*_{g1},...,x_{1n_g}$ denote a replicate sample.
4. Calculate the new set of p-values, pv^*_k, by applying the Cochran–Armitage trend test to each of the replicate samples, find the smallest, min pv^*, of the k p-values, pv^*_k calculated from the replicate sample.
5. Calculate the adjusted p-values, apv_k, for each k using the proportions of samples for which min pv^*_k is equal to or less than pv_k.

The authors conducted a simulation study comparing the bootstrap method with the permutation method of Farrar and Crump[46,47] and Heyse and Rom.[48] They reported the following simulation results: (a) the bootstrap method approximates nominal significance levels more closely than the permutation method, and (b) the bootstrap method has more power than the permutation method.

In the tests for the positive dose–response relationship in tumor incidence rates, FDA statistical reviewers currently use data of the concurrent control groups and comparable, historical control data to classify common and rare tumors, and adopt the following decision rule in their evaluation: a positive dose–response relationship is considered not to occur by chance of variation alone if the p-value is less than 0.005 for a common tumor, and 0.025 for a rare tumor. A tumor type with a background rate of 1% or less is classified as rare; more frequent tumors are classified as common.

The above FDA statistical decision rule for tests for a positive trend in tumor incidence has been developed based on recent studies using real historical control data of CD mice and CD rats from Charles River Laboratory and simulation studies conducted internally and in collaboration with NTP.[50,51] The FDA decision rule achieves an overall false positive rate of around 10% in a standard two-species and two-sex study.[50–53] The 10% overall false positive rate is seen by CDER statisticians as appropriate in a new drug regulatory setting.

The false negative error issue in animal carcinogenicity study, although equally important as the false positive error issue, has not received as much attention as has the false positive error issue. This may be in part because of the following two reasons:

1. This issue is less familiar to people. Statistically, the theory of the false negative error issue is more complicated than that of the false positive error issue. The false negative error is a function of alternative hypotheses one is interested in testing. The statistical distributions used in the evaluation of false negative errors are complicated and involve noncentrality parameters.
2. Because of the high cost involved in developing a new drug, the drug sponsor will pay more attention to false positive errors than to false negative errors.

As mentioned at the beginning of this section, the large false negative error that occurs in animal carcinogenicity study, is caused by the inherent limitations of small numbers of animals used and by the low incidence rates in the majority of tumors examined. Because of the above limitations, the power of statistical tests for positive dose–response relationship is going to be small. That is, the false negative errors are expected to be large. A study by Ali[26] shows that under the conditions he simulated (which assumed tumor incidence rates following Weibull models), the powers of the exact permutation trend test, the Peto prevalence test for trend, and some modified forms of Peto prevalence test are no more than 0.25. That is, the false negative errors are greater than 0.75. If the above simulation results reflect the general magnitudes of the power of statistical trend tests, then the false negative error issue should cause concern to investigators and be weighted at least equally with the false positive error issue in the overall evaluation of results of an animal carcinogenicity study.

Table 2.10 contains some of Haseman's[6] calculations of tumor rates that needed to be induced in the treated group in order to achieve certain levels of power in the Fisher's exact test at .05 and .01 levels of significance under

TABLE 2.10
Tumor Rates (%) Needed to be Induced in the Treated Group in Order to Achieve Levels of Power of 0.50 and 0.90

Spontaneous tumor rate in control (%)	$\alpha = 0.05$		$\alpha = 0.01$	
	Power = 0.5	Power = 0.9	Power = 0.5	Power = 0.9
0.1%	9.5%	15.8%	13.5%	20.5%
1.0	11.0	18.4	15.1	23.4
3.0	14.0	22.9	18.9	29.0
5.0	17.0	27.0	22.5	33.3
10.0	24.2	35.7	30.2	41.9
20.0	36.8	49.0	43.2	56.0
30.0	48.1	61.1	54.8	67.0

various assumed spontaneous rates in the control group (assuming 50 animals in the treated group and in the control).

Statistically, there are at least three ways to increase the power of tests to ensure that the overall false negative errors are not excessive. The most obvious way is to increase group sizes. However, the increase in power probably won't be significant unless the group size is drastically increased, say, from 50 to 250 animals per group. This approach to increasing power may not be financially or logistically feasible.

The second way to ensure adequate power in statistical tests of positive dose–response relationship in tumor rates is to administer to treated animals with dose levels that are high enough to induce tumors. As mentioned in Section II, the determination of a dose close to MTD for treating animals in the high dose group is an important, controversial, and complicated issue. Information about clinical signs, histopathological toxic effects, body weight gain, and mortality, as well as pharmacokinetic and metabolic data is needed for the evaluation of MTD.

Haseman used results of some NTP studies to emphasize the importance of using dose levels that provide an adequate tumor challenge to the treated animals. He found that half of the carcinogens tested in those studies would be judged as noncarcinogens if half of the MTDs were used as the highest dose. Under the current four-group design in which a medium group was added as a cushion for cases where the high dose used may be over MTD, it is feasible to take a greater risk of using the highest possible dose level to ensure adequate power in statistical tests.

The third way to increase power in statistical tests is to assume a larger overall false positive error. One may have to be willing to assume an overall false positive error in the 15% to 20% range in order to balance out the low power of statistical tests.

If one wants to control one of the two types of error to a small magnitude, then he or she has to pay the price for committing a large magnitude of the other type of error. In the general case, a statistical test is performed at a prespecified level of false positive error, usually .05, and a decision rule is derived to maximize the power (or to minimize the false negative error) of the test under the alternative hypothesis tested. However, because of the intertwining and conflicting relationship between the magnitudes of the false positive error and false negative error that one is willing to assume, the choice has to be determined by the cost-risk (or cost-risk-benefit) factor in new drug evaluation. For drug products, such as cancer and AIDS drugs that are intended for treating terminally ill patients, one may take a greater risk (false negative error) by taking a smaller overall false positive error. This will be especially true when there is no alternative drug available in the market. Alternatively, for drug products for treating common illnesses that can be treated with other available approved alternative drugs and that will be used by a larger population, one can be more cautious about the overall false negative error. To ensure that the false negative error is not excessive, one may have to assume a larger overall false positive error. It is true that limited resources should not be wasted by rejecting an effective drug, but for the protection of the health of the general public, it is equally important that drugs with carcinogenic potential should not be misinterpreted as safe and allowed to enter the market.

Although concurrent control groups are the most relevant controls in testing drug related increases in tumors in a study, there are situations in which historical control data from previous comparable studies can be useful in the overall evaluation of the results of the study. One of the situations is to use the comparable historical control information to define rare tumors (which have less effect on overall false positive error) and therefore can be tested at higher levels of significance. Another situation is to check if a marginally significant finding is really drug related or purely caused by chance of variation. A third situation is to use historical control data to check if a study was conducted properly.

In the first situation, a tumor is defined as rare if it was so classified by reviewing pharmacologists and pathologists, or if the background spontaneous incidence rate is less than 1%. In the second situation, the incidence rates of the treated groups are compared with the incidence rates of the historical control data. The significant finding will not be considered as biologically meaningful if the incidence rates of the treated groups are within the ranges of historical control incidence rates. In the third situation, a question about the quality of the study will be raised if incidence rates of tumors of the concurrence control of the study are not consistent with those in the comparable historical control data. "However, before historical control data can be used in a formal testing framework, a number of issues must first be considered."[6]

These issues include: the nomenclature conventions and diagnostic criteria used by pathologists and conducting laboratories; study durations; strains and species of animals used; and time (calendar year) when a study was conducted. It is important that the historical control data can be useful only if it is comparable with the concurrent control data. The comparability includes identical nomenclature conventions and diagnostic criteria, same species, strain and sex, same source of supplier, same testing laboratory, comparable survival and age at termination, comparable time frame of studies (within 5 years), and comparable food consumption and body weight gain.

FDA statisticians routinely perform tests for positive dose–response relationship (trend) in incidence rates in individual or pooled site/tumor combinations using the decision rule of testing common tumors at 0.005 and rare tumors at 0.025 levels of significance. Comparable historical control data, when available and reliable, are used to assist in classifying common and rare tumors, and in deciding if significant findings are biologically relevant. As mentioned at the beginning of the chapter, the adoption of the Bonferroni type of adjustment for the effect of multiple tests by FDA statisticians is based on a review of current literature, input received from consultations with outside experts, our own research, and our best scientific judgment.

To make sure that the false negative error committed is not excessive, statistical reviewers collaborate with the reviewing pharmacologists, pathologists, and medical officers to evaluate the adequacy of the gross and histological examination of control and treated groups, the adequacy of dose selection, and the durations of experiments in relation to the normal life span of the tested animals.

V. CARCINOGENICITY STUDIES USING TRANSGENIC MICE

The high cost (between $1M and $2M) and long time (a minimum of three years) needed to conduct a standard long-term *in vivo* carcinogenicity study, and the increased insight into the mechanisms of carcinogenicity because of the advances made in molecular biology have led to alternative *in vivo* approaches to the assessment of carcinogenicity. People also argue that genetically altered mice are better animal surrogates for human cancer because they carry some specifically activated oncogenes that are known to function in human and animal cancers. ICH has developed a document, accepted by the U.S. and other regions, entitled "Guidance on Testing for Carcinogenicity of Pharmaceuticals."[54] The guidance outlines experimental approaches to the evaluation of carcinogenic potential that may obviate the necessity for the routine use of two long-term rodent carcinogenicity studies, allowing sponsors either to continue to conduct two long-term rodent carcinogenicity studies or to use the alternative approach of conducting one long-term rodent carcinogenicity study together with a short- or medium-term rodent test. The short- or medium-term rodent test systems include such studies as initiation-promotion in rodents, transgenic rodents, or new-born rodents, which provide rapid observation of carcinogenic endpoints *in vivo*.

Studies using transgenic mice have become the most important alternative to carcinogenicity testing among the short- or medium-term rodent test systems recommended in the ICH guideline. Many new studies of known carcinogens and noncarcinogens from previous two-year bioassays but using transgenic rodents have been carried out by the National Toxicological Program (NTP) and by the International Life Science Institute (ILSI) to evaluate the specificity and sensitivity of alternative test systems. Different strains of transgenic mice (models) have been proposed and used in the alternative system of testing carcinogenicity of pharmaceutical and environmental chemical compounds. We also have seen and reviewed carcinogenicity studies of pharmaceuticals using transgenic mice submitted by drug companies. The following are the main strains (models) having been proposed and used in the studies mentioned above: (a) p53 +/− transgenic mice (with knockout of one of the two alleles of the tumor suppression gene p53), (b) Tg.AC transgenic mice (with genetically initiated skin to induce epidermal papillomas in response to dermal or oral exposure to chemical agents and act as a reporter phenotype of the activities of the tested chemicals), (c) rasH2 transgenic mice (with five or six copies of the stable human c-Ha-ras gene. These were first developed and patented in Japan), and (d) XPA −/− repair deficient mice (developed in Europe).

The standard study protocol described below has been used in the above studies:

1. Study duration: 26 weeks.
2. A positive control group with treatment of a known carcinogen such as p-cresidine, benzene, and TPA, in addition to the regular three or four treatment groups (negative control, low, medium, and high)
3. 15 to 30 animals per sex and treatment group.
4. Tissues and organs of p53 +/−, rasH2, and XPA −/− repair deficient mice died or terminally sacrificed are microscopically examined for neoplastic and nonneoplastic lesions.
5. In studies using Tg.AC transgenic mice, only data (incidence rates and weekly counts of papillomas observed over time) of tumor type of skin papillalomas are collected and tested for drug effects.

In studies using p53 +/−, rasH2, and XPA −/− repair deficient mice, tumor data and methods of analysis are similar to those of 2-year studies. However, methods for analyzing the data of weekly counts of skin papilloma in studies using Tg.AC transgenic mice are somewhat different from those for studies using the above models.

In general, the exact and asymptotic tests for trend and difference in tumor incidence for the traditional 2-year study can be applied to carcinogenicity studies using p53 +/−, or rasH2 or XPA −/− transgenic mice because the endpoints in these two types of study are the same.

Because the major differences in designs used, i.e., 15 to 30 animals per sex/treatment group and a small number of tumor types developed in animals in the new type of study using the above models, the decision rules used in the two-year studies may have to be modified in order to maintain a desirable level of overall false positive rate. Also because only 15 to 30 animals per sex or group are used, the power of the trend and pairwise comparison tests should be evaluated.

Carcinogenicity studies using Tg.AC transgenic mice are different from the traditional 2-year studies because skin papillomas (weekly incidence rates and weekly counts of the tumor) in areas inside and outside of topical application of the chemical are used as the endpoints of measuring the carcinogenic effect of a drug.

Incidence rates of skin papilloma (proportions of animals with the tumor) of different weeks can be analyzed separately by the same methods used in regular 2-year studies. For the data of counts of skin papillomas of different weeks, the nonparametric procedures, Jonckheere's test for trend and the Mann-Whitney test for pairwise comparison, can be used separately. Because the number of papillomas in the application area in an animal can be counted only up to a prespecified number, 20 or 30, there could exist a large number of observations with this value. The large number of tied observations could be a problem in applying the nonparametric procedures.

The above separate tests basing on data of individual weeks produce results difficult to interpret and ignore some important biological factors. A more recently developed method by Dunson et al.[55] uses data of papilloma counts of all time points in one analysis. This method separates the effects on papilloma into latency and multiplicity, and accommodates important features of the data, including variability in expression of the transgene and dependency in the tumor counts.

Because skin papilloma is the only tumor type used as the endpoint of testing the carcinogenic effect of a drug, the adjustment for multiplicity is no longer an issue. However, there are suggestions that the examination of only skin papillomas may not be sufficient in detecting a carcinogen in studies using Tg.AC transgenic mice.

VI. DATA PRESENTATION AND SUBMISSION

To facilitate statistical reviews, sponsors should present their data in the reports in such a way that the reviewers are able to verify the sponsors' calculations so as to validate their statistical methods as being appropriate to the way the data were generated, to trace back the sponsors' conclusions through their summaries and analyses to the raw data, and to reanalyze the data, if necessary, in order to explore alternatives or to gain greater insight into the relationships between various events of the studies.

In addition to reviewing the reports submitted by sponsors, statisticians at FDA also perform additional statistical analyses that they believe are appropriate and necessary to evaluate the analyses and conclusions contained in the reports. Therefore sponsors should make the raw data easily accessible in an appropriate format to the statistical reviewers. Statistical reviews are delayed when data are not accessible or not submitted in appropriate formats. To expedite the statistical reviews, sponsors are advised that the tumor data on computer readable forms be submitted with their original initial submissions of the hardcopy NDA or IND following the formats and specifications described in the FDA guidance for industry on electronic data submission.[2,4,56]

VII. CONCLUDING REMARKS

In designing an experiment, randomization methods should be used in allocating animals to treatment groups to avoid possible biases caused in animal selection. A sufficient number of animals should be used in the experiment to ensure reasonable power in the statistical tests used. In negative studies in which results of the analysis show no significant positive dose–response relationships in tumor incidence rates, a further evaluation on the validity of the designs of experiment should be performed to see if there are sufficient numbers of animals that lived long enough to get adequate exposure to the chemical and to be at risk of forming late-developing tumors, and if the doses used are high enough and close to the MTD to present a reasonable tumor challenge to the tested animals.

In the review and evaluation of methods of statistical analysis in an animal carcinogenicity study submission, the statistical reviewers in FDA examine the appropriateness of the statistical methods used by the sponsor and perform additional independent analyses to evaluate and verify the sponsor's conclusions. Appropriate statistical analyses of animal carcinogenicity study data should include the following areas.

The intercurrent mortality data should be evaluated first to see whether the survival distributions of the treatment groups are significantly different and the dose–response relationship in mortality is significant. Because the effects of differences in intercurrent mortality on number of tumor-bearing animals can be substantial, survival-adjusted methods should be used in tests for positive dose–response relationships in tumor incidence rates.

The determination of survival-adjusted methods to be used in tests for positive dose–response relationships in tumor incidence rates should be based on the contexts of observation of the tumors whose data are to be analyzed. The death-rate method and the prevalence method should be used to analyze data of tumors observed in fatal and incidental contexts of observation, respectively. However if the information about the contexts of observation of tumors is not available or is available but is considered as not accurate enough, then statistical methods such as poly-k, that do not require the information, should be used.

When the number of tumor occurrences across treatment groups is small, the test results of the death-rate method and the prevalence method that use the normal approximation are not stable and reliable. In this circumstance, exact permutation methods should be used to replace the above methods in tests for positive dose–response relationships in tumor incidence rates.

Controlling the overall false positive error and the overall false negative error to acceptable levels is the central element in the interpretation of study results. The control of the two types of error involves statistical and nonstatistical issues that require statistical as well as biological judgments. Therefore, it is important that an overall evaluation of the tumorigenic potential of a drug should be made based on knowledge of statistical significance of positive dose–response relationship and information of biological relevance.

To facilitate the FDA's statistical review, sponsors should present their data in the reports in such a way that the reviewers should be able to verify their calculations, to validate their statistical methods, and to trace back the calculations through their summaries and analyses to the raw data. The sponsors should make the raw data easily accessible in an appropriate format to the statistical reviewers. Statistical reviews are delayed when data are not accessible. Sponsors are advised that the electronic tumor data be submitted with their original initial submissions of the hardcopy NDA or IND.

ACKNOWLEDGMENTS

The authors thank Dr. William R. Fairweather and Dr. Judith L. Weissinger for their thoughtful comments and suggestions.

The views expressed in this chapter are those of the authors and are not necessarily those of the FDA and of Otsuka. The second author was formerly with the FDA.

REFERENCES

1. Fairweather, W.R., Statistical considerations in tumorigenicity study review (abstract), presented at the Drug Information Association Meeting, Toronto, Canada, July 12, 1988.
2. U.S. Department of Health and Human Services, *Guidance for Industry: Statistical Aspects of the Design, Analysis, and Interpretation of Chronic Rodent Carcinogenicity Studies of Pharmaceuticals*, Center for Drug Evaluation and Research, Food and Drug Administration, 2001.
3. Lin, K.K., Carcinogenicity studies of pharmaceuticals, In *Encyclopedia of Biopharmaceutical Statistics*, Shein-Chung Chow, ed., Marcel Dekker, New York, pp. 88–103, 2000.
4. U.S. Department of Health and Human Services, *Guidance for Industry: Providing Regulatory Submissions in Electronic Formats — NDAs*, Center for Drug Evaluation and Research, Food and Drug Administration, 1999.
5. Office of the Federal Register, Chemical carcinogens; a review of the science and its associated principles in Part II, Office of Science and Technology Policy, *Federal Register*, pp. 47–58. (Note: The paper was also published with the same title and authorized by U.S. Interagency Staff Group on Carcinogens in Environmental Health Perspectives, 67, pp. 201–282), 1985.
6. Haseman, J.K., Statistical issues in the design, analysis and interpretation of animal carcinogenicity studies, *Environ. Health Perspect.*, 58, 385–392, 1984.
7. Chu, K.C., Cueto, C., and Ward, J.M., Factors in the evaluation of 200 National Cancer Institute carcinogen bioassays, *J. Toxicol. Environ. Health*, 8, 251–280, 1981.

8. ICH, *SIC Dose Selection for Carcinogenicity Studies of Pharmaceuticals, ICH — SIC*, 1995.

9. Peto, R., Pike, M.C., Day, N.E., Gray, R.G., Lee, P.N., Parish, S., Peto, J., Richards, S., and Wahrendorf, J., *Guidelines for Simple, Sensitive Significance Tests for Carcinogenic Effects in Long-Term Animal Experiments, Long-Term and Short-Term Screening Assays for Carcinogens: An Critical Appraisal*, International Agency for Research on Cancer, Lyon, France, IARC Monographs Supplement 2, pp. 311–426, 1980.

10. Gart, J.J., Krewski, D., Lee, P.N., Tarone, R.E., and Wahrendorf, J., *The Design and Analysis of Long-Term Animal Experiments*, Vol. III, International Agency for Research on Cancer, World Health Organization, Lyon, France, 1986.

11. Cox, D.R., Regression models and life tables (with discussion), *J. Roy. Stat. Soc. Ser. B*, 34, 187–220, 1972.

12. Thomas, D.G., Breslow, N., and Gart, J.J., Trend and homogeneity analyses of proportions and life table data, *Comput. Biomed. Res.*, 10, 373–381, 1977.

13. Breslow, N., A generalized Kruskal–Wallis test for comparing K samples subject to unequal patterns of censorship, *Biometrics*, 57, 579–594, 1970.

14. Gehan, E.A., A generalized Wilcoxon test for comparing k samples subject to unequal patterns of censorship, *Biometrika*, 52, 203–223, 1965.

15. Cox, D.R., The analysis of exponentially distributed life-times with two types of failures, *J. Roy. Stat. Soc. Ser. B*, 21, 412–421, 1959.

16. Tarone, R.E., Tests for trend in life table analysis, *Biometrika*, 62, 679–682, 1975.

17. Bancroft, T.A., Analysis and inference for incompletely specified models involving the use of preliminary test(s) of significance, *Biometrics*, 20, 427–442, 1964.

18. Mantel, N., Chi-square tests with one degree of freedom; extensions of the Mantel–Haenszel procedure, *Biometrics*, 37, 763–764, 1963.

19. Dinse, G.E. and Haseman, J.K., Logistic regression analysis of incidental-tumor data from animal carcinogenicity experiments, *Fundament. Appl. Toxicol.*, 6, 44–52, 1986.

20. Dinse, G.E., Testing for trend in tumor prevalence rates: I. Nonlethal tumors, *Biometrics*, 41, 751–770, 1985.

21. Dinse, G.E. and Lagakos, S.W., Regression analysis of tumor prevalence data, *J. Roy. Stat. Soc. Ser. C*, 32, 236–248, 1983.

22. Lin, K.K. and Reschke, M.F., The use of the logistic model in space motion sickness prediction, *Aviat Space Environ. Med.* A9–A15, 1987.

23. Armitage, P., Tests for linear trends in proportions and frequencies, *Biometrics*, 11, 375–386, 1955.

24. Armitage, P., *Statistical Methods in Medical Research*, Wiley, New York, 1971.

25. Lin, K.K., Peto prevalence method vs. regression methods in analyzing incidental tumor data from animal carcinogenicity experiments: An empirical study, *1988 Proceedings of the Biopharmaceutical Section of the American Statistical Association*, American Statistical Association, Alexandria, VA, pp. 95–100, 1988.

26. Ali, M.W., A comparison of power between exact and approximate tests of trend of tumor prevalence when tumor rates are low, *1990 Proceedings of the Biopharmaceutical Section of the American Statistical Association*, American Statistical Association, Alexandria, VA, pp. 66–71, 1990.

27. Goldberg, K.M., An algorithm for computing an exact trend test for multiple $2 \times k$ contingency tables, Presented at Symposium on Long-Term Animal Carcinogenicity Studies, Washington, DC, 1985.

28. Mantel, N., Assessing laboratory evidence for neoplastic activity, *Biometrics*, 36, 381–399, 1980.

29. Ali, M.W., Exact versus asymptotic tests of trend of tumor prevalence in tumorigenicity experiments: a comparison of *p*-values for small frequency of tumors, *Drug Inf. J.*, 24, 727–737, 1990.

30. Dinse, G.E., A comparison of tumor incidence analyses applicable in single-sacrifice animal experiments, *Stat. Med.*, 13, 689–708, 1994.

31. Bailer, A. and Portier, C., Effects of treatment-induced mortality on tests for carcinogenicity n small samples, *Biometrics*, 44, 417–431, 1988.

32. Cochran, W., Some methods for strengthening the common χ^2 tests, *Biometrics*, 10, 417–451, 1954.

33. Bieler, G.S. and Williams, R.L., Ratio estimates, the delta method, and quantal response tests for increased carcinogenicity, *Biometrics*, 49, 793–801, 1993.

34. Woodruff, R.S., A simple method for approximating the variance of a complicated estimate, *J. Am. Stat. Assoc.*, 66, 411–414, 1971.

35. Chen, J.J., Lin, K.K., Huque, M.F., and Arani, R.B., Weighted P-value for animal carcinogenicity trend test, *Biometrics*, 56, 586–592, 2000.

36. Fairweather, W.R., Bhattacharyya, A., Ceuppens, P.P., Heimann, G., Hothorn, L.A., Kodell, R.L., Lin, K.K., Mager, H., Middleton, B.J., Slob, W., Soper, K.A., Stallard, N., Ventre, J., and Wright, J., Biostatistical methodology in carcinogenicity studies, *Drug Inf. J.*, 32, 401–421, 1998.

37. Mancuso, J.Y., Hongshik, A., Chen, J.J., and Mancuso, J.P., Age-adjusted exact trend tests in the event of rare occurrences, *Biometrics*, 58, 403–412, 2002.

38. Heimann, G. and Neuhaus, G., Permutational distribution of the log-rank statistic under random censorship with applications to carcinogenicity assays, *Biometrics*, 54, 168–184, 1998.

39. McConnell, E.E., Solleveld, H.A., Swenberg, J.A., and Boorman, G.A., Guidelines for combining neoplasms for evaluation of rodent carcinogenesis studies, *J. Natl. Cancer Inst.*, 76, 283–289, 1986.

40. Gart, J.J., Chu, K.C., and Tarone, R.E., Statistical issues in interpretation of chronic bioassays for carcinogenicity, *J. Natl. Cancer Inst.*, 62, 957–974, 1979.

41. Tarone, R.E., A modified bonferroni method for discrete data, *Biometrics*, 46, 515–522, 1990.

42. Fears, T.R., Tarone, R.E., and Chu, K.C., False-positive and false-negative rates for carcinogenicity screens, *Cancer Res.*, 37, 1941–1945, 1977.

43. Haseman, J.K., Response to 'Use of statistics when examining lifetime studies in rodents to detect carcinogenicity', *J. Toxicol. Environ. Health*, 3, 633–636, 1997.

44. Haseman, J.K., A reexamination of false-positive rates for carcinogenesis studies, *Fundam. Appl. Toxicol.*, 3, 334–339, 1983.

45. Salsburg, D.S., Use of statistics when examining lifetime studies in rodents to detect carcinogenicity, *J. Toxicol. Environ. Health*, 3, 611–628, 1977.

46. Farrar, D.B. and Crump, K.S., Exact statistical tests for any carcinogenic effect in animal bioassays, *Fundam. Appl. Toxicol.*, 11, 652–663, 1988.

47. Farrar, D.B. and Crump, K.S., Exact statistical tests for any carcinogenic effect in animal bioassays, II Age-adjusted tests, *Fundam. Appl. Toxicol.*, 15, 710–721, 1990.

48. Heyse, J.F. and Rom, D., Adjusting for multiplicity of statistical tests in the analysis of carcinogenicity studies, *Biometrical J.*, 30, 883–896, 1988.

49. Westfall, P.H. and Young, S.S., P-value adjustments for multiple tests in multivariate binomial models, *J. Am. Stat. Assoc.*, 84, 780–786, 1989.

50. Lin, K.K. and Rahman, M.A., Overall false positive rates in tests for linear trend in tumor incidence in animal carcinogenicity studies of new drugs, *J. Pharm. Stat.*, 8(1), 1–22, 1998a, with discussions.

51. Lin, K.K. and Rahman, M.A., *False Positive Rates in Tests for Trend and Differences in Tumor Incidence in Animal Carcinogenicity Studies of Pharmaceuticals under ICH Guidance S1B*, unpublished report, Division of Biometrics 2, Center for Drug Evaluation and Research, Food and Drug Administration, 1998b.

52. Lin, K.K., A regulatory perspective on statistical methods for analyzing new drug carcinogenicity study data, *Bio/Pharam. Q.*, 1(2), 18–20, 1995.

53. Lin, K.K., Control of Overall False Positive Rates in Animal Carcinogenicity Studies of Pharmaceuticals, presented at 1997 FDA Forum on Regulatory Sciences, December 8–9, Bethesda, Maryland, 1997.

54. ICH. *S1B Testing for Carcinogenicity of Pharmaceuticals, ICH — S1B, Federal Register*, Vol. 63, 1998, pp. 8983–8986.

55. Dunson, D.B., Haseman, J.K., van Birgelen, A.P.J.M., Staiewicz, S., and Tennant, R.W., Statistical analysis of skin tumor data from Tg.AC mouse assays, *Toxicol. Sci.*, 55, 293–302, 2000.

56. FDA. *Guideline for the Format and Content of the Nonclinical/Pharmacology/ Toxicology Section of an Application*, U.S. Department of Health and Human Services, Rockville, MD, 1987.

3 The FDA and the IND/NDA Statistical Review Process

Satya D. Dubey, George Y. H. Chi, and Roswitha E. Kelly

CONTENTS

I. THE FDA: WHY?

Food and drug laws have been a necessity to mankind since the beginning of civilization. Early Hebrew and Egyptian laws governed the handling of meat, Greek and Roman laws prohibited adding water to wine and short measures for grain and cooking oil, and in royal households, the "King's taster" protected the monarch from inferior or poisoned food. As civilization advanced, more complex protection became necessary. Apothecaries and food merchants of the Middle Ages organized as trade guilds to combat adulteration by inspecting spices and drugs. With the industrial revolution came an increasing use of chemicals, some of them harmful, such as poisonous food colors containing lead, arsenic, and mercury, and preservatives such as formaldehyde and borax. Such practices led the British parliament in 1860 to pass the first nationwide general food law of modern times.

The first general law against food adulteration in the United States was enacted in Massachusetts in 1784; gradually, other states passed a variety of food and drug statutes. As the country expanded, however, it became clear that a national law was needed. Many states had no laws or lacked enforcement. Products that met the requirements of one state could be illegal in adjoining states and variations in labeling requirements became intolerable. From 1879 to 1906 more than 100 food and drug bills were introduced in the U.S. Congress. The first advocates of Federal legislation were state officials who knew the problems and the weaknesses of existing controls. It was the leadership of one remarkable man, Harvey Washington Wiley, Head Chemist for the Department of Agriculture's Bureau of Chemistry, which finally made food and drug protection a function of the Federal Government.

With support and encouragement from various segments of the drug and food industries, state governments, women's groups, writers, business organizations, and a host of crusading individuals, Congress passed the first national legislation designed to control impure and unsafe foods and drugs: The Pure Food and Drug (Wiley) Act of 1906. The administration of the law was assigned to the Bureau of Chemistry, which was headed by Dr. Wiley. Under Wiley's direction the Bureau continued the development of scientific methods of analysis, worked out the legal procedures and techniques of inspection, and applied them in hundreds of hard-fought court cases. They won scores of judicial interpretations, which both strengthened the law and disclosed its weaknesses.

Laws and amendments following the Wiley Act have greatly increased the ability of the Federal Government to protect the U.S. consumer and to safeguard this nation's sources of food and drugs. It became quickly evident that this initial legislation did not have the necessary "teeth" to control many of the problems associated with the distribution and consumption of foods and drugs existing in the U.S. during the early part of the last century. For example, the Supreme Court ruled in 1911 that the law allowed for false and unproven therapeutic claims as long as all of the ingredients were properly listed. In the following year (1912) in an attempt to correct this omission, Congress passed the Sherley Amendment prohibiting "false and fraudulent label claims." However, this amendment did not prove effective, for it placed the burden of proof as to what constituted fraud on government prosecutors; a distributor only needed to demonstrate that he "believed" that the product produced the advertised effect in order to escape prosecution for fraud.

In an effort to increase the visibility of the organization and to raise needed revenues, the Bureau of Chemistry became the Food, Drug, and Insecticide

Administration in 1927. Four years later, in 1931, the name was changed to the Food and Drug Administration (FDA).

Motivated by the public clamor resulting from the infamous Elixir Sulfanilamide disaster, Congress passed the Food, Drug and Cosmetic Act in 1938. The Sulfanilamide incident resulted from the marketing of a medication containing diethylene glycol, a common component of antifreeze. The solution was prescribed as an antibiotic but produced fatal kidney failure that killed 107 people. This "elixir" was marketed without toxicological tests.

The Food, Drug and Cosmetic Act of 1938 greatly increased the power and responsibility of the FDA. Marking a basic change in the attitude of the Government to the regulation of drugs, the legislation required the preapproval of drugs by the FDA. In this new system, drug companies were required to submit evidence of drug safety. With this procedure the FDA had 60 to 180 days to review an application. Failure to disapprove within the time period would lead to marketing.

The 1938 law required that the drug manufacturers list additional warnings and descriptions for use of marketed drugs. In addition, the Act required factory inspection, gave prosecutors the added weapon of court injunctions as a regulatory weapon, and simplified the prosecution of false claims by eliminating the need to prove fraud.

Amendments to the 1938 Act and regulations issued by the FDA have further refined and improved the U.S. drug regulatory system. The Humphrey–Durham Amendment in 1951 gave the FDA the authority to define and label prescription drugs and prohibit refills.

Under this law, labeling was available on request but was not routinely shipped with the product. In 1960, the FDA issued regulations requiring that detailed information on indications, dosing, and safety be included with drug packaging and in sales literature.

In 1962, in a response to the Thalidomide tragedy, the Kefauver–Harris Amendment was passed, further increasing the regulatory authority of FDA. This amendment required for the first time that drug sponsors demonstrate the efficacy of a drug by providing substantial evidence from controlled trials. The Kefauver–Harris Amendment also eliminated the passive approval system by making it a requirement that the FDA approve drugs prior to marketing. The 1962 Amendment also required that adverse drug reactions be reported to the FDA, tightening Investigational New Drug Application (IND) provisions requiring informed consent, and gave FDA the authority to regulate advertising for prescription drugs.

In 1983, the Orphan Drug Act was passed to provide incentives for the pharmaceutical industry to develop drugs for relatively rare diseases. The 1984 Price Competition/Patient Term Restoration Act provides for increased patent protection to compensate for patent life lost during the approval process and simplified the approval of generic drugs. In responding to criticisms concerning the length of the review process, the FDA issued the "NDA Rewrite" in 1985, with new and revised drug regulations that were designed to improve the content and format as well as the processing of New Drug Applications (NDAs).

In 1987, recognizing the health crisis brought on by the AIDS epidemic, the Agency issued the "Interim Regulatory Procedures" (Federal Register Part VI, 21 CFR Parts 312 and 314, page 41516). These Interim procedures make it possible for more seriously ill patients to receive promising experimental drugs, while preserving appropriate guarantees for safety and effectiveness. These procedures reflect the recognition that the benefits of a drug need to be evaluated in light of the severity of the disease being treated; physicians and patients are willing to accept greater risks from products that treat life-threatening and severely debilitating illnesses than they would accept from products that treat less serious illnesses.

With this rule, the expanded availability of drugs for "immediately life-threatening conditions" can begin near the end of the second phase of human testing. In this way the drug would become available as soon as the initial safety evidence was on-hand and the proper dose had been determined (Phase I), and after some evidence of efficacy had been obtained (Phase II). Under these procedures, it is also possible that, with early evidence for efficacy and safety, drugs for "serious but not immediately life-threatening illnesses" can be approved for expanded use during Phase III trials. If FDA approval is gained on the basis of limited but sufficient evidence from clinical trials, it will usually be important to conduct postmarketing (Phase IV) clinical studies to extend knowledge of the drug's safety and efficacy, thus allowing physicians to optimize its use (21 CFR, Part 312.85, page 92).

In 1992, the Prescription Drug User Fee Act (PDUFA) authorized the agency to charge industry fees when submitting a new drug or similar application for review and the agency in return would adhere to new strict approval timelines and clearance of back-logs without compromising review quality. FDA primarily spent these new resources to hire additional personnel (a 56% increase in FDA review staff) to review human drug applications and to upgrade the information technology infrastructure supporting the human drug review process. The FDA's success in making the drug approval process more predictable, accountable, and scientifically sound, while making safe and effective drugs available to the public more quickly, was recognized in late 1997 when the FDA received the prestigious Innovations in American Government Awards, jointly sponsored by the Ford Foundation and Harvard University's John F. Kennedy School of Government. PDUFA contained a "sunset" provision for automatic expiration on September 30, 1997. However, PDUFA was deemed a success and reauthorized and extended through September 2002. This extension authorized the FDA to collect and spend fee revenues to accomplish increasingly challenging goals over the next five-year span. Because of the continued success of this program, PDUFA was again reauthorized for another five years in 2002. PDUFA III corrects some of the flaws of the previous acts and should provide FDA with sufficient resources to continue to meet the challenging goals and undertake pilot programs and new initiatives. Some of the PDUFA III goals require development of guidance documents and databases to track performance as well as the development of infrastructure and tools necessary to enhance electronic application receipt and review. An overview and comparison of the major goals of the PDUFA I–III and further details can be found at http://www. fda.gov/oc/pdufa3/2003plan/default.htm.

PDUFA I enabled the agency to reduce a 30-month average review time to 15 months, in large part because of the addition of almost 700 new employees in the drug and biologics review program. The FDA Modernization Act of 1997 (FDAMA) reauthorized PDUFA as well as enacting many FDA initiatives (http://www.fda.gov/opacom/7modact.html). It codified programs such as Vice President Gore's Reinventing Government, modernized the regulation of biological products to bring them in harmony with regulations for drugs, eliminated the establishment of license applications, eliminated the batch certification and monograph requirements for insulin and antibiotics, stream-lined the approval processes for drug and biological manufacturing changes, etc. It also codified FDA regulations and practices to increase patient access to experimental drugs and medical devices and to accelerate review of important new medications. The law also provided for an expanded database on clinical trials, which is accessible to patients. In the area of drugs, the law codified the agency's practice of allowing, in certain circumstances, one clinical investigation as the basis for product approval. This issue and the related Guidance document on "Providing Clinical Evidence of Effectiveness for Human Drug and Biological Products" are discussed in more detail later in the chapter. The act, however, does preserve the presumption that, as a general rule, two adequate and well-controlled studies are needed to establish a product's safety and effectiveness. Another noteworthy objective of FDAMA was to adequately fund and staff research. The Regulatory Science and Review Enhancement initiative actively encourages the submission of concept papers that explore approaches, methods, or data that can potentially enhance the quality or efficiency of the IND/NDA review process, or the design and evaluation of clinical or non-clinical protocols. The proposals are evaluated and funded at the Center level and support the Critical Path initiative as well as the professional growth of the staff.

Another recent major amendment to the Federal Food, Drug, and Cosmetic Act is the Best Pharmaceuticals for Children Act (BPCA) of early 2002, which concentrates on the improvement of the safety and efficacy of pharmaceuticals for children. It grew out of FDAMA, which granted six-month exclusivity to manufacturers who conducted studies of drugs in children. However, the pediatric exclusivity provision had a sunset date of January 1, 2002. By early 2001, the agency concluded that the pediatric exclusivity provision had been highly effective in generating pediatric studies on many drugs and in providing useful new information in product labeling. However, some categories of drugs and some age groups remained inadequately studied, which the enactment of BPCA seeks to rectify (see also: http://www.fda.gov/cder/pediatric/index.htm#bpca).

Many IND and NDA submissions now are nearly paperless. In 1997, the agency published a guidance that provided for the voluntary submission of regulatory records in electronic format (see: http://www.fda.gov/cder/guidance/2867fnl.pdf). In 1998, CDER issued a draft guidance for industry, "Providing Regulatory Submissions in Electronic Format — NDAs," which expanded on the earlier document. This guidance was finalized in January 1999 and has been the *modus operandi* since then. Additional draft and final guidance documents have been developed to further facilitate the paperless submission and review process.

The body of law currently defining the FDA's authority is comprehensive, providing a variety of controls required by the nature of the market, the product and attendant health risk. For many years, the Agency's job consisted almost entirely of inspections aimed at uncovering adulterated and impure products and exposing fraudulent labeling. However, in addition to this traditional monitoring role, the FDA today serves an important role as the "gatekeeper" for new drug technologies; it applies its substantial scientific resource base to the premarket evaluation and approval of new drugs, and to the postmarketing monitoring of drug labeling, advertising, and quality control.

The demand for the FDA's regulatory role in the marketing of drugs — as expressed in U.S. laws, amendments, and regulations — has evolved based on the needs of the drug industry, the public, the scientific community, the courts, and the Federal Government. As this brief historical description on the "Why" of FDA's existence illustrates, American drug laws and the FDA owe their existence to a fundamental belief that drug companies cannot be fully trusted to assure the safety and efficacy of their products. Unfortunately, there are enough examples in the past and present of dangerous and ineffective drugs on the market to perpetuate this mistrust. At the same time, it should be remembered that a combination of forces — scientific, regulatory, economic, medical, and legal — work together to assure the safety and efficacy of the American drug supply. None of these elements alone should be considered sufficient to provide the margin of control that the American public expects and demands.

A. THE FDA TODAY

The FDA has been described as the "principal consumer protection agency of the Federal Government." In fact, recent concerns about bioterrorism and growing incidences of preventable medical costs have widened the scope of responsibilities and provide greater challenges than ever. For more information on the wide range of responsibilities and activities at the FDA, the reader is referred to http://www.fda.gov.

In simplest terms, the provisions of the food and drug laws, the FDA's review and enforcement actions are intended to ensure:

- Food is safe, wholesome, and secure (from bioterrorism against the food supply).
- Drugs (both human and veterinary), biological products, and medical devices are safe and effective.

- Cosmetics are unadulterated.
- The use of radiological products does not result in unnecessary exposure to radiation.
- All of these products are honestly and informatively labeled.
- Counterterrorism initiatives focus on quickly responding to acts of terrorism and enhancing food security (see: http://www.fda.gov/oc/mcclellan/strategic_terrorism.html).

The FDA is an agency within the Department of Health and Human Services. It is administered by a Commissioner who is appointed by the Secretary of the Department of Health and Human Services. To perform its mission, the Agency is currently organized into seven centers, namely, the Center for Biologics Evaluation and Research, the Center for Drug Evaluation and Research, the Center for Devices and Radiological Health, the Center for Food Safety and Applied Nutrition, the Center for Veterinary Medicine, the National Center for Toxicological Research, and the Office of Regulatory Affairs.

The review and evaluation of efficacy and safety of drugs, a primary focus of this chapter, is the responsibility of the Center for Drug Evaluation and Research (CDER); CDER is currently divided into 12 offices:

Office of the Center Director
Office of Executive Programs
Office of New Drugs
Office of Management
Office of Medical Policy
Office of Information Management
Office of Compliance
Office of Information Technology
Office of Pharmaceutical Science
Office of Pharmacoepidemiology and Statistical Science
Office of Regulatory Policy
Office of Training and Communications.

B. THE OFFICE OF BIOSTATISTICS

The Office of Biostatistics (OB) is part of the Office of Pharmacoepidemiology and Statistical Science (OPaSS) and currently consists of the Immediate Office, three divisions of Biometrics, the Biologics and Therapeutics Statistical Staff, and the Quantitative Methods and Research Staff (QMRS). Each division of Biometrics provides comprehensive statistical and computational services to several medical divisions and to all programs of CDER. QMRS primarily supports the Office of Pharmaceutical Sciences. In addition, the newly formed Biologics and Therapeutics Statistical Staff is responsible for satisfying the needs of biological products in the therapeutic areas of oncology and internal medicine. The Office of Biostatistics employs more than 80 statisticians and support personnel. As stated at OB's website (http://www.fda.gov/cder/Offices/ Biostatistics/default.htm), OB serves CDER by

- Providing leadership, direction, and policy development on statistical, mathematical and computational aspects of review, evaluation, and research
- Providing independent and collaborative evaluations and reviews to all programs and disciplines of CDER in support of the scientific and regulatory review process
- Developing statistical and mathematical methods to enhance the drug and biologics review process in:
  - Pharmacokinetics; pharmacodynamics; bioequivalence;
  - Bioavailability testing;
  - Drug safety monitoring;
  - Analysis and risk assessment;
  - Chemical testing and evaluation; and
  - Product quality assessment and control
- Evaluation and utilizing analytic statistical and mathematical simulation software to enhance the drug development process.

In an effort to improve the quality and consistency of the advice to CDER decision makers and to industry in general, the Office has taken the lead in the development of several statistical guidance documents on specific scientific topics, most notably on ICH E9 and ICH E10, which promote the global effort of harmonizing science and diverse regulatory processes. Similarly, each final statistical review and evaluation report becomes a public document upon approval of the drug that represents the best thinking of the Office on the issues arising from each submission.

II. THE IND REVIEW

The Code of Federal Regulations (CFR) section 312.22 describes the purpose of IND reviews. It states that "FDA's primary objectives in reviewing an IND are, in all phases of the investigation, to assure the safety and rights of subjects, and, in Phase 2 and 3, to help assure that the quality of the scientific evaluation of drugs is adequate to permit an evaluation of the drug's effectiveness and safety." Further, "FDA's review of Phase 2 and Phase 3 submissions will also include an assessment of the scientific quality of the clinical investigations and the likelihood that the investigations will yield data capable of meeting statutory standards for marketing approval."

A schematic of the IND review process (Figure 3.1) is given below and can be found at http://www.fda.gov/cder/handbook/ind.htm. On the website, clicking on the individual boxes provides a more detailed description of each topic.

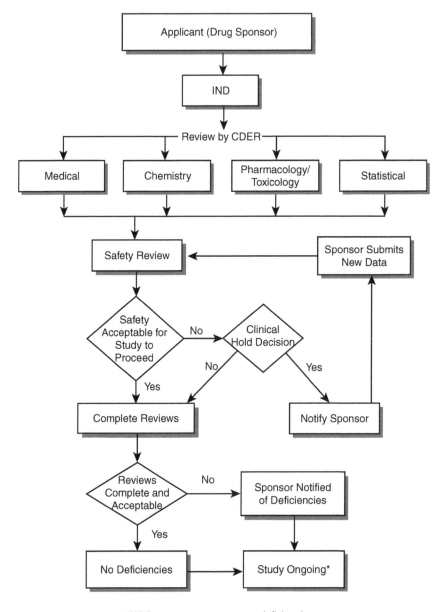

*While sponsor answers any deficiencies

FIGURE 3.1 IND Review.

As can be seen, statistics is but one scientific review area that provides input to the sponsor's drug development program, but it seems clear from the above stated purpose that a statistical review addressing the quality of evidence and likelihood of success of the study should be performed on many types of Phase 2 and 3 protocols, especially those of a confirmatory study meant to provide the primary source of evidence for efficacy. This is even more important under FDAMA, which requires that in general both the sponsor and the FDA abide by their prior agreements, including some agreements made during the IND phase. In particular, a "Special Protocol" is a Phase 3 protocol submitted after being discussed at an End-of-Phase-II meeting. A protocol with this classification requires a specific timeline for review and is considered binding if the requirements for the study are met.

CDER biostatisticians function as reviewers, consultants, and technical experts to their medical CDER colleagues in discussions on scientific/regulatory/ drug development issues associated with the sponsor's proposals and strategies to demonstrate either the efficacy, safety, or both of a new drug. The statistical reviewer does not work in a vacuum but can draw on the intellectual resources of the Office of Biostatistics to get answers and advice on successful approaches used in other medical areas that can be useful in constructive critiques of study protocols and other drug development strategies that rely on sound study designs and prospective data analysis plans. Formal reviews are undertaken for Phase 1, 2, or 3 protocols for which the study design, the methods of analysis proposed in the analysis plan, or the decision rules for declaring a successful study are proposed by the sponsor and CDER is asked for its position on such. Such reviews or critiques are documented and archived. CDER statisticians serve as consultants and technical experts also in general discussions with the medical review division and/or with the sponsor on approaches to studying a drug for a disease that is not well understood or characterized and where decisions need to be made for particular study designs, statistical monitoring procedures, or approaches to handling study withdrawals from treatment. Similarly, statistical input is needed when a range of potential statistical approaches may fit a particular study design, but none appears clearly best for the problem. CDER statisticians may perform independent research and carry out extensive simulations of different study scenarios to develop best approach strategies for a particular situation. Or, a sponsor may ask for CDER's position on a statistical approach that is to be applied to a series of future submissions. Such advice is provided to the sponsor early in the drug development program to maximize the chances of success of an individual clinical trial, of the collection of evidence from several studies to meet regulatory standards, and to minimize problem areas that otherwise might surface late in the IND and NDA program.

As the success of a NDA depends to a great extent on the success of the confirmatory (Phase 3) trials needed to establish the efficacy and safety claims, most of such protocols are reviewed. Protocols of open-label safety studies or non-comparative studies generally do not require a statistical review, because there are few statistical issues involved in planning these types of trials.

The success of a confirmatory trial on the other hand depends heavily on the appropriateness of the design, conduct, and analysis of the study. Critical issues include, but are not limited to, the appropriateness of the study design in relation to the study objectives, relevancy of primary endpoints, clarity of the decision rule for efficacy assessment, multiplicity and maintenance of type I error rate, sample size consideration, randomization plan, proposed conduct of the study, interim looks, alpha spending functions, missing data involving informative censoring, and planned methods of analysis including meta analyses for combining two or more studies. The primary consideration is whether the study, as planned in the protocol, will be capable of providing the desired quality and strength of evidence needed under the statutory requirements for the approval of the drug.

Many trials have failed because of design flaws such as improper choice of dose, insufficient power from an overestimation of effect size, lack of a clear clinical decision rule for efficacy assessment, lack of a proper statistical support structure for the proposed clinical decision rule, or failure to properly account for multiple testing (e.g., in post hoc subgroup claims). Similarly, planned interim analyses, in particular so-called administrative interim looks, present an opportunity for operational bias being introduced and warrant careful review. Design modifications based on interim data can also lead to an inflation of type I error rate and proper statistical methodology needs to be prospectively specified in the protocol to permit such design modifications without the associated inflation in type I error rate. In general, methods of analysis that properly take into consideration missing data, the different nature of censoring, competing risks, repeated measurements over time, multiple testing (including multiple treatment comparisons, multiple endpoint testing, repeated testing over time), etc., need to be carefully considered.

Some Phase 2 protocols may also require statistical review. This may be the case if the protocol proposes the use of a new or subjective measurement instrument or endpoint, a new design, or statistical method. In life threatening disease areas, such as oncology, where there is no treatment available, Phase 2 trials may be accepted as pivotal studies, and therefore would require an in-depth statistical protocol review during the IND stage. These studies rely on the outcome of a single arm and on surrogate endpoints, such as tumor response in lieu of survival, and may contain flexible designs with the option of combining results from Phase 2 and 3 studies. However, for non-life threatening conditions, a Phase 2 trial with a large sample size may also require a statistical review because there is the potential for the sponsor to change the intended use of the data at a later date (such as, presenting the results as if it had been planned as a Phase 3 study). It is important to clarify the goal of such studies within the drug development program. In general, a Phase 2 protocol should require a statistical review if it is intended to provide supportive evidence of efficacy, or to support an accelerated approval.

There are two additional kinds of protocols that may require statistical input. Both are applicable to life-threatening situations only. An Emergency IND allows for an investigational drug to be given to a specific patient who has exhausted all other treatment options, when time does not allow for submission of an IND application in the usual manner. A Treatment IND requests a specific treatment use of a drug in a defined group of patients with a serious or life-threatening disease who have no satisfactory alternative therapy when the drug has shown safety and preliminary efficacy results. The evaluation of a Treatment IND usually presents an additional challenge because of the short time frame available to review such a protocol.

In general, the statistical review of a protocol addresses almost all aspects of the study design, the hypotheses to be tested, and the proposed statistical analysis plan (see ICH E9). These include the randomization scheme, level of blinding, type of design and control, the proposed indication, patient entry criteria, primary and secondary endpoints, decision rule, multiplicity and maintenance of type I error rate, sample size and power, rationale for and plan of interim analyses and related infrastructure, standard operating procedures (SOPs), plan for design modifications (such as sample size re-estimation), methods of analysis, treatment of missing data and dropouts, sources of operational or methodological bias, handling of treatment-by-center interactions, and potential confounding of treatment effects due to design flaws. The evaluation may also address the role the study will play in the overall drug development plan, focusing on the goal of achieving substantial and robust evidence to support efficacy for the indication upon completion of the trial.

III. THE NDA REVIEW

Under section 505 of the Federal Food, Drug and Cosmetic Act, a drug sponsor is required to obtain prior approval from the FDA for the marketing of a new drug. The drug sponsor is required to submit a NDA, or an abbreviated NDA application (ANDA), to the FDA for review and approval, as well as amendments, supplements (SNDA) (e.g., new indications, or other labeling changes [21 CFR 314.70 (b)(3)]) and postmarketing reports [21 CFR 314.80].

When wishing to market a new molecular entity, the Code of Federal Regulations [21 CFR 314.50] states that the drug sponsor must submit a NDA. The NDA must contain seven technical sections [21 CFR 314.50 (d)]. The seven sections are: chemistry including manufacturing and control, nonclinical pharmacology and toxicology, human pharmacokinetics and bioavailability, microbiology, clinical data, statistics, and pediatric use. For electronic submission, the clinical and statistical sections are rolled into one and include the protocol, description and analysis of each controlled clinical study, and the documentation and supporting statistical analyses used in evaluating the controlled clinical studies. In addition, it contains a summary of information about the safety of the drug product and supporting statistical analyses used in evaluating the safety information.

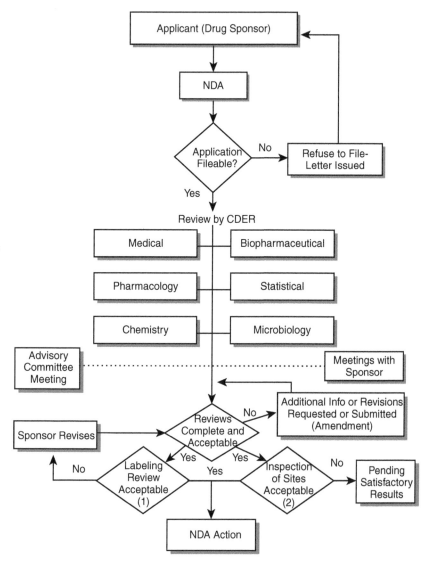

FIGURE 3.2 NDA Review.

(1) Labeling in this context means offical instructions for use

(2) Manufacturing sites and sites where significant clinical trials are performed

A schematic of the NDA review process (Figure 3.2) is given above and can be found at http://www.fda.gov/cder/handbook/nda.htm. On the website, clicking on the individual boxes provides a more detailed description of each topic. The nature of the NDA submission requires a multidisciplinary approach to drug review. This is reflected in the concept of a NDA review team, which consists of at least a project manager, medical team leader, medical officer, statistical team leader, statistical reviewer, pharmacologist, chemist, and microbiologist. The FDA's statistical reviewers review the clinical/statistical section of a NDA submission. In addition, statistical reviews may be required for stability studies (chemistry), PK/PD studies (human pharmacokinetics and pharmacodynamics), carcinogenicity studies (nonclinical pharmacology and toxicology) and pediatric data.

For a supplement to an approved drug, the drug sponsor is also required to submit an application for the changes desired [21 CFR 314.70, 314.71]. Just as in a NDA, the statistics section is reviewed. Statistical review of other sections may or may not be necessary depending upon the changes requested. For an abbreviated application, statistical reviews may be needed for stability studies and bioequivalence studies [21 CFR 314.94 (a) (9), (7)].

The NDA review process is very structured and is pressured by a tight time line. Therefore, only a few studies may be targeted for in-depth review. In addition to studies identified as pivotal by the sponsor, a reviewer may identify other key confirmatory trials or studies containing important issues that may impact on the efficacy claim of the drug in light of existing policies, prior agreements with the applicant, or possible concerns of the review divisions.

Federal regulations [21 CFR 314.101 (a) (1)] require that FDA will determine within 60 days of receipt of the NDA if it is sufficiently complete to permit a substantive review. For this purpose, a *45-day filing meeting* is scheduled upon receipt of a NDA submission. At this meeting the review team determines whether the application is reviewable and at least potentially approvable as submitted. If the submission is incomplete because it does not contain, on its face, the minimum information required under 21 CFR 314.50 or 314.94 (format and content of a NDA and ANDA, respectively), the provision 21 CFR 314.101 (d) (3) allows for the refusal to file of the application. Refusal to file decisions may also be made under other provisions of 21 CFR 314.101 (d). A simple criterion for judging fileability is whether each reviewer can proceed with his/her review of the NDA or ANDA submission without undue delay because of lack of necessary data or information, and whether it is potentially approvable as submitted. At times, communication with the sponsor may be needed to clarify whether any obvious deficiencies can be remedied in time. In most cases, the NDA should be fileable. If the NDA is fileable, a decision is made whether to classify it as a priority or standard application. A priority application requires the Center to make a decision regarding approvability within six months. The time line for a standard submission is ten months.

The primary purpose of a NDA review is to provide a detailed assessment of whether the application meets the current established statutory standards for pre-market approval. Such standards include safety, efficacy, and data quality. Each evaluation of a clinical trial provides a reviewer with the opportunity to evaluate the methodology used by the sponsor in terms of its appropriateness, potential bias, and sensitivity; to apply more proper methods if needed; and to arrive at an overall assessment of the strength of evidence to ensure that the correct interpretation of the results is made. If the drug receives a positive review, recommendations for proper labeling, which includes adequate directions for use, and secondary labeling claims need to be addressed. The review may also assure that potentially misleading or unsubstantiated statements do not appear in the label.

The comprehensive review of a confirmatory study may begin with a review of the study protocol for an examination of the planned study design, conduct of the trial, data sets to be analyzed, and method of analysis, as well as protocol amendments and correspondence between the applicant and FDA. Deviations from the original plans may involve changes in objectives, method of selection of subjects, nature of the control group, primary endpoints, safety variables, event adjudication criteria, methods of analysis, unplanned interim analyses, and more. Changes that were not discussed in protocol amendments or in correspondence may have introduced potentially major sources of bias. The impact of such changes on the quality of the data, integrity of the trial, the results of the primary efficacy endpoint and especially on the overall strength of evidence need to be assessed and quantified if possible.

Keeping the protocol and any modifications or deviations in mind, the review of the actual trial can be addressed. On the surface, the principal objective of a confirmatory study is often fairly simple, namely, it is to demonstrate that the drug shows a certain clinical benefit for a certain target population. However, such an objective needs to be translated in terms of a clinical decision rule that involves one or more primary endpoints, some secondary endpoints and an appropriate statistical support structure. The statistical support structure should reflect the clinical decision rule, test statistics, proper allocation of α to maintain the overall Type I error rate, adequate power, etc. Therefore, some of the major points that need addressing in the review of a confirmatory trial are:

1. Can the design address the principal objective of the study?
2. Is the randomization successful?
3. Is the planned level of blinding maintained throughout?
4. Are patient characteristics and demographics those of the intended treatment population?
5. Is the clinical decision rule compatible with the design?
6. Is the clinical decision rule consistent with the desired indication or clinical claim?
7. Is the clinical decision rule supported by the appropriate statistical support structure?
8. In a non-inferiority trial, is the non-inferiority margin defined appropriately?
9. If an interim analysis was planned, is there any deviation from the interim analysis plan?
10. Is there any modification to the design, conduct, and analysis of the trial after an interim analysis?

11. What is the frequency and distribution of each reason for loss to follow-up?
12. Are there major compliance issues with the study?
13. Do the data sets permit duplication of the sponsor's results?
14. Do the data sets permit independent analyses?
15. Are the statistical assumptions underlying the proposed primary analysis met?
16. What patient data sets are evaluated (e.g., ITT or intent-to-treat)?
17. Are the findings robust?
18. Are results consistent with subgroup adjustment?
19. Is there potential for Type I error inflation due to multiple comparisons, multiple testing of primary endpoints, repeated testing over time, etc.?
20. What sources of bias have been introduced and can their effect be quantified?

Beyond these and many other considerations, the overall *strength of evidence* presented by a given confirmatory trial is of crucial importance and can be assessed by considering features such as:

- Overall quality of the trial, good trial conduct, quality of key data elements
- Sample size and power of the study
- The number of centers involved
- The number of studies involved (where appropriate)
- The number of endpoints for various clinical events
- Observed treatment effect size and its associated significance level
- Internal consistency of the results across centers, various subgroups and clinically relevant endpoints
- Robustness of the results relative to a variety of alternative analyses.

An important issue in a NDA is *robustness* of the statistical evidence. Robustness of statistical evidence can be demonstrated in several ways. In a single study, robustness of statistical evidence can be shown when various appropriate statistical methods yield similar conclusions. Moreover, when the intent-to-treat analysis and the evaluable patient analysis yield similar results, they provide robust statistical evidence of effectiveness. Additionally, when the best case analysis and the worst case analysis produce similar p-values and confidence intervals, robust results are realized. Robustness is also demonstrated in being able to show that the effectiveness of a new drug is reproducible in multiple studies. If the p-values and confidence intervals are homogeneous among themselves to an extent that they are considered statistically equivalent and the respective confidence intervals are fairly consistent, the results of the statistical analyses are considered robust.

A. BIAS

Bias is a very fundamental issue in evaluating the robustness of statistical evidence. In a clinical trial, bias refers to the consequence of any design feature, property of the study treatment, characteristic of the disease, intentional or unintentional conduct, or decision that results in a systematic exaggeration of the treatment difference either in favor or against the study treatment in a show-a-difference trial. It also refers to the consequence of a systematic dampening of the treatment difference in favor of the study treatment in an active control, non-inferiority, or equivalence trial. Bias affects the estimate of the true treatment effect and may lead to drawing incorrect conclusions regarding the overall effect of the study treatment. This is especially important in an active control non-superiority trial where it is crucial to obtain an unbiased estimate of the effect of the active control.

Randomization is the standard procedure used in clinical trials to achieve balance in both known and unknown important baseline covariates and prognostic and demographic factors between the treatment and the control arms. However, there are still many potential sources for bias in a randomized controlled clinical trial. These sources include confounding, operational bias during trial execution, evaluation bias in outcome measurements, and unblinding. In any given situation, bias could come from one or more of these sources.

Blinding is the most important technique for controlling *operational bias*. A confirmatory trial should be blinded at the study level. If necessary, special blinding techniques should be considered at the individual patient level and the investigator level. The aim is to minimize the likelihood of unblinding by the individual patients, the investigators, evaluators or raters, or the study personnel, and to minimize its impact in the event of actual unblinding.

In a controlled clinical trial, even randomization and blinding may not fully protect against *structural bias* resulting from flaws in the design. Design flaws can occur and are not infrequent. Thus, properties of the study treatment, types of treatment administration, nature of the disease, objectives of the trial, and other pertinent information should be well understood to ensure that the design of the trial is not flawed. Structural bias has the potential to invalidate the results of the entire trial.

Even a randomized controlled trial that is blinded and has no design flaws can still have *statistical bias* introduced at the final analysis stage. Statistical bias can arise as a result of the method of analysis, the manner in which patients or data are excluded from the data set, or the manner in which missing data are being handled. This kind of statistical bias can sometimes be fairly subtle.

An important principle in the analysis of clinical trial data is the so-called intent-to-treat principle. The intent-to-treat principle simply espouses the view that the primary analysis should be performed on the outcome measures from all of the randomized patients. When there is no other source of bias, such as design flaws, then the intent-to-treat analysis should provide an unbiased estimate of the treatment effect if there are no patient exclusions and no missing data.

When the outcome measure is not available from all of the randomized patients, efficacy subset analysis is likely to provide biased estimates of the treatment effect. To reduce the impact of missing data, it is recommended that a confirmatory trial should attempt complete follow-up on all missing primary response data from dropouts or others, and provide better documentation of reasons for dropping out and missing primary response data. This will minimize the impact of bias and may provide the basis for determining the proper method of handling the missing data.

In view of the various potential sources of bias in a clinical trial, it is important for a confirmatory trial to consider adopting appropriate measures at the design stage to minimize the impact of potential biases.

B. Combination Drug Policy

The evaluation of a combination drug product presents special challenges. The federal regulations [21 CFR 300.50] on fixed combination prescription drugs states that "Two or more drugs may be combined in a single dosage form when each component makes a contribution to the claimed effects and the dosage is such that the combination is safe and effective for a significant patient population requiring such concurrent therapy as defined in the labeling for the drug."

The regulations continue to discuss other special cases where a fixed combination can be considered. In general, from the efficacy perspective, one needs to ensure that the combination drug is superior to its individual components. This is interpreted to mean that the combination has to be statistically significantly better at the pre-specified level of α than each of the individual components.

C. Review of Safety Data

Currently, the statistical contribution to this area is limited but growing. The analysis of safety data is quite different from the analysis of efficacy data. Safety analyses are generally not pre-specified in the protocol and involve numerous outcome variables (i.e., lab results, adverse events), which raises the multiplicity problem and protection of the Type I error. Thus, a significant finding in a safety analysis is difficult to interpret and becomes dependent on the results observed in other trials. The focus of the analysis may be viewed as hypothesis generating rather than hypothesis testing because most studies are not of sufficient size to achieve statistical significance when comparing incidence rates of safety variables between treatment groups. It is important, however, to identify a "signal" and compare results across trials. Consistency of findings may be more important than the size of the p-value. Other than for comparative safety claims, descriptive statistics may suffice and consistency of results may outweigh the magnitude of p-values. Data mining and visualization methods are currently used more as browsing tools than for statistical decision making. Confidence intervals of adverse event rates, especially when they are narrow, provide useful information for regulatory decision purposes.

D. EVIDENCE OF EFFECTIVENESS FROM A SINGLE STUDY

The added rigor and size of contemporary clinical trials have made it possible to rely in certain circumstances on a single adequate and well-controlled study, without independent substantiation from another controlled trial, as a sufficient scientific and legal basis for approval. Information on evidence of effectiveness derived from a single study can be found at http://www.fda.gov/cder/guidance/1397fnl.pdf.

A *large multi-center study* may meet the requirement. If no single study site provided an unusually large fraction of the patients and no single investigator or site was disproportionately responsible for the favorable effect seen, the study's internal consistency lessens concerns about lack of generalizability of the finding or an inexplicable result attributable only to the practice of a single investigator. If analysis shows that a single site is largely responsible for the effect, the credibility of a multicenter study is diminished. Further confidence is gained if there is *consistency across study subsets.* Frequently, large trials have relatively broad entry criteria and the study populations may be diverse with regard to important covariates such as concomitant or prior therapy, disease stage, age, gender, or race. Analysis of the results of such trials for consistency across key patient subsets addresses concerns about generalizability of findings to various populations in a manner that may not be possible with smaller trials or trials with more narrow entry criteria.

Multiple studies in a single study, such as properly designed factorial studies, may be analyzed as a series of pairwise comparisons representing, within a single study, separate demonstrations of activity of a drug as monotherapy and in combination with another drug. This model was successfully used in ISIS II, which showed that for patients with a myocardial infarction both aspirin and streptokinase had favorable effects on survival when used alone and when combined (aspirin alone and streptokinase alone were each superior to placebo; aspirin and streptokinase in combination were superior to aspirin alone and to streptokinase alone). This represented two separate (but not completely independent) demonstrations of the effectiveness of aspirin and streptokinase.

In some cases, a single study will include several important, prospectively identified primary or secondary endpoints, each of which represents a beneficial, but different, effect. Where a study shows statistically persuasive evidence of an effect from *multiple endpoints involving different events*, the internal weight of evidence of the study is enhanced. For example, favorable effects on both death and nonfatal myocardial infarctions in a lipid-lowering, postangioplasty, or postinfarction study would represent different, but consistent, demonstrations of effectiveness, greatly reducing the possibility that a finding of reduced mortality was a chance occurrence. In contrast, a beneficial effect on multiple endpoints that evaluate essentially the same phenomenon and correlate strongly, such as mood change on two different depression scales or SGOT and CPK levels postinfarction, does not significantly enhance the internal weight of the evidence from a single trial. Moreover, although two consistent findings within a single study usually provide reassurance that a positive treatment effect is not due to chance, they do not protect against bias in study conduct or biased analyses. For example, a treatment assignment not well balanced for important prognostic variables could lead to an apparent effect on both endpoints. Thus, close scrutiny of study design and conduct are critical to evaluating this type of study.

In a multi-center study, a very low *p*-value indicates that the result is highly inconsistent with the null hypothesis of no treatment effect. In some studies it is possible to detect nominally statistically significant results in data from several centers, but even where that is not possible, an overall *statistically very persuasive finding* and significance level mean that most study centers had similar findings. Preventive vaccines for infectious disease indications with a high efficacy rate (e.g., point estimate of efficacy of 80% or higher and a reasonably narrow 95% confidence interval) have been approved based on a single adequate and well-controlled trial.

Caveats: While acknowledging the persuasiveness of a single, internally consistent, strong multicenter study, it must be appreciated that even a strong result can represent an isolated or biased result, especially if that study is the only study suggesting efficacy among similar studies.

When considering whether to rely on a single multicenter trial, it is critical that the possibility of an incorrect outcome be considered and that all the available data are examined for their potential to either support or diminish reliance on a single multicenter trial.

E. THE STATISTICAL REVIEW AND EVALUATION REPORT

CDER statistical reviewers write a Statistical Review and Evaluation Report of the reviewed NDA to document their conclusions regarding the effectiveness of the drug based on the data submitted in the NDA. The report discusses the strength of evidence relative to the established statutory standards of effectiveness and data quality, any unresolved issues, and gives final recommendations on the evidence.

The Statistical Review and Evaluation Report is an official document and is submitted to an electronic archival in CDER. When a NDA is approved, the report becomes part of the public record documenting the FDA's positions about the product. It then becomes available (minus any redacted materials) for public use on the FDA website.

F. STATISTICAL NDA REVIEW TEMPLATE

The Office of Biostatistics implemented a Statistical NDA Review Template that is being used to document statistical findings in a structured, organized format, so that all statistical reviewers follow a similar structure for the report.

Review standards define workable guidelines, which ensure that all key review areas are addressed. The Template promotes consistency in review practices so that all relevant information is adequately reflected and essential results of evaluations are relayed in an organized order of presentation. Template use allows flexibility in intellectual execution of the review while requiring minimal adherence to prescriptive methods of documenting findings and conclusions.

This tool serves as a guide in review development and fosters effective communication among a range of audience disciplines. Reviewers are encouraged to summarize overall findings from detailed discussion of individual study reports by distilling this information into the concise, clear summation of an Executive Summary (www.fda.gov/cder/Offices/Biostatistics/default.htm).

The statistical reviewers are currently required to follow this Template to achieve consistency of the statistical review reports with respect to the format.

G. ADVISORY COMMITTEES

The FDA has 30 Advisory Committees organized along product lines and body systems (e.g., cardiovascular, gastrointestinal products, etc.). The members of each committee are (rotating) non-FDA experts in the disease areas who are convened periodically to give advice on some of the Agency's most difficult and/or complex review issues. The members of an advisory committee complement the Agency's scientific expertise by bringing cutting-edge research, patient and patient caregiver concerns, and industry and consumer advocacy viewpoints to the table for discussion (http://www.fda.gov/cder/handbook/advisory.htm). Both the sponsor of the particular submission and the FDA reviewers present their best case for consideration before the committee. However, during the open public hearing session, any person may make a presentation of scientific fact or personal experience.

H. TRANSPARENCY

The content of this chapter is intended to make the IND and NDA review process transparent to outsiders, especially drug sponsors who are actively interested in the review approach of CDER reviewers. The scope of the review process as outlined here aims at helping drug sponsors understand the process clearly and inspiring them to develop IND and NDA submissions smartly and efficiently. This approach is consistent with the concept of *transparency*, which is one of the operating principles of the FDA.

I. CONSISTENCY

The NDA Review Template and the Statistical Review and Evaluation Report, as described, are aimed at achieving consistency among statistical reviewers across medical review divisions and multiple disease areas on fundamental issues.

Again, this approach addresses the idea of *consistency*, which is another operating principle of the FDA.

IV. CONCLUSION

Industry and the FDA must, out of necessity, work closely together in conscientiously maintaining and strengthening the public trust in the safety and efficacy of the nation's drugs. It should be prominently noted that without voluntary efforts by a majority of drug sponsors to meet and exceed the requirements of the law, the FDA would never have enough staff or resources to enforce its requirements. It is the responsibility of the FDA and industry statisticians to work together to ensure that drugs are marketed only after rigorous scientific evidence has demonstrated that they are both safe and efficacious. The American public demands and expects this type of professional dedication.

Researchers in the Office of Biostatistics (OB) have been active in producing, presenting and publishing papers on the various aspects of regulatory statistical research. The list of publications is a long one and even a brief summary of these papers is beyond the scope of this chapter; they are published in pertinent statistical and scientific journals. Readers are encouraged to review these published papers with a view to extending, enlarging, as well as enhancing their perspectives and gaining greater insights into our evaluation process of the IND/NDA submissions. In this connection, a list of selected publications by OB statistical scientists is available on the website.

V. DISCLAIMER

The authors are solely responsible for the views expressed in this chapter and these views do not necessarily reflect the official position of the FDA on this matter.

FURTHER READING

Guideline for the Format and Content of the Clinical and Statistical Sections of an Application, U.S. Department of Health and Human Services, Public Health Service, FDA, July 1988.

International Conference on Harmonization (ICH), Guidance on Statistical Principles for Clinical Trials (E9): Federal Register, Vol. 63, No. 179, September 1998.

International Conference on Harmonization (ICH); Choice of Control Group in Clinical Trials (E10): Federal Register Vol. 64, No. 185, September 1999.

Anello, C., FDA statistical program: an overview, *Encyclopedia of Statistical Sciences*, Vol. 3, Kotz, S. and Johnson, N.L., eds., Wiley, New York, pp. 39–43, 1983.

Anello, C. and O'Neill, R.T., Does research synthesis have a place in drug regulatory policy? Synopsis of issues: assessment of safety and postmarketing surveillance, *Clin. Res. Regul. Aff.*, 13, 13–21, 1996.

Anello, C., O'Neill, R., and Dubey, S., Multi-clinic trials: a U.S. Regulatory perspective, *Stat. Methods Med. Res.*, 14(3), 303–318, 2005.

Cui, L., Hung, H.M.J., and Wang, S.J., Modification of sample size in group sequential clinical trials, *Biometrics*, 55, 853–857, 1999.

Chi, G.Y.H., A design problem in ulcer prevention trials, *Proceedings of the Biopharmaceutical Section*, American Statistical Association, Alexandria, VA, pp. 100–105, 1985.

Chi, G.Y.H., Multiple testing: multiple comparisons and multiple endpoints, *Drug Inf. J.*, 32(Suppl.), 1347s–1362s, 1998.

Chi, G.Y.H. and Liu, Q., The attractiveness of the concept of a prospectively designed two-stage clinical trial, *J. Biopharm. Stat.*, 9, 537–547, 1999.

Dubey, S.D., The role of statisticians in the efficacy and safety evaluation of new drugs, In *Statistics in the Pharmaceutical Industry*, Marcel Dekker, New York, pp. 87–105, 1981.

Dubey, S.D., FDA statistical programs: human drugs, In *Encyclopedia of Statistical Sciences*, Kotz, S. and Johnson, N.L., eds., Wiley, New York, pp. 43–48, 1983.

Dubey, S.D., Robust statistical evidence for establishing effectiveness of new pharmaceuticals, *Proceedings of the Section on Biopharmaceuticals*, American Statistical Association, Alexandria, VA, pp. 292–299, 1990.

Dubey, S.D., CANDAs and the statistical review: past present and future, *J. Appl. Clin. Trials*, 1, 42–47, 1992.

Dubey, S.D., Statistical reporting of clinical trials in new drug applications, *Clin. Eval.*, 20(Suppl. VI), 41–53, 1992.

Dubey, S.D., Meta-analysis: its role in new drug applications and AIDS drug studies, *J. Clin. Res. Regul. Aff.*, 10, 13–33, 1993.

Dubey, S.D., The FDA and the IND/NDA statistical review process, In *Statistics in the Pharmaceutical Industry*, 2nd ed., Buncher, C.R. and Tsay, J.Y., eds., Marcel Dekker, New York, pp. 93–105, 1994.

Dubey, S.D., Adjustment of p-values for multiplicities of intercorrelating symptoms, In *Statistics in the Pharmaceutical Industry*, 2nd ed., Buncher, C.R. and Tsay, J.Y., eds., Marcel Dekker, New York, pp. 513–527, 1994.

Dubey, S.D., Food and Drug Administration (FDA), In *Encyclopedia of Biostatistics*, Armitage, P. and Colton, T., eds., Wiley, New York, pp. 1539–1552, 1998.

Sankoh, A.J., Huque, M.F., and Dubey, S.D., Some comments on frequently used multiple endpoint adjustment methods in clinical trials, *Stat. Med.*, 16, 2529–2542, 1997.

Lindberg, S.R. and Ellenberg, S.S., Food and drug administration, In *Encyclopedia of Biopharmaceutical Statistics*, Chow, S.C., ed., Marcel Dekker, New York, pp. 379–385, 2003.

Peace, K.E., *Statistical Issues in Drug Research and Development*, Marcel Dekker, New York, 1988.

Liu, Q. and Chi, G.Y.H., On sample size and inference for two-stage adaptive designs, *Biometrics*, 57, 172–177, 2001.

Huque, M.F., Dubey, S.D., and Fredd, S., Establishing therapeutic equivalence with clinical endpoints, *Proceedings of the Biopharmaceutical Section*, American Statistical Association, Alexandria, VA, pp. 46–52, 1989.

Huque, M.F. and Dubey, S.D., A meta-analysis methodology for utilizing study-level covariate information from clinical trials, *Commun. Stat. Theor. Method.*, 23, 377–394, 1994.

Huque, M.F., Al-Osh, M., and Dubey, S.D., P-values, evidence and multiplicity considerations for controlled clinical trials, In *Encyclopedia of Biopharmaceutical Statistics*, Chow, S.C., ed., Marcel Dekker, New York, pp. 696–706, 2003.

Jin, K. and Chi, G.Y.H., Application of bootstrap in handling multiple endpoints, *Proceedings of the Biopharmaceutical Section*, American Statistical Association, Alexandria, VA, pp. 150–155, 1997.

Jin, K. and Chi, G.Y.H., Clinical decision rules and statistical support structures — a novel approach to handling the multiple endpoints problem, *Proceedings of the Biopharmaceutical Section*, American Statistical Association, Alexandria, VA, pp. 56–62, 1998.

Chi, G., Jin, K., Chen, G., and Cui, L., Some statistical issues of relevance to confirmatory trials, In *Advanced Medical Statistics*, Liu, Y. and Fang, J.Q., eds., World Scientific Publishing Co., Singapore, pp. 523–580, 2003.

Nuri, W.A. and Dubey, S.D., Testing for treatment effects against placebo in multicenter trials, *Proceedings of the Section on Biophamaceuticals*, American Statistical Association, Alexandria, VA, pp. 118–123, 1996.

CDER Guidance documents, MaPPs, CFR statements, FDAMA regulations, or ICH documents can be located at.

www.fda.gov/oc/pdufa3/2003plan/default.htm

www.fda.gov/oc/mcclellan/strategic_terrorism.html

www.fda.gov/opacom/7modact.html

www.fda.gov/cder/mapp.html

www.fda.gov/cder/guidance

www.fda.gov/cder/regulatory

www.fda.gov/cder/pediatric/index.htm#bpca

www.fda.gov/cder/guidance/2867fnl.pdf

www.fda.gov/cder/handbook/ind.htm

www.fda.gov/cder/handbook/nda.htm

www.fda.gov/cder/guidance/1397fnl.pdf

www.fda.gov/cder/handbook/advisory.htm

www.fda.gov/cder/Offices/Biostatistics/default.htm

www.fda.gov/cder/Offices/Biostatistics/publications.htm

4 Clinical Trial Designs

C. Ralph Buncher and Jia-Yeong Tsay

CONTENTS

I. INTRODUCTION

Designing clinical trials of pharmaceutical products shares many characteristics with other types of scientific study. General principles of experimental design applied to other types of scientific studies also apply to clinical trials, i.e., to reduce experimental error in the data collection and to avoid bias in the decision making. The unique characteristic of clinical trials is that the experimental units are human beings, commonly called subjects — and usually sick ones at that. Modern clinical trials must be designed in such a way that the participants can be well informed about the conduct, purpose, and reasonable risks and benefits of the trial, and that the welfare of each participant remains more important than carrying out the trial as designed. The Declaration of Helsinki,[1] item 5 of Basic Principles states " ... Concern for the interests of the subject must always prevail over the interests of science and society." The basic purpose of the trial is to obtain pharmaceutical information that is applicable to the people who will take the drug in the future. In short, the design must be such that the interests of the individual are balanced with the interest of the group.[2] Generally speaking, the clinical trials must meet the requirements of "Good Clinical Practice" as described in ICH Guideline E-6 (http://www.ich.org).

A century ago volunteers were given diseases such as yellow fever and malaria in experimental conditions, and some of these persons lost their lives. This predictable loss of life of a few of the volunteers resulted in the saving of the lives of thousands of other persons because of the more rapid scientific advances made from those experimental studies. However, acceptable research behavior and government regulations such as FDA/guidelines/guidance (http://www.fda.gov/cder/guidance) and EMEA guidance (http://www.emea.eu.int), have drastically changed because of greatly improved mortality rates, changing moral concepts, and also as a reaction to some prior abuses in clinical trials. Suffice it to say that at the current time in the United States and other countries with comparable research philosophies, a primary characteristic of all clinical trials is a concern for the safety of the volunteer participants. The general principle of informed consent, that all participants will be fully informed of the characteristics of the trial, is now universally accepted, although efforts to make it work better continue.[3,4]

Each class of drugs generates unique characteristics for clinical trials. For example, antibacterial drugs tend to have an action that can be measured in days and safety that can be measured in months, while a cardiovascular drug produces an action measured in months and safety measured in years. This chapter will discuss some of the fundamental characteristics of all clinical trials and leave to the later chapters the specific characteristics within a few of the unique fields.

II. CLINICAL TRIAL DESIGN

A. TREATMENT COMPARISON (CONTROL)

The first characteristic of clinical trials is that any clinical trial of the drug must be controlled in the scientific sense of having some comparison, called control, for the results of the drug under study, preferably a comparison provided in the same clinical trial, i.e., concurrent control. A common type of control in many therapeutic areas is a placebo control, a type of study in which at least some of the study participants receive a preparation with the physical appearance of the drug but none of its pharmacological properties. This type of trial is considered ethical in those instances where there is no standard treatment and where placebo is well known to cure a high proportion of persons, e.g., pain relief or mood enhancement. Chapter 9 provides more information on analgesic trials.

A study may also be controlled through the use of a positive control for the disease under study, particularly if the trial is in patients with life threatening disease such as cancer (see Chapter 6 for details and relevant statistical issues). An example would be an antibiotic or an oncology drug known to be effective, which could be used in instances where it would not be ethical to deny treatment to participants. Sometimes a trial may have placebo and active controls simultaneously for the purpose of internal validation or assessing relative efficacy and safety compared with a drug in the market. Another type of concurrent controlled trial is the dose–response trial using different doses in the same trial for comparison. Other control possibilities that are much less frequently used are historical controls and no control.

B. MASKED EVALUATION (BLINDING)

Another characteristic of the clinical trials is that all evaluations must be made without bias. Painful experience has proven that patients and clinical evaluators have subjective opinions and views of life that can affect the outcome in most trials. These potential biases must be thwarted by proper experimental design. The most common design technique, called blinding, is to make the study subjects and evaluators in a clinical trial act as if they were blindfolded or masked as to the identity of which medication is which in the trial. These trials are most commonly called "double-blind," short for double-blindfold, although "double-masked" is a preferable term by some.[5] This is accomplished by making the medications look exactly alike and be alike in all characteristics that might be observed, save only the chemical differences.

Moreover, the labeling must be done in such a way that a person having access to the complete set of labels would not know which medication is which and therefore could not tell which medication would be given to the next participant. This is usually accomplished by numbering the medications sequentially (1, 2, 3, 4,…) and having separate codes, which are usually stored in a secured place like a fire-proof locked cabinet and available only in an emergency situation, to describe which number is equivalent to each medication.

Each container of medication used in interstate commerce must be labeled with the contents, but the labels used in pharmaceutical trials are generally a variety of sealed labels such that one can only determine the medication by breaking the seal (often glue sealed by heat). If the label is opened, it cannot be resealed again. Obviously, the labels are also made so that holding them up to the light does not permit reading what is inside. Thus, return of the sealed labels is one important piece of evidence that no one has discovered which medication was taken by which patient. Clearly, the degree to which the placebo matches the active medication and other characteristics of the trial also contribute to the proof that no one knew which medication was which.

Most trials are double-blind or double-masked in the sense that neither the participant nor the evaluating clinical personnel knows which medication is which. It is also possible for trials to be single-blind. In the more common single-blind situation the clinician in early trials knows which is the study medication and which is the placebo, to be able to more knowledgeably monitor progress of the trial and side effects, but the participant in the experiment does not know which medication is which. In some single-blind situations — for example, when the medication cannot be blinded, as in the comparison of a surgical treatment and a drug treatment — the patient is aware of which treatment is which but the evaluating clinical personnel are "blindfolded." Again, this is a single-blind trial.

Notice that sometimes when two treatments (say, A and B) cannot be made identical or are given with different timing of the doses, a technique, called double-dummy, can be used to conduct a double-blind rather than single-blind trial. In this case, each treatment will have an active version and a placebo version. Then each subject will take either the set of active A and placebo B, or the set of active B and placebo A. Finally, some studies are done on an open-label or unblinded basis — for example, when all concerned are aware that an experimental drug is being used for collecting long-term safety information.

C. RANDOMIZATION

Randomization is a process of assigning subjects to treatment groups using an element of chance to avoid bias. Randomization serves four important purposes. (1) It avoids known and unknown biases on the average in the assignments to treatment groups. (2) It balances known and unknown prognostic factors on the average. (3) It helps convince others that the trial was conducted properly. (4) It is the basis for the statistical theory that allows us to calculate probabilities.

In general, patients are assigned to treatments based on a randomization schedule. There are many ways of allocating drug names to the labels numbered in order. While many methods are suggested in textbooks and pamphlets, those who frequently randomize use a random permutation schedule. Random permutations are the most general scheme for randomization, and they can be tailored to almost any design requested.

Consider the numbers 1, 2, 3, and 4. There are 24 different orderings of these four numbers, e.g., 1, 2, 3, 4; 1, 2, 4, 3; 1, 3, 2, 4, and so on through to 4, 3, 2, 1. If four random numbers are generated, then the rank of the magnitude of these numbers can be considered as an ordering. For example, suppose the random numbers were 378, 842, 103, and 927, then these random numbers, considering their ranks from smallest to largest, would have generated the permutation 2, 3, 1, 4. Because each rank had an equal chance of occurring in each position, each of the 24 possible orders would have had an equal opportunity of being chosen.

To apply the random permutation technique to choose two persons to receive the active drug and two to receive the placebo, one decides before starting that numbers 1 and 2 will be active drug, for example, and 3 and 4 will be placebo. The random permutation then chooses which persons will receive which drugs. The extension of this schedule to larger sizes should be obvious. The schedule can be done by hand with ease in small trials, programmed into a computer, or found in software packages. However, the pharmaceutical regulatory agency expects "The randomization schedule should be reproducible (if the need arises)" as stated in the ICH Guideline E-9. Using software packages to generate the randomization schedule is now the standard practice in the pharmaceutical industry.

To avoid bias or a confounding effect, a randomization technique, called stratification, is commonly used in clinical trials.[6] For multicenter trials, the randomization is mostly stratified by study center, so that within each center subjects are randomly assigned to treatments in a prespecified proportion between treatments and most commonly in equal proportion. In this way center effect will not be confounded with the treatment effect and can be accounted for by a proper statistical analysis model. Stratification sometimes is performed for demographic and prognostic factors also. For example, if gender or severity of disease has a potential impact on the effect of the treatment, these factors may be stratified in the randomization to ensure proper balance in these factors. In general, randomization should not be stratified for more than three factors, particularly when a trial may include centers with low recruiting capability.

Changes over time during the course of a designed trial are always a possibility. For various reasons, a trial may even stop before all patients have been entered. The statistician can make the design more robust against these contingencies by randomizing the sample in blocks that are complete (i.e., all treatments are included in the same block) and balanced at the end of each block. For example, in a three-arm trial (i.e., three different treatment groups), using blocks of six patients each would guarantee the desired balance at the end of every sixth patient. In this way, randomization is carried out within each block, which is one form of "restricted randomization." In like manner, in the 200-patient study with two drugs, one could create blocks of size 4 or 6 (or even 8 or 12 with one smaller block) so that the study would be balanced at the end of each of these blocks. Sometimes, one also randomizes the block sizes to protect against investigators guessing the final treatments in a block. One caveat of using random block sizes is that with so many different disciplines of personnel involved in the clinical trial operations, there is an increased chance of mis-randomization that may cause serious consequences, such as invalidity of the results or high financial cost for correcting the problem. Therefore, the risk/benefit ratio for using random block sizes should be carefully considered.

There could be one or multiple blocks per center in a multicenter trial. Of course, one should not tell any investigator or relevant staff of the study about the block size, and given the complexities of the usual trial and sophistication of the blinding they will not be able to guess it accurately.

Statisticians have rejected alternatives to randomization for decades, although there is an active field of research in useful modifications to strict randomization. For example, Royall[7] examined ethical and scientific dilemmas in randomized clinical trials and urged statisticians to improve the statistical methodology of nonrandomized clinical trials when randomization is not ethically or practically feasible. An excellent source is the December, 1988 issue of Controlled Clinical Trials (volume 9, number 4), which features a number of articles about randomization, mostly written by John M. Lachin.

An area of research that is still developing is unequal randomization. Do the two or more groups have to have the same number of patients? This type of clinical trial is not unusual outside of the pharmaceutical industry.

Thus, if the group is somewhat convinced that treatment One is better than treatment Two, it is sensible to randomize so that more patients end up on the better treatment which is thought to be treatment One. One such simple schedule is the play-the-winner rule.[8] If treatment One results in a success, then treatment One is also used on the next patient. When treatment One results in a failure, then treatment Two is used on the next patient. If this process is continued for the whole trial, the result is that more of the patients will have used the better treatment. Some of the literature in this field is found under the title of biased coin or adaptive randomization.[9] Although these designs are of great interest to theoreticians and are very useful in certain instances, they are not used very much in the pharmaceutical industry. The schedules are more difficult to use and introduce problems when trying to convince others of the efficacy of the product, and standard designs are usually adequate.

Another area undergoing rapid development is called "adaptive designs." More and more commonly, designs are being used that may change after the initial batch of observations is made. These are modernizations of sequential statistical, group sequential, and interim analysis designs.[10-13] They are driven by the desire to make timely decisions in the middle of a clinical trial, rather than the more expensive and time-consuming task of completing one study and then starting a new one. See Chapters 13 and 14 for details in this area.

III. STATISTICAL DESIGN

The actual design of a trial that explains which patient receives which drug (called "treatment" in the jargon of design of experiments) can be classified in one of two general categories. The trial may be a parallel design in which each patient receives one and only one treatment (although that treatment may be given at more than one dose), or a crossover design in which the same patient is given two or more different drugs. In this latter case, the patient serves as the patient's own control for treatment comparison, because the comparison of treatments is made within the patient.

Some time ago, crossover designs were considered among the best in pharmaceutical research. The theoretical advantage of a smaller sample size with a crossover design was emphasized along with the advantage of making comparisons within patients, which is especially appealing to clinicians. Problems with crossover designs are also important. Suppose there is an adverse effect found 1 week after the end of the study. How do we know which drug, if either, should be held responsible? As an extreme example, if ten patients died after a crossover study, all we would know is that each took each medication. On the other hand, in a parallel study, we might know that five patients were on placebo and five on the test drug, or that nine patients were on the test drug and only one was on placebo. Clearly the parallel design offers us potentially more information about side effects. The advantages and disadvantages of crossover designs are discussed more completely in Chapter 21 with regard to bioavailability studies. The U.S. Food and Drug Administration[14] recommends the use of two-treatment crossover designs for bioequivalence studies.

All the usual designs available in the statistical design of experiments are also candidates for pharmaceutical trial designs — for example, the completely randomized design, in which all patients are divided into the group on the new drug and the group on the comparison treatment, is very commonly used. Another very commonly used design is the randomized block design in which groups of patients are put together in such a way that patients in a "block" resemble each other more than they resemble patients in other blocks. For example, in a study of pain one might use as a blocking factor the type of operation, the gender of patients, the degree of severity of the pain, or some combination of all three. In each case the goal is to reduce variation by putting together those patients who are similar in a block and then allocating the treatment within that block. The extreme example of this design is the matched pair design, in which two persons are selected who are very similar, and then drug and placebo are randomly allocated one to each member of the pair.

Latin square designs are also frequently used if their size is small enough. A Latin square is a type of randomized block design in which there are two simultaneous blocking factors. Thus, patients could be blocked on degree of pain in three classifications and in three classifications of type of operation. Frequently the second blocking factor is the time period in which the drugs will be given. For example, in a study of the pain of rheumatoid arthritis, one could design three different levels of impairment and then have three pain relievers (new drug, placebo, and positive control) given for 1 week each over a total of 3 weeks of treatment. This is also another example of a type of crossover trial.

Efficient experimental designs defined according to certain statistical optimality criteria are desirable in pharmaceutical research. However, most frequently the optimal criteria, for which there is a theory already developed, impose some assumptions that are found to be hard to meet in the clinical setting. Therefore, these designs are little used in clinical trials. There is an opportunity for a great deal of statistical research using current optimality criteria as well as developing new optimality standards to suggest the most efficient designs that will also accomplish the necessary goals of practical research. Among the latter are robustness against frequently encountered problems of clinical trials, balance with respect to all important factors, and the challenge of convincing others of the correctness of the interpretation of the results of the trial. Simpler designs lead to obvious interpretations; complex designs lead to statistical interactions, extraneous but important variables, other unavoidable realities of practical research, and difficult interpretations.

Any of the designs with blocking can be incomplete in the sense that not all of the treatments are used in each of the blocks. The usual goal is to balance these incomplete blocks in such a way that the number of treatments within a block is the same in all of the blocks and each treatment appears with each other treatment an equal number of times.

An interesting example of this variety involved the use of three analgesic drugs that were self-administered by pregnant women during labor pains.[15] There were three analgesic mixtures: 50% nitrous oxide and 50% air, 75% nitrous oxide and 25% oxygen, and 0.5% trichlorethylene and 99.5% air. The usual randomized block experiment would have each patient (the blocking factor) use each analgesic in random order. The constraint was that patients were not expected to be able to use more than two of the analgesic mixtures during their labor pains. The design selected was to have each of 150 women use two mixtures such that each of the three pairs of drugs was compared by 50 randomly selected women. Moreover, the 50 women were subjects in a crossover design so that 25 had the first mixture followed by the second, while the other 25 had the second mixture first followed by the first mixture. Each subject was asked, "Which was more effective in relieving the pain of uterine contraction?" in order to evaluate the pair of analgesics. The results showed that the 50% nitrous oxide mixture was the weakest and the other two were about equally effective.

This design is a balanced incomplete block design because each block is missing one analgesic and the blocks are balanced for all possible combinations. This example is mentioned to suggest that the standard designs mentioned are only the simplest of samples out of a vast design warehouse. The simplest designs have the advantage of being easier to finish successfully in practical situations and often become the ultimate sophistication in clinical trials.

IV. PHASES OF CLINICAL TRIALS

When drug development leaves the laboratory and reaches the clinical stage, it has a set of phases of clinical trials to traverse. Sometimes the precise phase is vague so it is difficult to differentiate one phase from another. This is because a trial may have several different goals in the protocol, or the goal of a trial may be multiple, among other reasons.

A. PHASE I

When the study drug is first time tested, we need to know how the body reacts to the drug, including the processes of absorption, distribution, metabolism, and excretion (ADME) of the drug in the body over a period of time, i.e., to do a pharmacokinetic trial. We also need to know to what dose level can humans tolerate the drug, i.e., to find the maximum tolerated dose (MTD) in a dose-ranging trial. All these trials are Phase I trials and usually are done in 20 to 80 normal healthy volunteers in the setting of a special clinical facility. Sometimes study drugs for certain diseases are likely to be more toxic, e.g., AIDS and oncology drugs are in this category. It is considered unethical to expose healthy volunteers to such toxic drugs. In this case, the trials are conducted in patients with the underlying disease.

B. Phase II (See Ref. 16)

Phase II clinical trials are usually the initial phase of clinical studies that involve patients/subjects who have the disease or condition to be treated, diagnosed, or prevented, except in some therapeutic areas like oncology or AIDS. Sometimes Phase II trials are classified into two categories: Phase IIA and Phase IIB.

Phase IIA clinical trials are usually conducted by highly trained clinicians called clinical pharmacologists who make the study of therapeutic medications their specialized area in medicine. In these trials information concerning degree of safety and the effectiveness of the drugs in humans is obtained in a selected population of 100 to 300 subjects who have the disease or condition to be treated, diagnosed, or prevented. Usually, these trials are sufficient to select the optimal dose or doses of the drug for usual clinical use. Also, the common side effects on a subjective basis, e.g., dizziness and nausea, are discovered, as are common biochemical side effects, e.g., changes in liver enzymes or sodium levels.

Phase IIB clinical trials are those of well-controlled trials to evaluate safety and efficacy in subjects who have the disease or condition to be treated, diagnosed, or prevented. These trials usually represent the most rigorous demonstration of efficacy.

There are interesting design problems associated with these early drug trials. Kaitin et al.[17] provide some useful insights. Since the audience for these trials is small and more specialized, we have not devoted much space to them. Instead, we shall discuss general problems of trials and several of the problems encountered in later drug trials.

C. Phase III

Typically Phase III trials are multicenter trials in populations of 500 to 3000 (or more) subjects for whom the medicine is eventually intended. The Phase III clinical trials that prove the effectiveness and safety of the medication are the ones which provide the further detailed comparisons to verify the earlier results from Phase II, thus frequently called confirmatory trials. In addition, less common side effects are discovered during these larger and more extensive trials. For a number of reasons, Phase III trials are usually conducted by general clinicians or specialists in a particular clinical field, rather than by those specifically trained in clinical trials. First, there is the desire to use the drug in a more typical environment rather than in the highly controlled situation of a clinical pharmacologist in a research-oriented setting. Likewise, one must find clinicians who have larger numbers of patients in order to provide the numbers of drug-recipients necessary to verify efficacy and safety. Finally, it must be pointed out that later clinical trials are rarely of as much scientific interest as the earlier trials, and thus do not as frequently lead to medical journal articles, the basic currency of a "publish or perish" scientific standard.

The clinicians who do participate are motivated by other factors. These factors include financial benefits for the participants and investigators, access to a drug that would not be available outside the research program, the opportunity and status of participating in a research program, and doing a favor for an old friend. Clearly the research design must be robust against any biases that could creep into a study because of these reasons for participating in it.

Some clinical trials are conducted after submission of the NDA, but before the product's approval and market launch. This type of trial is called Phase IIIB. These trials may supplement earlier trials or seek different kinds of information like quality of life measures or other information for marketing promotion.

D. PHASE IV AND PHASE V

One of the issues that makes drug approval at the FDA difficult, is the question of safety. Sometimes a question of a side effect from phase III trials is not completely resolved and additional information is needed. Sometimes after a drug is approved and used by thousands or even millions of people, some side effects that were not known at the time of approval may be discovered. An alternative is to do studies of side effects after the drug is approved for marketing. Frequently, the FDA needs further information on a safety issue at the time of NDA approval and requires the sponsor to commit some clinical trials to provide further safety information. Also, the sponsor may want to do postmarketing studies to collect additional details of safety and efficacy information or further information on drug–drug or drug–demographic interaction, or to evaluate formulation, dosages, treatment duration, etc. These postmarketing studies are generally called Phase IV studies. In fact, postmarketing studies that are primarily observational or nonexperimental are frequently called postmarketing surveillance or simply called Phase V studies.[16] The observational studies are not randomized clinical trials and fall more into the realm of epidemiology than biostatistics.

V. STUDY PROTOCOL

Before any clinical trial is carried out by a pharmaceutical company, the details of the study are first agreed to and expressed in a written document called the study protocol. Generally speaking, the protocol is a document that describes the study objectives, design, methodology, statistical consideration, entrance and exclusion criteria, and other organization of a trial. At most pharmaceutical companies, the study protocol is the joint effort of the clinical scientists, the biostatisticians, others with a concern in the study, and the investigator. A general discussion for pharmaceutical trials is found in Ref. 18.

The protocol includes information on the objectives of the study as well as details of the study. The objectives should be stated as precisely as possible, e.g., "This study will investigate whether the new drug causes weight loss in diabetic patients of ages 45 to 65 when compared with an identically appearing placebo." The details include the study design (e.g., 8-week parallel trial, control treatment, blinding, randomization); the criteria for inclusion of patients into the study, including how patients will be diagnosed for the disease being treated; criteria for exclusion of patients from the study; the clinical and laboratory procedures that will be carried out with each patient; the description of the drug treatment schedule (doses of drugs, route of treatment); description of laboratory and other tests; the criteria that will be used to measure efficacy; and the planned statistical analysis that has to be very specific for primary parameters and other statements about how the study will be carried out.

In the statistical methods section, the statisticians describe how the sample size was derived and how they will analyze the data. The statistical procedure for primary analysis has to be clearly described in great detail, including what level of significance is to be used. If an interim analysis will be performed, it is critically important to describe when it will be done, by whom, and what methods will be used for the analysis, particularly how the Type I error rate will be controlled and who will have access to the results. The procedure to handle missing data should be stated. Finally, the protocol contains the method of eliciting information about adverse events and the course of action to be taken if adverse events are reported. The set of case report forms that will be used for this study is usually attached to the protocol as an appendix.

In summary, the protocol contains all of the directions that can be written out explaining how to do a study. The challenge is to maintain a balance between completeness and brevity. The protocol must be long enough to contain meaningful comments on each of the points just mentioned. On the other hand, if the protocol gets to be too long, then it is unlikely that the investigator and other personnel involved with the study will carefully read the details of the protocol. In that case, the investigator and co-workers are likely to violate some of the requirements specified in the protocol. The statistician then has a difficult time trying to analyze the data and interpret the results.

Studies are reviewed by an Institutional Review Board, which considers the ethical issues in the study. Some larger and longer pharmaceutical studies may also have a Data Safety and Monitoring Board (DSMB) or Independent Data Monitoring Committee (IDMC) that is concerned with patient safety and dissemination of interim analysis information to protect the integrity of the trial. As stated above, more and more frequently, studies are reviewed before completion in an interim analysis. Information on this topic can be found in Chapters 13 and 14.

REFERENCES

1. Declaration of Helsinki, *BMJ*, 313(7070) 1964, 7 December 1996 (http://www.cirp.orh/library/ethics/helsinki/).
2. Buncher, C.R., Principles of experimental design for clinical drug studies, In *Perspectives in Clinical Pharmacy*, Francke, D.E. and Whitney, H.A.K. Jr., eds., Drug Intelligence, Hamilton, IL, pp. 504–525, 1972.

3. Simel, D.L. and Feussner, J.R., Clinical trials of informed consent, *Control. Clin. Trials*, 13, 321–324, 1992.
4. Lasagna, L., Informed consent revisited: commentary, *Scrip Mag.*, 121, 21, March, 2003.
5. Ederer, F., Patient bias, investigator bias, and the double-masked procedure in clinical trials, *Am. J. Med.*, 58, 295–299, 1975.
6. McEntegart, D.J., The pursuit of balance using stratified and dynamic randomization techniques: an overview, *Drug Inf. J.*, 39, 293–308, 2003.
7. Royall, R.M., Ethics and statistics in randomized clinical trials, *Stat. Sci.*, 6, 52–88, 1991.
8. Wei, L.J., Exact two-sample permutation tests based on the randomized play the winner rule, *Biometrika*, 75, 603–606, 1988.
9. Simon, R., Adaptive treatment assignment methods and clinical trials, *Biometrics*, 33, 743–749, 1977.
10. Lan, K.K.G. and DeMets, D.L., Group sequential procedures: calendar versus information time, *Stat. Med.*, 8, 1191–1198, 1989.
11. Wang, S.J., Hung, H.M.J., Tsong, Y., and Cui, L., Group sequential test strategies for superiority and non-inferiority hypotheses in active controlled clinical trials, *Stat. Med.*, 20, 1903–1912, 2001.
12. Liu, Q., Proschan, M.A., and Pledger, G.W., A unified theory of two-stage adaptive designs, *J. Am. Stat. Assoc.*, 97, 1034–1041, 2002.
13. Lan, K.K.G., Conditional power: a Bayesian approach, *Int. Chin. Stat. Assoc. Bull.*, 43, July, 2000.
14. FDA. *Guidance: Statistical Procedures for Bioequivalence Studies Using a Standard Two-Treatment Crossover Design*, Division of Bio-equivalence and Division of Biometrics, Center for Drug Evaluation and Research, Food and Drug Administration, Rockville, MD, 1992, July 1.
15. Stewart, E.H., Self-administered analgesia in labor with special reference to trichlorethylene, *Lancet*, 2, 781–783, 1949.
16. Ganter, J., Glossary of clinical trials terminology, *Appl. Clin. Trials*, 11, 22–32, 2002.
17. Kaitin, K.I., Phelan, N.R., Raiford, D., and Morris, B., Therapeutic ratings and end-of-phase II conferences: initiatives to accelerate the availability of important new drugs, *J. Clin. Pharmacol.*, 31, 17–24, 1991.
18. ICH E-6, *Guideline for Good Clinical Practice*, 1996 (http://www.ich.org).

5 Selecting Patients for a Clinical Trial*

C. Ralph Buncher and Jia-Yeong Tsay

CONTENTS

---

* "Patient" and "subject" are used almost interchangeably in this chapter, although some publications make a distinction between them. For instance, *Applied Clinical Trials* (*ACT*) house style requires that article submissions make the FDA and ICH distinction between patients (persons under physician's care for a particular disease or condition) and subjects (individuals who participate in a clinical trial, either as recipient of the investigational product or as a control) as indicated by Toby Jane Hindin, Editor-in-Chief, *ACT* (2004).[24]

OVERVIEW

Statisticians know that patients who are randomly allocated to two or more groups are supposed to have equal characteristics on the average, and thus an inference from the study will validly compare two treatments. If the two groups remain equal in the characteristics during the trial, then there is no bias in the resulting outcomes since other factors or covariates will be equal in the groups.

On the other hand, if the studies, like many cardiovascular studies in the past, only include male patients for instance, then any inference about females is based on extrapolation and thus is not directly based on the data collected in the trial. In this chapter, we try to describe some of the possible biases that exist in selecting the patients who actually take part in the trials. For example, one concern is that if a drug has been shown to be effective in patients aged 21 to 75, should it also be approved for the same indication in those over age 75? Should it be approved for children based on these results in adults? Should it be approved for pregnant women if they were excluded from the studies? Even if the medication was not specifically studied in and approved for a subgroup of the population, individual physicians still have the problem of choosing a treatment for their specific patients, so-called "off-label use." Moreover, if Doctor A takes care of patients of a different ethnicity than those who were in the trials, do the results of the published studies still apply to those patients? This is an important issue in global drug development to market a drug in a new region with a different population as shown in ICH E-5 Guideline (1998).[1]

Several themes are intertwined in this chapter. For the clinician-investigator, the concern is whether there will be enough patients willing to take part in the trial to fulfill the sample size requirement calculated by the statistician. For the clinical monitor, the concern is to decide whether the investigator, or investigators in a multi-site study, will be able to obtain an adequate supply of the desired patients in the desired time frame. For the statistician, one concern is whether the patients entered into the study will be representative of the population desired. All of these concerns focus on whether there are enough candidates available for the trial and whether a sufficient and representative number of them will actually take part in the trial. Among other factors, these decisions involve the subjects' attitudes towards clinical research, the inclusion and exclusion criteria in the protocol, the content and implications in the Informed Consent, and the investigator's ability to resolve the situations that arise during a clinical trial. The challenge for the statistician is to understand the biases that are operative in selecting those patients who actually participate in the studies. This greater insight will often suggest statistical comparisons that will illuminate the results of a clinical trial.

The focus of pharmacology in the 20th century was to characterize the effects in the average patient. In the 21st century, the focus will continue to shift to finding and characterizing those patients in whom the medication works and those in whom it does not work. Can one describe the differences in those patients who will show an important side effect? Whether the basis for the difference is genetic or environmental, the more one understands, the more effective will be the use of the medication.

Most studies provide only limited information about the non-participants. A couple of exceptions are Siminoff et al.[2] and Mengis et al.[3] which describe patients in breast cancer trials and Phase III leukemia trials, respectively.

Subject recruitment and retention is quite a challenge in clinical trials. Jean Sullivan[4] characterizes four types of barriers to success in subject recruitment and retention and provides extensive discussion in each category of the barriers. To improve subject accrual to clinical trials, the barriers to recruitment and retention need to be identified and overcome accordingly. For further advice on Good Recruitment Practice in clinical trials, see Joan F. Bachenheimer.[5]

Michael Weintraub and José F. Calimlim described some of their experiences in obtaining patients for clinical trials in the following excerpts from Weintraub and Calimlim:[6]

Part A: The Outpatient by Michael Weintraub
Part B: The Inpatient by José F. Calimlim

This chapter provides some actual observations on what happens with patient selection between the time a trial is designed and the time study patients are started on medication.

We know that pregnant women and often women who may become pregnant during a trial have frequently been excluded from clinical trials. Persons addicted to illegal drugs have also been excluded. An important concern then becomes apparent when a clinician wishes to treat patients in one of these groups and discovers that no or few studies have ever involved persons in these classifications.

One example of the lack of representativeness is the use of geriatric patients in research articles. Geriatric patients are underrepresented among patients in clinical trials. For example, Morley et al.[7] showed that the percentage of articles on humans that included subjects over 65 years of age grew from perhaps 12% in 1966 to 15% in 1986 while discharges from short-stay hospitals of the same persons increased from 17 to 31% in 1986. In addition we note that geriatric patients take more medications than do younger patients and yet are used in trials far less than their share of consumption of the final product.

Major studies find the description of patient recruitment to be an important part of the study characterization. For example, the methods, strategies, costs, and effectiveness of recruitment for the Lung Health Study have been explained in detail.[8]

PART A: THE OUTPATIENT BY MICHAEL WEINTRAUB

I. INTRODUCTION

Patient selection affects many aspects of a clinical trial. It determines whether or not the clinical trial can be carried out and how long it will take to complete. It will affect the outcome of the trial and thus will directly influence the regulatory agency. The selection process will also affect the clinician's ability to generalize the findings of the study. Ultimately, then, selection of patients for a trial can even influence drug utilization. This section deals with outpatient populations having chronic conditions.

The patients who end up in clinical trials may represent only a small percentage of the theoretical universe of available patients. Usually the analysis will not suggest that extrapolation from the study sample was unjustified.

In the University of Rochester Rheumatology Unit, the names of patients and their diagnoses are kept in a coded card catalog. It is possible, then, to retrieve quickly a list of all patients having the diagnosis of rheumatoid arthritis. We knew from experience that the diagnosis recorded on the cards should not be accepted as final, since further investigations often reveal a second disease or, with the passage of time, a revised diagnosis may be made but not recorded in this file. Also, the diagnosis appearing on the card may have been based on the physician's clinical impression rather than on the rigid criteria needed in our clinical trial.

For these reasons we hired a medical student to do a feasibility study before beginning the trial, and convinced the sponsoring pharmaceutical company to pay for it. The student reviewed the records and entered diagnostic information on a standard form, assisted the investigators in contacting the patients and finding out whether they still met the diagnostic criteria, and set up appointments for interviews and examinations. The initial survey of the card file provided 300 patient names and unit numbers. The charts of 150 of these patients were not available for review. Several of the patients had died. Of the 150 patients whose charts were available, 101 were rejected after screening for the following reasons:

40% had not been seen for more than five years.
10% did not meet the diagnostic criteria.
10% had recently been examined in the clinic and were reported to be in remission or without symptoms.

10% were judged by the rheumatologist caring for them to be unable to respond to therapy other than surgical replacement of joints.

10% had drug toxicity akin to that expected from the study drug.

10% were considered unable to follow the protocol reliably.

Only 49 patients (16% of the initial sample) remained to be interviewed and examined. As mentioned more completely elsewhere,[9] 31 patients were removed from consideration for participation because:

eleven did not have disease activity great enough to warrant their inclusion.

seven had concurrent disease not evident from the charts of screening, including:

two with abnormal liver chemistries (SGOT, SGFT, and LDH).

two with asymptomatic gastric ulcers demonstrated by a screening upper gastrointestinal (GI) series.

one who revealed after long discussion that she had frequent nausea and vomiting with or without drug therapy.

one with an asymptomatic aortic aneurysm.

one with renal stones.

four were found unacceptable for reasons pertaining to the protocol, viz.

one in whom pregnancy was diagnosed by the radiologist (before he began the upper GI series).

two who were taking other nonsteroidal, anti-inflammatory drugs not noted in their records and were doing well on them.

one who had been scheduled for joint replacement.

four declined to participate because of inconvenience or distance to the clinic.

five refused outright to participate in the study.

The reasons they gave were interference with their work, with family responsibilities, or with their "life style." Only one patient gave toxicity as the reason, and that was prompted by pressure from her husband, who feared that she might develop an ulcer and be unable to participate in the enjoyment of his retirement. (This patient later entered an open-label study of the same drug and did, in fact, develop a duodenal ulcer.)

II. THE SELECTION PROCESS AND GETTING ENOUGH PATIENTS TO DO THE STUDY — LASAGNA'S LAW AND ITS COROLLARIES

"Lasagna's Law"[10] teaches us that the incidence of the disease under study will drastically decrease once the study begins. It will not return to its previous level until the completion of study (if completion occurs before the investigators retire). There are obvious and valuable public health aspects of this law, but it has an undesirable impact on the conduct of clinical trials. The following discussion examines how Lasagna's law operates to diminish acceptable candidates for participation in a clinical trial.

A. The Many Become the Few

One can never know whether there will be enough patients for a clinical trial simply from investigators' estimates of how many patients will meet the diagnostic criteria. Physicians have selective memory of how many patients of a particular type they see. Their interest in the study may cause them to overestimate the number of suitable patients available. Files are frequently out of date or lost. Patients move, retire, die, or recover. Ideas change over time as to what constitutes the disease entity under study.

B. The Few Become the Fewer

The diagnostic strictures imposed by the clinical trial decrease the number of available patients even further. In clinical practice the diagnostic criteria need not be as rigid as those laid down by, for example, the American Rheumatism Association, the pharmaceutical industry, or the Food and Drug Administration. In clinical practice, the special tests required to fulfill the stringent criteria are neither done nor necessary. Patients with variations on the theme of the disease are included under the basic rubric because such fine distinctions will not often affect therapy. If in studies, however, only the strictest criteria are used, one ends up with the purest-of-the-pure sample, and this distillate will be very small. It is rarely considered that such a refined population may not provide an adequate or fair test of the study medication. Data based on such a purified sample may not apply to the population at large but may fulfill certain internal or regulatory needs.

C. Avoiding the Lazarus Trap

Once the diagnosis is assured, investigators must make a judgment on disease activity, the stage of disease, and the severity of the disease. An optimum selection would include patients with enough disease present to show a good response to medication but not so much disease that they are unable to respond or have irreversible changes — "burned-out" disease. The latter patients would not be suitable for participation in a clinical trial because inclusion of their data could cause a Type II error and a rejection of an active medication. Requiring a drug to show its efficacy in patients in whom no other medication has been of value is what has been called the "Lazarus Phenomenon." Including too many Lazaruses will bias the study against the drug.

D. All God's Children Get Sick from Time to Time

The next major problem of the selection process is the presence of concurrent disease that has been apparent from the very outset, before the pre-drug-screening tests. Although some diseases obviously require exclusion, what about past conditions that mimic the expected toxicity of the study drug? In the clinical trial of the nonsteroidal agent, the possibility of gastrointestinal toxicity with the study drug alerted us to the need for obtaining the history of such disease in prospective participants. Who should be rejected — patients who had an ulcer two years ago? five years ago? ten years ago? Then, too, sick people frequently have other diseases. Some diseases often coexist with, or result from, therapeutic measures used in the disease under study. These are important determinants of a patient's suitability for inclusion in a clinical trial. Yet if everyone who has the merest touch of another disease is excluded, the study population will shrink even further. The question of what constitutes serious renal, hepatic, or cardiovascular diseases also must be raised. Many diseases and laboratory test changes; e.g., cataracts, pulmonary changes, electrocardiographic "abnormalities," hypertension, adult onset diabetes, decreased creatinine clearance, and increased globulins may occur as part of the natural course of aging. Too often clinical logic does not function in the elimination criteria for studies of drugs brought to Phase II. The standard exclusions are used indiscriminately without any modification based on the disease process, the type of medication, toxicity shown in preclinical testing, or the toxicity demonstrated during Phase I trials.

E. THE FEW BECOME THE ROCK-BOTTOM FEWEST

Both Bloomfield[11] and Lasagna[10] have pointed out the therapeutic effect of looking for study participants. As discussed above, the reasons why potential study participants disappear once a clinical trial begins are quite mundane. The main reason is the rigor of diagnostic criteria. Another is that the patient's disease changes; he/she may have had enough active disease during the initial review but improves before the trial gets underway, or during the run-in period, especially if the disease is cyclic. Then, as Joubert et al.[12] have observed, during the screening period potential participants frequently are found to have laboratory pseudo abnormalities in the form of meaningless deviations from normal values — cholesterol levels that are too low, minor electrocardiographic variations, or even spurious laboratory vagaries. In the study under discussion, we made sure that only patients with "cast-iron stomachs" and no laboratory abnormalities would participate, i.e., whose upper GI series results were negative despite high doses of aspirin/prednisone, and gold therapy.

Many times the abnormalities that show up in laboratory tests are caused by illnesses unrelated to the disease under study, or to necessary therapeutic intervention. It is more difficult to decide whether to include this latter group in a trial. For example, in the first study we found a patient with increased liver enzymes, probably induced by aspirin. She of course, was excluded from participation. Similarly, aspirin therapy, especially if the patient takes aspirin intermittently, can result in the shedding of large numbers of renal epithelial cells into the urine. These may be disturbing to the person examining the urinary sediment. Asymptomatic, serious illnesses may be discovered in patients being screened for a clinical trial. We found two patients with asymptomatic ulcers and one with an aortic aneurysm in the NSAID study. At this point in the selection process, investigators may turn their faces to the heavens and, like Job, cry, "What else, Lord, what else?"

F. NEED YOU ASK?

There are other burdens. In the first study a young woman who had assured us that she was practicing birth control became pregnant. Fortunately, the radiologist was astute enough to question the patient about her menstrual period before performing the upper GI series, and found she had missed her last period, which should have occurred between the screening interview and the time for the x-ray.

Next the question arises: How will the patient's other therapy effect the outcome of the trial? A certain amount of standard therapy must be permitted in many current clinical trials for ethical reasons. One could not, in good conscience, deprive patients suffering from serious rheumatoid arthritis of all their usual therapy. Investigators must learn a lesson from the early trials of L-dopa, when patients whose anticholinergic therapy was discontinued regressed to the point of severe Parkinson's disease and required months to return to even baseline status.[13.] Conversely, drugs that obviously interfere — ones capable of causing adverse effects similar to those expected from the study medication — should be discontinued. Competing agents should also be stopped. Other, nondrug treatment modalities can be handled in a variety of ways. For example, ancillary therapy can be forbidden, standardized or measured and included in the analysis. Background therapy can be categorized (none, minimal some, or maximal) by a set of rules and participants in each classification that will minimize the differences between groups.[14]

G. PARTICIPANT PSYCHOLOGY: CAPRICIOUS AND INTELLIGENT NONCOMPLIERS

Psychological factors play an important role in the physician's assessment of who should participate in a clinical trial. Physicians make judgments about the patient's ability to adhere to the protocol according to the patient's past demonstration of understanding prescription directions. "Capricious compliers" should not be included in clinical trials, since they vary their medication intake from day to day, according to ideas not necessarily founded on pharmacokinetic or pharmacodynamic theory. On the other hand, "intelligent noncompliers" — patients who stop medication for rational reasons — should be included if they can be relied upon to notify the study physician.[15] Patients who accurately report adverse effects may also be known to physicians and would be valuable participants in a clinical trial. The important psychological attributes of participants in a trial are stability coupled with flexibility.

When considering the ethical aspects of the participant selection process, physicians must also analyze the psychological factors that enable a patient to make a reasoned judgment about participation in a clinical trial. The ideal participants would be patients who will carry through the clinical trial and actively interact with the investigators rather than being passive experimental subjects.

H. "Not Unless I Can Be in the Placebo Group, Doctor"

Finally, there are some patients who meet the diagnostic and disease activity criteria, pass the screening tests, can respond to the study drug, and take the correct amount and type of other treatment but who refuse outright to participate. These are rare, however, in studies of treatments for chronic diseases. Patients with active rheumatoid arthritis despite therapy often will want to participate in a study that offers any hope of relief, no matter how remote. However, in a study such as the trial of a postoperative analgesic discussed by Dr. Calimlim, more patients decline to participate.

Some of the obstacles to participation mentioned by patients in our study may actually have been veiled but valid refusals. Problems with the clinic schedule, travel arrangements, and "cure" during run-in periods may give the patient ways to decline participation without outright refusal. Healthy volunteers often find alterations in life style the most disrupting aspect of participation in a clinical trial,[16] and perhaps this is an important deterrent to some patients as well. Fear of toxicity is another. However, in a test of how well the patients in this study recalled the information given them during the consent procedure, we found that very little of the toxicity data was retained.[9] Perhaps because of anxiety about their disease and desire to participate in the study, patients did not really listen to the discussion of the negative aspects of the trial. Other, less anxious patients may have listened and refused to participate.

I. The Selection Process and Regulatory Requirements

The choice of the target population must be made so that the drug has a fighting chance. I would like to term this "Lazarus versus Grendel." As previously discussed, too many "Lazarus" patients can cause even the best-designed study to reject an active, valuable drug. One must balance the availability of fresh, barely treated, or even untreated patients with the ethically and practically more sound practice of seeking difficult responders to participate in initial studies. This is the "Grendel," or worthy opponent, principle. (A lesser opponent than the terrible monster Grendel would not have truly tested Beowulf's courage, diminishing his heroic credentials.) In the trial discussed here, we elected to use patients with active disease despite full doses of standard therapy, but not patients with end-stage or nonresponsive disease, even if they met the criteria for pain and disease activity. If the drug works in tough but treatable ("Grendel") patient populations, one can say, "Great: We have an active valuable agent." If, however, it fails in the improper ("Lazarus") patients, it does not mean that the drug could not be effective in less severely ill patients.

J. Between a Rock and a Hard Place

Another goal of clinical trials related to the regulatory process is toxicity monitoring. The selection process exerts an influence on this goal also. Screening out every patient who has ever had, or could have, a particular sort of problem leaves a small, select group providing little indication of possible serious toxicity. If, for example, patients likely to develop gastrointestinal disease are included and each toxicity does occur, is it worse than if gastrointestinal lesions appear in patients who have been carefully screened for any possible predisposing factor or presence of disease? If, on the other hand, such toxicity does not occur, can one then assume that it will not occur in the average patient? If all patients are included in a study without any sort of clinical logic being applied, then we will end up including patients who already have some disease ("toxicity") before treatment with the study drug. The results will then make the drug look falsely toxic. Such patients may participate in late (Phase III) studies, where the goals are different and information on general usefulness is being sought. If included earlier, they must be equally distributed among the treatment groups.

III. PATIENT SELECTION PROCESS AND SCIENTIFIC MERIT OF PUBLICATIONS

A. GENERALIZATION OF DATA TO OTHER PATIENT POPULATIONS

In following the rigorous selection process outlined above, who finally enters the study? Does this patient population have any relationship to that seen in actual practice? The answer, of course, is that there are many important differences between study populations and patients in general, and these differences decrease our ability to apply the study results to any other population. Patients in a clinical trial are usually fairly homogeneous in terms of diagnostic criteria, other treatments, and duration and severity of disease; in clinical practice the population is much more heterogeneous. Diagnostic criteria are much more stringent with study patients than with patients in general whose disease may be more severe or more treatment resistant. Study participants may tolerate adverse reactions because of perceived benefit for the more severe illness. Patients in studies have often been referred to specialists, whereas in actual practice more patients are treated by primary care physicians. Patients participating in Phase II studies usually live in large cities, frequently those with university medical centers and academic investigators, whereas in actual practice there is a mixture of population densities, and physicians are less likely to be academic investigators. Patients in studies may have less restriction on their time; they may be retired, disabled, unemployed, or work for a benevolent company. Patients in clinical trials tend to adhere closely to therapeutic regimens and are good observers. This is not necessarily the case among the general population of patients.

B. ETHICS AND EXTRAPOLATION

Ethical considerations may also affect the patient selection process and the scientific merit of publication. Racial, social, and economic factors have frequently been offered as an important distinction between patients who participate in a trial and those who do not. Participation by patients who stand to benefit themselves or for the societal good from the research should be fostered.

In obtaining consent from our patients we found that much of the material on adverse effects was forgotten.[9] Two thirds of the patients could not remember at the end of the study ever having been told that they could get an ulcer from the medication, despite having been told five times about the ulcerogenic activity of the drug, having been given the written patient information form to take home on two occasions, having had an upper GI series, and having been questioned every two weeks about gastrointestinal symptoms. One third of the patients incorrectly noted that they had been told that this drug was safer than any other drug for rheumatoid arthritis. Only one third of the patients reported apprehension about the side effects of the new drug before the study started. This apprehension soon disappeared, however.

We keep our patient information form short and to the point. They are written in what we hope is an easily understood style, although, considering the socioeconomic status and educational level of the patients, much more complex material should have been easily understood. Actually, when tested, our patients retained material contained in the information form, rejecting from memory only the material on adverse effects.

An "add-on" study, in which test medication is added to the patient's current treatment, is frequently more ethical but presents serious difficulties for a clinical trial. Add-on studies alter the target population, in many cases making it broader and making the study more feasible. However, there will be less room for improvement in each individual patient (part of the Lazarus dilemma mentioned above). The resultant decreased experimental sensitivity and decreased patient responsiveness should be taken into account in the creation of "power curves" needed to determine the number of patients who should be in the study. The studies will be "dirtier," that is, there is likely to be an increased incidence of adverse drug reactions and less clear cut response attributable to the new agent. Data from add-on trials are easier to apply to the patient population at large. The ethical nature of the add-on studies, as well as the ability to be practical and to extrapolate to the general population, probably outweighs the drawback of results that are harder to interpret.

C. WHAT, ME WORRY?

Why should investigators and monitors in the pharmaceutical industry worry about patient selection processes and the effect on extrapolation? The most important reason relates to the possibility of achieving a true result from the study and a valid estimate of common toxicity. In addition, medical students have increasingly been trained in the critical evaluation of the literature. Physicians will downgrade studies in which the selection process appears to have biased the outcome, or in which the selection process was so rigid as to preclude extrapolation to their patient population. Then they will be less likely to use the drug except in selected patients. Regulatory bodies carefully analyze the study population's characteristics. Labeling restrictions (or even approval) may thus be affected by participant selection.

IV. IMPROVING THE SELECTION PROCESS

Bloomfield[11] recommended that investigators should check records and do formal pilot studies, assessing the availability and suitability of the patient population at hand for participation in a clinical trial and if the protocol is workable. Investing a small amount of time and money in such prestudy surveys will save the concerned parties much grief. Sponsors, investigators, and regulators must remain flexible in determining selection criteria. Small changes in the criteria may make vast difference in patient availability without materially influencing the outcome of the study or its extrapolatability. For example, in a study of a new hypnotic agent, slightly increasing the age limits for entry resulted in a large increase in potential participants, facilitating completion of the trial.

A corollary of the "flexibility" recommendation is to tailor the criteria to the institutions. Clinical trial logic must be applied at all stages of the process of patient selection — the diagnostic criteria, the prognostic criteria, the distribution of patients in the treatment groups, and the decisions made about adverse effects. In some areas the patient population may have certain demographic, diagnostic, or therapeutic idiosyncrasies, which would not deleteriously affect the outcome of the study but, if included, might improve the availability of patients.

These comments are intended to be an argument against many large, multicenter trials. The latter studies tend to be carried out by "data gatherers" instead of investigators. The necessary patient selection judgments are the province of the investigator on the scene. I believe that data gatherers do not have the time, the training or the inclination for these tasks.

V. AVOIDING STUDIES THAT RESEMBLE FINE SCOTCH (AGED IN THE CASK)

Another suggestion for rapid completion and for statistically and clinically significant results is to start all patients in the study at the same time whenever possible. This avoids long drawn-out studies during which the quality of the data deteriorates as investigator interest wanes. Additionally, starting patients as a group decreases "improvement bias" noted in rheumatoid arthritis studies.[17] Given the cyclic pattern of many chronic diseases, such as rheumatoid arthritis, patients often enter studies during an exacerbation. They then would be expected to get better with time, no matter what their treatment (regression toward the mean). Assigning treatment and starting all patients at one time, generally after a delay during which patients are selected for the study, diminishes improvement bias. Some patients will have passed the worst of the exacerbation, and others will be at some middle point.

The procedures used in obtaining consent can also be improved. We allow patients to bow out gracefully for whatever reasons they advance. We do not attempt to convince a patient to enter a clinical trial, and if a patient asks for more time to decide, we do not contact them again. They must contact us if they later decide to participate. Whenever possible in our studies, an investigator not associated with the daily care of the patient obtained the consent after discussing the pros and cons of entering the study. (This is a safeguard that cannot be used when physician/data gatherers conduct clinical trials.) Patients may feel constrained to participate when their own physicians are the ones obtaining consent. We have found that group discussions are an effective way of informing participants about a study. Potential participants gather together and are given information on the study and possible adverse effects. They ask questions and hear the concerns of others that might not have occurred to them. Video tapes, interactive computer programs, readability testing, and other newer methods for improving communication have been applied to the consent process.

Discussion, worry, and thought about patient selection are often left completely to the investigators. Pharmaceutical industry monitors should continue involvement after the inclusion and exclusion criteria have been established. Once the design and protocol have been established, the patient selection process may be the single most important determinant of the outcome of a clinical trial. Proper monitoring of patient selection becomes increasingly important now that physicians in nonacademic centers are taking part in multicenter clinical trials with standardized protocols imposed upon them. They may have neither the expertise nor the experience to assess the influence of patient selection on the outcome of studies. They may fail to realize how their entering a patient into a clinical trial could affect the outcome because they see only a small portion of the patients in the study. Patient selection problems are less likely when investigators trained in clinical pharmacology or having wide experience in performing clinical trials are involved in the design and management of a study.

Precise or quantitative data of the impact of patient selection on the outcome and extrapolatability of a study do not now exist. Although the population in the study discussed above had an incomplete response to standard treatment and differed from the population of arthritis patients as a whole, we were able to demonstrate significant drug effects. How one uses the information from that study in making a therapeutic decision or a regulatory decision is a difficult problem. More thinking and research is needed in this area.

PART B: THE INPATIENT BY JOSÉ F. CALIMLIM

I. INTRODUCTION

The term *clinical trial* covers a wide variety of different activities. To many people outside medicine it implies something exciting and dramatic and possibly dangerous, involving the early administration of a new drug to man. There are clinical trials of that kind, but the majorities are more mundane but no less important.[18]

It is not easy to generalize about clinical trials in new drugs because applications vary so widely. On the one hand, the drug concerned might offer the first effective treatment for a hitherto untreatable form of cancer, and on the other hand it might be a new substance for the treatment of pain. Obviously the approach to these two problems would be very different. However, there are some basic principles which apply throughout this type of work.

Before a drug is offered for a clinical trial a great deal of work has been done on it and a lot of money has been spent. If the drug is reasonably safe in animal and Phase I clinical trials in man, and has an action which might be useful in the treatment of pain, it will probably be accepted for study by a clinical investigator. If the secondary trials turn out successfully and no serious toxicity is observed in man, analytical and descriptive papers on the drug then go back to the Food and Drug Administration for approval. If the proof of the efficacy and safety is acceptable, the pharmaceutical company will be given permission to market the drug.

We take the need for clinical trials to be self-evident. It is impossible to conceive of a modern civilized society without the benefits of modern drugs. Development and assessment of new analgesics is not possible without clinical trials. We do not think that many people would deny this general case as long as trials are carried on with utmost safety and efficiency.

In some clinical trials the use of placebo is essential.[19] The drug can only be assessed on the basis of what the patient tells the doctor or observer about the pain. The pain is often lessened somewhat by a tablet that does not contain any active ingredients (a "placebo effect"); therefore, a comparison of no treatment with the active tablet might give a false positive result because of this effect. Here it is necessary to compare the active tablet with a placebo.

It is more difficult to generalize about the role of the patient in the trial of new drugs. If the drug is for the treatment of a serious condition, it is easy to find patients who are unresponsive to established drugs. A new drug is usually offered to patients who are in this position. But for new drugs with unproven efficacy to relieve pain, it is a little bit more difficult to obtain patient participation. In these circumstances a heavy responsibility falls upon the clinical investigator conducting a clinical trial for the patient's safety.

The first step in an analgesic clinical trial is to choose which kind of pain to study, a choice determined in part by the goal of the research.[20] Two kinds of pain have been studied in assaying analgesics: experimentally induced and clinical pain. Experimental pain now has few protagonists, partly because with the institution of double-blind procedures it was found that many of the most famous experiments involved bias and cuing, and partly because assay of the therapeutic value of a drug is appropriately done against clinical pain.

The next decision to be made is what kinds of subjects to utilize. In studies of clinical pain, the subjects will be patients of some sort. As with experimental pain, they also will be volunteers, although the factors which influence their participation and understanding are likely to be different.

If one works with outpatients, some special difficulties arise. One can never be certain that they take their doses when and as directed.[21] Their interest and cooperation cannot be actively and continuously engaged.

If inpatients are selected, the next choice is between acute and chronic patients. Acute postsurgical pain and its relief have been the subject of many reports.[22] The meaningfulness of much of this work is evaluated subject to the diversity of etiologies and preoperative as well as postoperative surgical states. Postsurgical patients are also, to a varying and not altogether predictable extent, still recovering from the anesthesiologist's marvelous bag of tricks. Postoperative pain has been described as "the most frequent and neglected painful state in the hospital situation." Many others, including intelligent and informed patients, have echoed this sentiment, but postoperative pain relief is still too often left to the junior physician's "cautiously administered opiate and the balm that comes from time alone."

Most civilized men today surely concede that there is need for the relief of postoperative pain on humanitarian grounds alone. There are, however, other obvious reasons for mitigating the discomfort of the patients. These include the need to promote deep breathing and cooperation with the physiotherapist and the desirability of early mobilization to avoid deep venous thrombosis.

For clinical trials to be of any value, one must be able to extrapolate the results to the general population for whom the drug is designed. For extrapolation to be valid there must be a relationship between the study sample and the population from which it was selected.

This discussion is an attempt to examine the degree of selection and attrition due to protocol and other factors that occurred in the course of obtaining 100 consenting volunteers completing a single-dose postsurgical analgesic study.[22] An attempt is also made to compare the study population and the population from which it was selected.

II. DESCRIPTION OF THE STUDY

The protocol was written for a study intended to evaluate the efficacy of three analgesic treatments and a placebo administered in single-doses in double-blind fashion for postoperative pain. Subjects were postoperative surgical patients. Surgical procedures of potential participants were classified as: general superficial surgery, gynecological surgery, plastic surgery, dental surgery, and superficial neurosurgical procedures. Excluded from the study were: cardiovascular, thoracic, and abdominal surgical procedures.

There were several criteria for admission to the study. Patients must have been 21 to 65 years old, weighing 120 to 200 lb. Patients whose medical or surgical history was consistent with a reasonable suspicion of gastrointestinal, liver, or urinary disease that might interfere with the absorption, metabolism, or excretion of medications were excluded.

Acceptable patients were those who had not participated in any other drug studies in the past three weeks, who had recovered from a surgical procedure sufficiently to request and receive oral analgesic medication during the first three postoperative days, who had at least a moderate degree of pain after surgery, and who did not have history of tolerance to analgesic medication.

Permission to visit patients for discussion of the study was obtained from the patients' physicians prior to the operation.

III. SELECTION PROCESS

A. SCHEDULE SURVEY AND SCREENING

Survey of the daily elective surgical schedule for the duration of the study showed a total of 8027 patients potentially available. This number was reduced by 39% (3103) because of patients not screened due to unavailability during appointed hours of interview for various reasons such as late admissions, being worked up by staff, referral to specialty clinics, or out on pass. This left 4924 patients available for screening. Preliminary exclusion eliminated 4254 or (86%) of these. Only 670 patients were thus available for interview, i.e., only 8% of the total number of patients originally available for the study.

B. PRELIMINARY EXCLUSIONS

The reasons for preliminary screening exclusions are described in Table 5.1. 45% or 1921 were excluded because of age. Of these, 1232 were below 21 years and 689 were over 65 years. The lower age limit, 21 years, was the legal age of majority in New York State at the time of the study. The upper age limit was chosen arbitrarily. Age was thus a major factor for excluding 45% of the number available for screening.

Insufficiency of postoperative pain excluded an additional 1155 or 27%. Some patients do not require postoperative pain relief even after major operations. The scheduled surgical procedures included diagnostic curettage

TABLE 5.1
Reasons for Preliminary Exclusion

Below 21 or above 65 years	1921 (45%)
Insufficient postoperative pain	1155 (27%)
Excluded surgical procedures	718 (17%)
No physician consent	337 (8%)
Short-term admissions	123 (3%)
Total	4254

and superficial gynecological surgery, superficial general surgery, and excisions of small lesions, gingivectomy, some simple eye and nose surgery, and endoscopies, procedures in which pain is often mild postoperatively.

Some of the surgical procedures that were excluded were gastrointestinal resections, open heart surgery, spine fusions, and facial or mandibular surgery, where oral administration may be ineffective or inappropriate in the early postoperative period. These made up 718 exclusions or 17%. The remaining were excluded for miscellaneous reasons, e.g., admitted in the morning for scheduled surgery and sent home later in the afternoon. Such patients numbered 123 or 3%. A considerable number of patients (337 or 8%) were not included in the study because some attending surgeons had not consented to let us interview their patients for the study.

C. CHART SCREENING AND PATIENT INTERVIEW

After these preliminary exclusions, only 670 (or 14% of the total initially available) were left for screening and interview (Table 5.2). This number was cut further by such factors as patients not being available for interview at designated time, surgery canceled, or surgical procedure changed to a less painful one (e.g., laparotomy to laparoscopy) so that there was insufficient postoperative pain.

Twenty-one patients were in this group. The charts of the remaining 649 patients were screened and reviewed in detail prior to interview with emphasis on the past and present history and physical findings together with the available laboratory reports. This brought about rejection of an additional 258 patients prior to interview. Thus 391 patients were left to be interviewed.

D. REASONS FOR REJECTION PRIOR TO INTERVIEW

There were several reasons why we rejected these 258 patients prior to interview after review of their charts. Many had multiple medical problems unrelated to the indication for surgery (Table 5.3). Some were underweight or overweight. Allergy or sensitivity to the drug was also reported but not observed. Others were too apprehensive, high-strung, and agitated; or overly concerned about the loss of a particular organ such as breast, uterus, testis, etc. Active peptic ulcer disease,

TABLE 5.2
Patients Available for Interview

Patients not screened	21
Patients screened	649
Total	670
Patients interviewed	391 (60%)
Patients rejected before interview	258 (40%)
Total	649

TABLE 5.3
Reasons for Rejection Prior to Interview

Multiple medical problems	82	31%
Overweight or underweight	60	23%
Sensitivity to study medication	28	11%
Emotional overlay	20	8%
Chronic analgesic intake	17	7%
Active peptic ulcer disease	16	6%
Psychiatric history or illness	10	4%
Language problems	8	3%
Multiple allergies	6	2%
Physical impairment (deaf, blind)	4	2%
Refused surgery	4	2%
Mental retardation	3	1%
Total	258	—

chronic intake of analgesics, and psychiatric illness or history thereof added to the exclusions. Language problems were also encountered, as were physical impairments (blindness or deafness) and mental retardation. Some patients refused surgery. A few reported severe multiple allergies to drugs and were excluded on that account.

This left 391 patients interviewed (Table 5.4), of which 53 were interviewed but rejected. Some of these patients who were interviewed and rejected at this stage were found to have had incomplete or absent workups. Old records were not available for evaluation prior to interview, so that in the process of patient interview other exclusion criteria were noted which were not known prior to

TABLE 5.4
Patients Interviewed

Number of patients interviewed	391
Number interviewed but rejected	53
Reasons for rejection	
Multiple allergies	14
Medical problems	13
Very apprehensive	13
Overweight	7
No relief from study drug	3
Language problem	3
Patients asked for consent	338
Patients consenting	246 (73%)
Patients not consenting	92 (27%)

interview. Such patients were therefore rejected from the study. There were various reasons for such rejections. Some patients had multiple allergies and sensitivity to drugs. Others had medical problems. Quite a few were excessively apprehensive. Problems of overweight and language were also encountered. Still others claimed no relief with one of the study drugs on the basis of previous use. These patients were interviewed and rejected but the explanation of the purpose and process in conducting the drug study were not discussed.

Two hundred and forty-six patients (73%) consented to participate in the study; 92 (27%) did not consent. There were various reasons given for refusing to consent (Table 5.5). The majority of patients about to undergo surgery develop varying degrees of anxiety and tension related to the extent of surgery and its attendant risks. For many patients the prospect of pain still remains a dreaded specter, so that relief or avoidance of pain is one of the primary concerns of patients after surgery.

A major reason for not consenting (71%) was the preference for a parenteral pain medication for fast, effective relief. The effectiveness of parenteral agents like morphine and meperidine has been assisted by the introduction of recovery room and intensive-care areas; it is now feasible for the anesthesiologist to routinely administer narcotics intravenously to achieve an immediate effect. Lowenstein et al.[23] demonstrated that surprisingly large doses of narcotic can be given intravenously to pain-free individuals without dangerous cardiopulmonary depression, but in practice, adequate analgesia from parenteral agents frequently leads to impaired respiratory function and pulmonary sequelae. Some patients cannot decide whether to participate or not. Others graciously refuse consent after a member of the family present during the interview has commented or made a subtle indication of disagreement during the interview. Others refuse without offering any reason. In another study (unpublished) which did not include a placebo in the protocol, the nonconsenters were much less common (13%), with 396 patients interviewed. Perhaps the presence of a placebo in a study may be a factor that influences nonconsenting. In another clinical trial in progress which includes a placebo, there is already a 17% nonconsenting rate among 123 patients interviewed.

Of the 338 patients ultimately interviewed in this study (which is only 4.2% of the total number of patients originally available), we thus had a group of

---

TABLE 5.5
Reasons for Not Consenting

Prefers intramuscular medication	65 (71%)
Cannot decide	10 (11%)
Study drugs not effective in past	9 (10%)
Family refuses	5 (5%)
No reason	3 (3%)
Total	92

TABLE 5.6
Reasons for Nonmedication

Consenting patient	
Not medicated	146
Data not available	12
Difference	134
Insufficient pain when oral medication allowed	47 (35%)
Oral medication not permitted then discharged day 1	35 (26%)
Oral medication not permitted days 0, 1, 2, 3	29 (22%)
Dropped from study by request of patient or surgeon	10 (7%)
Medical complications after surgery	9 (7%)
Surgery canceled	4 (3%)
Total	134

246 patients who consented to participate in the study, underwent surgery, and were followed closely up to the third postoperative day. One hundred were medicated; 146 were not. Data on 12 patients who were not medicated were not available, leaving 134 patients whose various reasons for nonmedication can be analyzed (Table 5.6). About 35% of patients were pain-free during the study hours (8:00 a.m. to 6:00 p.m.). Some patients (26%) were kept off oral intake during the immediate postoperative period and were subsequently discharged on the first postoperative day. These were usually patients who had superficial or relatively simple gynecological procedures such as an abdominal tubal ligation. Some patients (22%) were kept off oral intake more than 72 hours postoperatively, thereby going beyond the time limits set in our protocol. Some patients (7%) had medical complications after surgery and had to be taken off the study. A similar number (7%) were dropped from the study by request of the patient or the surgeon. Some had surgery canceled (3%).

IV. COMPARISON OF CONSENTERS VERSUS NONCONSENTERS

We decided to compare the 246 consenting patients and the 92 who did not consent out of the total 338 interviewed. Age, sex, social class, and anticipated pain severity after surgery were the bases for comparison. This seemed important to do in view of the need to extrapolate the results of the analgesic study. The mean age of the consenting group was 35, while the mean age of the nonconsenting group was 41, a statistically significant difference ($p < .001$). There was a slight trend to a higher percentage of women in the consenters (76.3%) than in the nonconsenters (65.4%), but this difference was not statistically significant.

TABLE 5.7
Comparison among Consenters

	Medicated (%)	Not Medicated (%)	Significance
Age	—	—	NS
Sex: female	67	83	$p = .01$
Social class (housewives excluded)	—	—	NS
Anticipated Pain Severity after Surgery			
Moderate	37	54	—
Severe	50	41	$p = .02$
Very severe	13	5	—

We coded Hollingshead's occupational categories as follows: high social class — higher executives and major professionals, proprietors of medium businesses ($35,000 to $100,000); middle social — lesser professionals to semiprofessionals and farmers ($24,000 to $35,000); and lower class — clerical and sales workers and unskilled employees. The housewife category was removed to reduce sensitivity to the difference in gender distribution. There was no significant difference between the two groups in the proportions of high, middle, and low social classes.

V. COMPARISON AMONG CONSENTERS

We then compared the 100 consenters who were medicated and the 134 consenters who were not medicated (Table 5.7). Data was not available from the other 12 consenters. There was no significant difference between the two groups in the distribution of age and social class. However, there was a significant and unexpected difference in regard to sex. More females tended not to be medicated ($p = .01$). As expected, there was a difference in the pain severity of the operation, in that a significantly greater proportion of the patients with operations deemed prior to the surgery to be more painful were medicated than was the case for the other operations. The p value of the chi-square statistic was .02.

VI. SUMMARY

Initially most exclusions are for administrative reasons such as nonavailability during times of interview due to late admissions, patients undergoing referrals to specialty clinics or being worked up by other members of the staff, which reduced the pool by almost 40% in this example. At the next stage, 86% were eliminated, almost three fourth of which were due to age and insufficient severity of pain after operations, which were the two major reasons for preliminary exclusions. Most of the rejections prior to or at interview were due to concurrent medical problems, being overweight or underweight, or having allergies or possible sensitivity to study medication.

At the consent stage, most of the patients who refused reported doing so because they preferred parenteral medication. After consenting, it was mainly administrative reasons, degree of pain, or denial of oral intake that resulted in failure to provide data. The only statistically significant difference between consenters and nonconsenters was the factor of age.

VII. CONCLUSIONS

The patients who end up in clinical trials may represent only a small percentage of the theoretical universe of available patients. Nevertheless, in this study the analysis did not suggest that extrapolation from the study sample was unjustified.

REFERENCES

1. ICH E-5 Guideline., Ethnic factors in the acceptability of foreign clinical data, 1998 (see website: http://www.ich.org).
2. Siminoff, L.A., Zhang, A., Colabiaanchi, N., Sturm, C.M., Saunders, M.A., and Shen, Q., Factors that predict the referral of breast cancer patients onto clinical trials by their surgeons and medical oncologists, *J. Clin. Oncol.*, 18, 1203–1211, 2000.
3. Mengis, C., Aebi, S., Tobler, A., Dahler, W., and Fey, M.F., Assessment of differences in patient populations selected for or excluded from participation in clinical Phase III acute myelogenous leukemia trials, *J. Clin. Oncol.*, 21, 3933–3939, 2003.
4. Sullivan, J., Subject recruitment and retention: barriers to success, *Appl. Clin. Trails*, 13, 50–54, 2004.
5. Bachenheimer, J.F., Good Recruitment Practice: working to create the bond between study and subject, *Appl. Clin. Trials*, 13, 56–59, 2004.
6. Weintraub, M. and Calimlim, J.F., Selecting patients for a clinical trial, In *Statistics in the Pharmaceutical Industry*, 2nd ed., revised and expanded, Buncher, C.R. and Tsay, J.Y., eds., Marcel Dekker, New York, pp. 117–141, 1994, chapter 6.
7. Morley, J.E., Vogel, K., and Solomon, D.H., Prevalence of geriatric articles in general medical journals, *J. Am. Geriatr. Soc.*, 38, 173–176, 1990.
8. Lung Heath Study Research Group, *Controlled Clin Trials*, 14(Suppl.), 1S–79S, 1993.
9. Hassar, M. and Weintraub, M., Uninformed consent and the healthy volunteer: An analysis of patient volunteers in a clinical trial of a new anti-inflammatory drug, *Clin. Pharmacol. Ther.*, 20, 379–386, 1976.
10. Gorringe, J.A.L., Initial preparations for clinical trials, In *Principles and Practice of Clinical Trials*, Harris, E.L. and Fitzgerald, J.D., eds., Livingston, Edinburgh, pp. 41–46, 1970.

11. Bloomfield, S.S., *Conducting the clinical drug study, Proceedings of the Institute on Drug Literature Evaluation*, American Society of Hospital Pharmacists, Washington, DC, 1969, pp. 147–154.

12. Joubert, P., Rivera-Calimlim, L., and Lasagna, L., The normal volunteer in clinical investigation; How rigid should selection criteria be? *Clin. Pharmacol. Ther.*, 17, 235–257, 1975.

13. Yahr, M.D., Duvoisin, R.C., Schear, M.J., Barrett, R.E., and Hoehn, M.M., The treatment of Parkinson's disease with levodopa, *Arch. Neurol.*, 21, 343–354, 1969.

14. Taves, D.R., Minimization: A new method for assigning patients to treatment and control groups, *Clin. Pharmacol. Ther.*, 15, 443–453, 1974.

15. Weintraub, M., *Capricious compliance and intelligent noncompliance, Patient Compliance*, Vol. 10, Lasagna, L., ed., pp. 39–47, 1976.

16. Hassar, M., Pocelinko, R., Weintraub, M., Nelson, D., Thomas, G., and Lasagna, L., The free-living volunteer's motivation and attitudes toward pharmacologic studies, *Clin. Pharmacol. Ther.*, 21, 515–519, 1977.

17. Miller, R. and Willner, H.S., The two part consent form: A suggestion for promoting free and informed consent, *N. Engl. J. Med.*, 290, 964–966, 1974.

18. Fleiss, J.L., *The Design and Analysis of Clinical Experiments*, Wiley, New York, 1986.

19. Dollery, C.T., Problems in clinical trials, *Adv. Sci.*, 23, 508–511, 1967.

20. Murphee, H.B., Methodology for the clinical evaluation of analgesics, *J. New Drugs*, 15, 15–22, 1966.

21. Mainland, D., The clinical trial: Some difficulties and suggestions, *J. Chron. Dis.*, 11, 484–496, 1960.

22. Calimlim, J.F., Wardell, W.M., Lasagna, L., and Gillies, A.J., Analgesic efficacy of an orally administered combination of pentazocine and aspirin, with observations on the use and statistical efficiency of global subjective efficacy ratings, *Clin. Pharmacol. Ther.*, 21, 34–43, 1977.

23. Lowenstein, E., Hallowell, P., Levine, E.H., Daggett, W.M., Austen, W.G., and Lauer, M.B., Cardiovascular response to large doses of intravenous morphine in man, *N. Engl. J. Med.*, 281, 1389 1969.

24. Hindin, T.J., From the Editor — You say potato I say potatah: let's sort the whole thing out, *Appl. Clin. Trials*, 13, 12 2004.

6 Statistical Aspects of Cancer Clinical Trials*

T. Timothy Chen

CONTENTS

I. CANCER TREATMENT PROGRESS

In the 1930s, less than 20% of cancer patients were alive 5 years after diagnosis. In the 1940s, the figure was about 25%, and in the 1960s it was about 33%. Today about 40% of cancer patients will be alive 5 years after diagnosis. If we compared with a similar control population, then the 5 year relative survival rate was 48.9% for patients diagnosed in 1974–1976 and 49.8% for patients diagnosed during the period 1980–1985.[1] In the past three decades, good progress in treating cancer has been made in acute lymphocytic leukemia in children, Hodgkin's disease, Burkitt's lymphoma, Ewing's sarcoma, Wilms' tumor, rhabdomyosarcoma, choriocarcinoma, testicular cancer, ovarian cancer and osteogenic

---

* This work has been produced by the author in his capacity as a Federal Government employee, as part of his official duty, and hence this work is in the public domain and is not subject to copyright.

sarcoma. However, for other common cancers, effective treatments have not been found.

Debates about whether we had really made progress in fighting against cancer since the passage of the National Cancer Act in 1971 were kindled several years ago.[2] The observation that the proportion of deaths from cancer has increased progressively in the last 60 years has led to the conclusion that we are losing the fight against cancer. The progress against cancer is demonstrated clearly from examination of cohorts of men and women between 20 and 44 years of age.[3] As a result of debates, several measures of progress against cancer were examined and many recommendations about the modification or expansion of the current information base were made.[4]

More than 60 anticancer drugs have received FDA approval for marketing in the United States. More than 40 of these had their INDs (Investigational New Drug Application) sponsored by the National Cancer Institute. Currently, nearly 100 new drugs and 70 new biologics are under active clinical investigation.

New improved methods of treating cancer are being actively pursued in all types of cancer. To establish the effectiveness of a new treatment, appropriate clinical trials have to be carried out. Statistical methods are used in design, conduct, analysis, and reporting to ensure the validity and efficiency of cancer clinical trials.

II. BENEFIT TO RISK RATIO

Because an antineoplastic drug usually produces toxicity to normal cells as well as killing cancer cells, we always have to consider the efficacy and toxicity together in obtaining a favorable benefit to risk ratio in cancer treatment. In other words, an oncologist would want to make sure that the new drug can produce a net benefit when compared with no treatment or current standard treatment. The net benefit can result from a large improvement in efficacy with a small worsening in toxicity or from a large reduction in toxicity with a small decrease in efficacy. The ideal situation will be both an improvement in efficacy and a decrease in toxicity. Of course, how much the improvement in efficacy can balance out the harm of increasing toxicity is usually subjective and ambiguous.

When determining efficacy, the decision can be framed as accepting a treatment if it is good, or rejecting a treatment when it is not good. There are two types of error in this decision framework. The false negative error (Type I) is the error of misclassifying a good treatment as not good. The false positive error (Type II) is the error of misclassifying a bad or not so good treatment as good. There are costs or consequences associated with these two kinds of error. Usually in early clinical trials of a drug, we will tolerate a larger false positive error rather than a large false negative error.

In the process of developing a new treatment, the type and stage of cancer and the usefulness of the current standard treatment have to be considered in the estimation of the net benefit and the decision of whether to accept a new treatment.[5,6] Suppose the current treatment is not very effective for a certain type and stage of cancer, then the risk of using another ineffective drug is not so relatively high. In this situation, patients are willing to accept a larger false positive error or a larger variation for the estimation of net benefit. This kind of situation can be found in chronic lymphocytic leukemia in blast crisis, metastatic renal cell or germ cell cancer, Hodgkin's disease refractory to MOPP/ABVD, postmenopausal hormone refractory metastatic breast cancer, or advanced stage lung cancer. Some AIDS clinical trials are in this class.[7]

In other types and stages of cancer (e.g., previously untreated testicular cancer and Hodgkin's disease) the current treatment is very effective. Therefore, estimation of net benefit of the new treatment should have a higher precision, both false positive and false negative errors should be very small, and the new treatment should be compared with the current standard through a randomized controlled clinical trial.

In the above discussion, the risks of false positive and false negative errors are determined relatively according to the disease. This is reasonable from the treatment decision point of view. But from the perspective of scientific progress, the magnitude of errors should be small. Some large scale postmarketing studies could fulfill this purpose.

III. TRIAL ENDPOINTS

In cancer clinical trials, the efficacy endpoints include overall survival, quality of life, complete and partial response rate and duration, and time to progression. Overall survival is measured from the date of registration or randomization to the date of death or last follow-up. In the latter case, the observation is censored because the patient is still alive. Quality of life consists of many components including disease related symptoms and can be measured through a validated psychosocial instrument.[8,9] Complete response denotes the total disappearance of tumor lesions under clinical and diagnostic staging. The duration complete response is measured only for complete responders from the date of response to the date of relapse or last check-up. In the latter case, the observation is censored because the patients is still in remission. Time to progression is measured for all eligible patients from the date of registration or randomization to the date of relapse (for responders) or the date of progression (for nonresponders) or the date of death (before relapse or progression). In early stage cancer after complete surgical removal of cancer (adjuvant setting), time to progression is called disease-free survival, which is the time from study entry to relapse or death, with patients alive without relapse considered as censored.

The toxicity endpoints include the following major categories: blood or bone marrow toxicity, clinical, clinical hemorrhage, infection, gastrointestinal, liver, kidney, bladder, alopecia, pulmonary, heart, blood pressure, neurologic, skin, allergy, fever, metabolic, and coagulation. Within each major category, there are subcategories. For each subcategory, the grade of toxicity ranges from 0 to 4. Grade 0 means none or normal; grade 4 is life-threatening.[10]

In recent years many hematopoietic growth factors have been tested in cancer patients. The usefulness of these agents is measured by shortened duration of neutropenia or hospitalization, reduced episodes of febrile neutropenia, or delivery of more intensive chemotherapy. Other chemoprotectors are used to reduce incidence of nephrotoxicity and ototoxicity.

IV. PHASE I CLINICAL TRIAL

Drugs for treating cancer have to demonstrate effectiveness in tumor cell lines before actual testing in humans. The initial clinical evaluation of a new drug, biologic, or radiotherapy technique is called a Phase I trial, which evaluates dose, schedule, toxicity, pharmacology, and early evidence of clinical activity. The goal of a phase I trail is to arrive at a recommended dose with the minimum number of patients receiving either biologically inactive or toxic doses.

The patients selected for Phase I clinical trials are in those categories of cancer with no effective treatment at present. Patients should have good performance status and normal organ function. Hopefully, they might receive some benefit in using the investigative agent. The purpose of doing a Phase I trial is to find a dose that will cause dose-limiting toxicity in acceptable percentages of patients under a given method of administration for a fixed number of cycles.

The dose-limiting toxicity is usually defined as any grade 3 or 4 toxicity. The maximum tolerated dose (MTD) is usually defined as the dose that produces dose-limiting toxicity in 30% of patients. Many cytotoxic agents are observed to have a steep dose–response relation; therefore, the MTD estimated in a Phase I study will be the dose used in Phase II trials. Because a Phase I trial is a preliminary step for a Phase II trial, the requirement of statistical precision of dose determination is not high. Usually the dose can be further fine-tuned in a Phase II trial. The MTD is usually not disease-site specific. In general, pediatric patients have a different MTD from that of adults.

The usual starting dose in humans is one-tenth of the $MELD_{10}$ (mouse equivalent of the LD_{10}, dose with 10% drug-induced deaths) in mg/m^2 of body surface area, unless that dose is toxic in any species tested. The doses of drugs for human testing are usually selected by modified Fibonacci method. The second dose level is twice the starting dose. The third dose level is 167% of the second, the fourth dose level is 150% of the third, the fifth dose level is 140% of the fourth, and each subsequent dose level is 133% of the preceding dose.[11]

Because it is possible that the starting dose could be far away from the MTD and many patients will be exposed to a subtherapeutic dose, a pharmacokinetically guided dose selection scheme was proposed.[12] This approach builds upon a pharmacodynamic hypothesis that similar biological effects (e.g., toxicity) would happen at similar plasma levels in mice and man. For many agents, the area under the curve for plasma concentration versus time ($C \times T$) of the MTD for humans is found to be fairly close to the $C \times T$ for mice at the LD_{10} if calculated in mg/m^2 equivalents ($MELD_{10}$). Therefore, $C \times T$ of $MELD_{10}$ is considered as an upper limit, and the ratio F of $C \times T$ (MELD$_{10}$) to $C \times T$ (starting dose in men) is used to guide dose selection. One method takes the second dose as $\sqrt{F}$ times the starting dose, and the third dose is twice the second dose, then follows the modified Fibonacci scheme. The other method continues to double the dose until $0.4F$ times the starting dose is exceeded and then the modified Fibonacci scheme is followed. Another use of preclinical toxicological information is in choosing a higher entry dose than one-tenth of MELD$_{10}$. All these methods have a potential of reducing overall completion times by 25%.[12]

Drugs with high schedule-dependency in preclinical models will use the existing optimal schedule. For drugs without particular schedule dependency, two extremes of schedules (e.g., single bolus dose per course and 5-day continuous infusion) are generally examined.[10]

The usual dose-finding is carried out through a dose-escalation and de-escalation procedure. (1) Three new patients are studied at a dose level at the first stage. (2) If none experience dose-limiting toxicity, then the next higher dose is used for the subsequent group of three patients. (3) If two or more experience dose-limiting toxicity, then the MTD has been exceeded and three more patients are treated at the next lower dose (if only three patients were treated previously at this dose). (4) If 1/3 experiences dose-limiting toxicity at the current dose, then three more patients are accrued at the same dose at the second stage. If none of these three experiences dose-limiting toxicity, then the dose is escalated. Otherwise the MTD has been exceeded and three more patients are treated at the next lower dose (if only three patients were treated previously). (5) The MTD is the dose level where 0/6 or 1/6 experience dose-limiting toxicity with the next higher dose having at least 2/3 or 2/6 experience dose-limiting toxicity.

In the above procedure, we require new patients at each dose level. Sometimes at very low doses, we could re-enter a patient at a higher dose level and include this patient in the analyses of both dose levels. For higher doses, this kind of intrapatient escalation of doses could confound the result because of possible cumulative toxicity. The toxicity that occurs to these re-entered patients could either be caused by the higher second dose or the cumulated total dose. Therefore, if intrapatient escalation is used in high doses, then the patient is only included in the analysis of the first dose level.

Storer[13] proposed other single- and two-stage designs and the methods of estimating MTD. The different designs were compared through computer simulation by assuming logistic dose–toxicity curves. The results indicated that there is little difference among the two-stage designs because of the small sample sizes.

A Phase I study usually has a pharmacokinetic component to understand the absorption, distribution, metabolism, and excretion of the drug in humans. If the variation of pharmacokinetic behavior is too large for a drug among the patient population, then some kind of adaptive dosing can be used to control a patient's plasma concentration within a desirable range.[14] This approach has the potential of maximizing response and minimizing toxicity. Its usefulness is under investigation.

V. PHASE II CLINICAL TRIAL

After a MTD is determined, the drug at that dose and schedule is carried forward to get a better estimate of antitumor activity in a Phase II trial that will evaluate drug, biologic, or radiotherapy techniques in single modality or combined modality regimens. The definition of a Phase II trial in cancer clinical trials is different from that of a Phase II clinical study defined by the FDA in drug development. The Phase II cancer clinical trial usually requires fewer than 100 patients, whereas FDA Phase II trials require several hundred patients.[5]

From past experience, efficacy of a drug is disease-site specific; therefore, a Phase II trial is limited to a specific type of cancer. The kind of cancer to be tested is determined through preclinical animal data and the data collected in the Phase I clinical trials. Patients should have good performance status and normal organ function.

Because cancer drugs can be cross-resistant — that is, a drug can be less effective as a second-line treatment than as a first-line treatment — a new drug should be preferably used as a first-line treatment. The phenomenon of cross-resistance is caused by similar drug actions; when some tumor cells are refractory to a certain drug, they are going to be resistant to a similar-action drug. Therefore, a Phase II trial is preferably done in patients who have not been previously treated if there is no effective treatment at the present for this particular type of cancer. If we use previously treated patients, the efficacy could be low, and we cannot differentiate it from background noise.

For certain categories of cancer at early stages, there are some very effective treatments. A Phase II trial will usually be first done in patients with the late stage of these kinds of cancer where the existing treatment is not so effective and then later in patients with the early stage cancer. A phase II trial should not diminish a window of opportunity for patients to get effective treatment.[15]

The response variable for a Phase II trial is usually tumor response rather than survival; the tumor response can be determined in the first few months of treatment and it usually has good correlation with survival within a specific type of cancer. In order to obtain precise evaluation of response, the patients should have measurable disease that can be measured through diagnostic tools.

For solid tumors, response includes both complete and partial response. For leukemia, the response includes only complete remission because it is known that only complete remission is related to long-term survival.[16] In order to qualify as a response, the tumor reduction should be long-lasting, usually one month.

The design of a Phase II trial is based on one-sample binomial statistics with the probability of success being the probability of achieving a response. From the current treatment results, both desirable and undesirable response rates are specified. We would like to reject the drug as not promising if it is unlikely that it has the desirable response rate (the false negative error is small), and to accept a drug as promising if it is unlikely that it has the undesirable response rate (the false positive error is small). Because we prefer not to miss any promising drug, the false negative error should not be greater than the false positive error.

The trial is carried out in two stages[17] so that if a drug is not promising, the trial can be terminated early at the end of the first stage. This two-stage design and other multistage designs[18] are examples of a broad class of drug screening procedures.[19] This approach to Phase II trials is identical to sampling inspection in the industrial quality control setting.

For example, a Phase II trial for a new agent in nonsmall cell lung cancer can have the following two-stage design. For the first stage, 12 patients are enrolled. If there is no response (complete or partial) in these 12 patients, then the study is terminated and the agent is rejected. If there is at least one response, then 25 more patients are enrolled in the second stage. If there are less than four responses in 37 patients, then the agent is rejected; otherwise, the new agent will be deemed promising. This design is based on the current treatment result for nonsmall cell lung cancer; the response rate of 20% is desirable and 5% is undesirable. The false negative and positive rates are limited to 0.10. This design has the minimum expected sample size (23.5) when the agent has a response rate of 5%.[17]

Phase II trials usually are repeated in at least two different centers. Response rates from two trials could be different because of several reasons: patient selection, different evaluation and response criteria, intra- and inter-evaluator variability or bias, and protocol compliance. Whether a drug will enter into a Phase III trial depends not only on the tumor response observed in Phase II trials, but also on its toxicity, dose–response relationship, and cross-resistance with other active agents.

In the situation where there is more than one new agent, a randomized Phase II trial can be carried out. The sample size used here is about the size of a usual Phase II trial and the comparison will not be as precise as a Phase III trial. The advantage of a randomized Phase II trial is that the results for the several new agents can be compared within the same patient population and protocol procedure.

VI. PHASE III CLINICAL TRIAL

A. GENERAL CONSIDERATION

After a drug or treatment regimen has been shown to have promising antitumor activity, it may progress forward to a Phase III trial. A Phase III trial compares the experimental treatment(s) with a standard control treatment. The purpose of a Phase III trial is to demonstrate that the new treatment is either better than or equivalent to the standard control. The response variable for a Phase III trial is usually the overall survival or the quality of life.

Sometimes instead of concurrent control, historical control data are used in comparison. The validity and usefulness of this approach is very limited.[20] The historical controls have to be the patients treated in the same institution in the past few years with the same enrollment criteria and evaluation procedure. The baseline comparability of historical control patients and current patients can never be demonstrated beyond reasonable doubt. The usefulness of statistical adjustment is based on the validity of the model assumptions and the inclusion of all major prognostic variables.

In a Phase III cancer clinical trial protocol, the purposes of the trial have to be very clearly defined. For each stated purpose, the data collection procedure should be thought through and described in the protocol. The statistical techniques of analyzing these data need to be planned and stated in the statistical consideration section of the protocol.

The data collected should be valid and reliable. To be certain about its validity and reliability, unequivocal documentation must be provided. Overall survival is very reliable if every patient is followed until death. The response, progression, and relapse status are less reliable because of the limitation of diagnostic techniques or clinical evaluation. To ensure that these data are reliable, a uniform and unbiased follow-up, standardized supportive care, secondary treatment, and method of evaluation for all treatment groups are very important.

Treatment regimens need to be defined specifically. For chemotherapy, the dose, schedule, route of administration, and dose modification because of toxicity have to be described clearly. For radiotherapy, the dose, schedule, and field size should be similarly specified. For surgery, the incision margin and number of nodes to be sampled need to be specified. The quality of treatment delivered should be monitored very closely to maintain the protocol compliance. The purpose of doing quality control is two-fold: to ensure that patients get optimal treatment and to minimize variation in the treatment outcome.

The eligibility criteria of patients must be determined very carefully. Here we need to strike a balance between more and less stringent criteria. Usually good performance status and normal liver and kidney function patients can show maximal difference between the treatments in a trial. However, limiting the patient eligibility also limits the applicability of the trial result. Therefore, it usually is better to enroll all the patients who could benefit from the treatment and are healthy enough to receive the treatment.

Case report forms including prestudy, flow sheet, pathology, surgery, and radiotherapy should be designed with extra care so that only necessary and useful information is collected. If too much information is required, then the quality of data will deteriorate.

B. RANDOMIZATION

In a Phase III trial, a randomized trial will provide the best design.[21] The purpose of randomization is two-fold: (1) randomization will provide a theoretical foundation for the validity of the statistical analysis of the trial data; and (2) randomization will render the treatment groups comparable regarding unknown and known prognostic factors, and also reduce the bias in assigning patients to treatments. The actual process of randomization is usually done through a centralized statistical office.

The randomization scheme is usually not unrestricted randomization, but the sample sizes of the treatments are constrained to be equal. More desirable is block randomization with a block size of four to eight patients with blocks nested within each clinical center. With each block there is equal assignment of patients to each treatment. The purpose of doing this is to ensure that the final numbers of patients on the treatments are almost equal. The information about block size should not be revealed to avoid bias in the enrollment of patients.

The time of randomization should take place as close as possible to the time of beginning different treatments.[22] For example, the protocol can have the same induction regimen, but two different intensification regimens. The patients should be registered twice: once before induction, the second time for randomization before intensification. This approach will minimize the possible bias in the eligibility determination for intensification and control the variability of number of patients on the two intensification arms. The statistical analysis to compare the two intensification arms can be restricted to those patients who were randomized.

C. STRATIFICATION

Usually some important prognostic factors can be identified before a trial. In this case, it is advisable to stratify patients by these prognostic factors, and then randomize within each stratum. The purpose of stratification is two-fold: (1) to make the result of the study more convincing, and (2) to increase the efficiency of statistical analysis.

Peto et al.[23] stated that stratified randomization is not necessary for a large trial because the probability is high that the balance among important prognostic factors can be achieved by unrestricted randomization. However, a stratified randomization is similar to an insurance policy to insure against the unlikely event of unbalanced distribution of patients among the important prognostic factors. If this event happens, an adjusted analysis may not alleviate the doubt because the statistical adjustment usually depends on model assumptions.

If one wants to balance patient assignment on many prognostic factors, some kind of dynamic allocation scheme can be considered.[24] For a multicenter clinical trial, it is always desirable to balance treatments at each institution because there is usually an institutional effect on the trial outcome.[25]

D. SIZE OF THE TRIAL

The size of a trial depends on the degree of precision we would like to have about the estimate of the treatment difference. This is related to the width of the confidence interval for the treatment difference, or to the Type I and Type II errors of differentiating two hypotheses for possible values of the treatment difference. In a clinical trial, the sample size determination is usually done through the latter approach because the two types of error are usually not equally serious, and therefore not symmetric. However, there is a natural connection between the confidence interval approach and the hypothesis testing approach. In the analysis and report of the study, a confidence interval will provide more information than just a p-value. A p-value is the result of comparison of the observed difference with only one value of the hypothetical difference. A confidence interval or a standard error of the observed difference provides information about the whole range of values of the hypothetical difference. If the main variable is the overall survival, then the difference between treatments can be formulated in terms of the hazard ratio. If the main variable is the tumor response, then the difference between treatments can be formulated in terms of the odds ratio. If the main variable is a normal, continuous one, then the difference between two treatments is just the mean difference.

If the purpose of the trial is to show that a new treatment T_1 is better than the standard control treatment T_0, then we specify as the null hypothesis that the two treatments are the same, and try to use data to reject this null hypothesis. Because the likelihood of observing a treatment advance is not great (according to the past history of cancer clinical research), we want to control the Type I error α, which is the probability of rejecting the null hypothesis when it is true. The Type I error is specified as 0.05. We also specify an alternative hypothesis, which says the difference between the two treatments is a certain amount. We would like to control the Type II error β, which is the probability of not rejecting the null hypothesis when the alternative hypothesis is true. The Type II error is usually specified between 0.1 and 0.2 (i.e., the power is between 0.9 and 0.8). We usually specify the treatment difference in the alternative as a clinically meaningful difference, or the minimum difference we would like to detect. This value is usually subjectively obtained and usually is a compromise between what is really important and what can be done. If this value is too large then the study will not have enough power to detect a smaller difference.

For a one-sided alternative and normally distributed data, assuming that the variance of both treatments are the same, the formula to obtain the required number of patients for each treatment is $n = 2\tau^2/\delta^2$ where $\tau = (z_{1-\alpha}) + (Z_{1-\beta})$ and $\delta = (\mu_1 - \mu_0)/\sigma$. The z_P is the value of the normal deviate corresponding to the P point of the cumulative standard normal distribution. The value δ is the difference in means divided by the standard deviation. The value of τ is determined by the Type I and Type II errors. For a two-sided alternative, α should be replaced by $\alpha/2$. Note that the total sample size required for the trial is $4\tau^2/\delta^2$.

For binomial response data, the formula for n is similar with $\delta = 2(\arcsin\sqrt{p_1} - \arcsin\sqrt{p_0})$. The arcsine transformation of the square root of the observed proportion stabilized the standard deviation as $1/2\sqrt{n}$. A more accurate formula for the sample size to compare two binomials has been published.[26]

For the survival data, the formula for n is again similar with $\delta = \ln(\lambda_0/\lambda_1)\sqrt{2}/\sqrt{(1/p_1 + 1/p_0)}$. Here we make the assumption that the distribution of the survival data is exponential with hazard rates λ_0 and λ_1, and p_i $(i = 0, 1)$ is the proportion of actual events (deaths) for the ith treatment at the time of data analysis. This expected proportion of events p_i is a function of total accrual time (M), the further follow-up time (L) after the termination of accrual, and the hazard rate λ_i. Assuming a Poisson patient arrival over M, and all patients are observed till the end of the further follow-up time L, then p_i is

$$1 - \frac{\exp(-\lambda_i M)\exp(-\lambda_i L)(\exp \lambda_i M - 1)}{\lambda_i M} \tag{6.1}$$

The reason that δ is more complicated is because the sufficient statistic is the number of events and not the number of total enrollments for exponential data with censoring. The formula for n can be rewritten as

$$\frac{\tau^2}{(\ln(\lambda_0/\lambda_1))^2} = \frac{n p_0 p_1}{p_0 + p_1} \tag{6.2}$$

In the design of a Phase III trial comparing overall survival, an appropriate follow-up period should be allowed after the closure of enrollment so that the number of expected events under the alternative hypothesis will be np_0 and np_1 at the time of the final analysis.[27,28]

If the follow-up period is long enough, then p_0 is very close to p_1. The right hand side of the above formula would be very close to one-fourth of the total number of events in the trial. The total number of events in the trial is $4\tau^2/(\ln(\lambda_0/\lambda_1))^2$. If α (one-sided) is 0.025, β is 0.2, and the alternative of $1.5\lambda_1 = \lambda_0$ (a 50% improvement in median time to event) is to be detected, then the total number of events in the trial should be 192. If the follow-up period is not long enough, and p_0 is not close to p_1, then the total number of events should be greater, but not more than 110% of $4\tau^2/(\ln(\lambda_0/\lambda_1))^2$. For example, in a Phase III trial of stage IIIA and IIIB inoperable nonsmall cell lung cancer with vinblastine and cisplatinum followed by radiation therapy as the control, the experimental treatment could be vinblastine and cisplatinum followed by radiation therapy with concurrent carboplatin. If the accrual rate is 6.2 patients per month, and the control arm has a median survival of 15.5 months, then the study design should have an accrual period of 3.5 years (260 patients) and a follow-up period of 1.5 years in order to have 208 as the total number of events in the trial at the end of 5 years.

If the purpose of a Phase III trial is to show that the new treatment is equivalent to the standard control, then we have to define the term "equivalency." Some will define equivalence as within 10% of the control mean or an odds or hazard ratio between 0.9 and 1.1. Because the observed difference has variation, the definition will further require that the 95% confidence interval for mean ratio, odds ratio, or hazard ratio must be within the interval of 0.9 and 1.1. This kind of requirement is very stringent. If the true ratio is close to either 0.9 or 1.1, then the sample size would have to be very large to have the 95% confidence interval within the interval of (0.9, 1.1). Therefore, an equivalency trial usually requires more patients than a trial to prove superiority.

Sometimes a new treatment has less toxicity than the standard control and we are willing to "accept" the new treatment if it is not more than 10% inferior in efficacy. This kind of trial is also called an equivalency trial but it is different from the trial described in the previous paragraph. Here we only require that the lower limit of the confidence interval be greater than 0.9 and we set no bound for the upper limit. Again, the sample size will depend on how close the true efficacy ratio is to the value of 0.9. If we are willing to carry more risk, then the sample size will not be as large as the true equivalency trial in the previous paragraph. This trial is very similar to a superiority trial except the null value is shifted from 1 to 0.9.[29] To obtain a size for this kind of equivalency trial, one usually takes 0.9 as the null value and as the alternative value, the Type I error associated with the null value at 5% and the Type II error can be between 5 and 20%. This kind of design can be interpreted as a test that places a greater burden upon a new treatment to prove it is not more than 10% inferior in efficacy.

The expected accrual rate should be considered in the design. If a trial takes more than 4 years to complete, then the treatments being compared could become obsolete as the trial progresses and the investigator could lose interest in enrolling patients. Therefore, a Phase III trial is usually done by a cooperative oncology group. Sometimes for a rare cancer, the trial is done through an intergroup mechanism that pools several oncology groups together. This kind of pooling of resources makes sure that the trial can be finished in a reasonable amount of time. During the progress of the trial, accrual rate should be monitored to ensure it is not too far from the expected rate.

To compare survival or disease-free survival for two treatments, sometimes the comparison is done in terms of proportion of patients without event (survived, or survived and free of disease) at a specified time. If the sample size is calculated for comparison of two proportions, it is larger than that for the comparison of two exponential curves.[30] Because the final test is usually a logrank test that compares the entire survival curves, the latter sample size is preferable unless the exponentiality assumption is grossly untrue.

If patient compliance or loss to follow-up could become major problems in the conduct of a trial, an allowance should be provided in the sample size calculation.[31] The sample size requirement based on the logrank statistic without the exponentiality assumption has been derived under very general conditions that include cure rate models.[32,33]

E. DATA ANALYSIS

Because randomization provides a theoretical basis to carry out statistical analysis, the analysis of the trial should include all the randomized patients. However, some ineligible patients could also get randomized by mistake. If they do not belong to the patient population for which the treatments question is being asked, they can be excluded from the analysis. In rare instance, patients may cancel their registration before the treatment begins and are not included in the analysis. Other than these, all patients should be included in the analysis. This approach is called "intent-to-treat" analysis because we intend to treat all eligible patients according to the randomly assigned treatments. Those patients who do not comply with the protocol are called inevaluable patients; they are included in the intent-to-treat analysis in the groups into which they were randomized.

Because strict adherence to the protocol treatment is not easy when it is used in everyday practice, and we would like to find out in a Phase III trial what would happen if we used the treatments in a general patient population, doing intent-to-treat analysis will provide an answer close to the general practice. Also treatment could affect early death and early dropout and compliance; therefore, excluding these inevaluable patients in the analysis will not provide a fair comparison of the total treatment effect. Including all randomized eligible patients also minimizes the possibility of biased exclusion because cancer trials usually cannot be blinded to the patients or to the investigators. Of course, if there is no bias involved, then the analysis excluding inevaluable patients could provide additional useful information.

There has been tremendous development in the statistical methods for censored survival data since 1960. For the estimation of survival distribution, the product-limit estimator[34] is widely used in clinical trials whereas the life table method is mostly used in epidemiology.[35,36]

For comparing two treatments, one method used was an extension of the Wilcoxon rank statistics.[37,38] Later, another method used treated data as a series of 2 × 2 tables, as an extension of the Mantel–Haenszel test, and is now called the logrank test.[39,40] Both methods were shown to be in a class of weighted-sum statistics.[41,42] The logrank test has the benefit of being easily extended to cover the stratified analysis, and hence has been used extensively in the meta-analysis of cancer clinical trials.[43] The logrank statistic and its variance estimate can be used to calculate the hazard ratio estimate and its standard error.[44]

In analysis, the data of the major endpoints should be analyzed both unadjusted and adjusted by the stratifying factors. The adjusted analyses can be carried out through stratified analyses[39,45] or a regression model.[46–48] If a prognostic factor is ordinal or numerical, and the relationship between the response and the prognostic factor can be approximated by the regression model, the regression approach will provide a better test for the treatment effect.

If there is a statistically significant difference between the treatments, then it is appropriate to show that there is no qualitative interaction between treatments and known prognostic factors. This can be tested by a statistical procedure[49] and by a tabulation of means or medians of the major endpoints by treatments within patient subgroup.[50] This kind of tabulation to show there is no qualitative interaction will provide more credence for the conclusion. If there is no statistically significant difference between the treatments in the overall analysis, then subset analysis should not be done. Any intended subset analysis should be prespecified in the protocol and the sample size should be adequate within the subset. Any unprespecified subset analysis can only be used as hypothesis generating and any finding should be confirmed by another trial.

There is some controversy about using a one- or two-sided test. However, after using a two-sided test in a clinical trial, if we reject the null hypothesis of no differences, we will usually conclude that the new treatment is better than the control or the new treatment is worse than the control. Because we will not just conclude they are different, one-sided p-values are more relevant if we use the p-value as a strength of evidence to support our conclusion. Therefore, in order to be consistent in drawing conclusions after either a one-sided or two-sided test, a one-sided p-value of 0.025 should be seen as providing strong evidence.

Sometimes a better survival for responders than the survival for non-responders is used to argue for the efficacy of a new treatment in an uncontrolled single arm trial. This argument is not valid for two reasons.[51] First, the better survival for the responders could be from favorable prognostic status and not treatment. Second, the responders have to survive long enough to get a response. A randomized controlled trial is almost always needed to demonstrate the efficacy of a new agent beyond any reasonable doubt.

F. INTERIM ANALYSES

In the progress of a cancer clinical trial, if a new treatment has shown its superiority early, then a proper procedure should be in place to terminate the trial so that more patients will get the new effective treatment. Similarly, if the new treatment is worse than the standard control, the trial should be terminated early so that fewer patients will be exposed to the ineffective new treatment. However, if the interim analyses are carried out many times at the 5% significance level, the overall significance level is much larger than 5%.[52] Because the false positive result is quite common, interim analysis has to be carried out carefully so that the overall significance level (Type I error) stays at 5% (see Chapter 14).

For a large Phase III trial, the data monitoring procedure and stopping rule should be specified in the protocol and a data monitoring committee should convene periodically to decide whether to terminate the trial early. The members of this committee are privy to see the unblinded interim analysis results, whereas in semiannual oncology group meetings the reporting of interim analysis is blinded and the overall survival and toxicity results are usually pooled across treatments. The purpose of blinding the interim results is to safeguard the progress of the trial.

In doing interim analyses one controls the probability of making a wrong conclusion (Type I error) at 5% if the treatments are equally efficacious. Because the wrong conclusion can be reached at any interim analysis, the sum of (spending) probabilities of making wrong conclusions should total 5%. Lan and DeMets[53] proposed several use functions to spend this 5% in the process of the trial. Once a use function is specified as a function of the information fraction accrued in a trial, interim analysis can be carried out at any time with incremental error probability determined from the use function.

Originally, interim analyses were proposed to be carried out at fixed time intervals with an equal number of events (information time) in each interval. Pocock[54] proposed a procedure that uses the same critical value for each interim standardized test statistic. O'Brien and Fleming[55] proposed a procedure that uses different critical values for each interim standardized test statistic and that these critical values are inversely proportional to the square root of the number of events. This procedure is more conservative in the early looks; therefore, the power is reduced very little as compared with a fixed size trial. Because many cancer trials are analyzed before the semiannual oncology group meeting, it was shown that both procedures for repeated logrank analyses are quite robust if carried out at equal intervals of calendar time rather than information time.[56] Pocock[57] showed that there is not much gain in efficiency or ethical benefit in doing more than five interim analyses.

Because any testing procedure can be converted into a confidence interval, interim tests can be converted into repeated confidence intervals.[58] The width of the interval is z_P times the standard error of the observed treatment efficacy ratio where z_p is the critical value for the interim standardized test statistic. The repeated confidence intervals can be used for early decisions about any prespecified treatment efficacy ratio, not just the value of one.

Because the interim analysis is making an inference with incomplete data, the assumption of uninformative censoring is a critical one. Using early results to predict the long-term outcome, we assume that the early trend will continue. It is prudent to have sufficient follow-up before terminating a trial. A subsequent analysis for the long-term result is appropriate in many cases.

Sometimes early termination is carried out to conserve patient resources when the two treatments are quite similar. Lan et al.[59] proposed a stochastic curtailing procedure to terminate a trial in this situation. They compute a conditional probability of not rejecting the null hypothesis given the current observed data and the alternative hypothesis is true. If this probability is very high, then the trial can be terminated. The complement of this procedure can be used to terminate a trial when the two treatments are very different; however, it is more conservative than the group sequential approach.

VII. TRIAL REPORT

After the data set is analyzed, a paper should be written for peer review. Some guidelines have been suggested for writing up a report.[60] The following has been proposed by Simon and Wittes[61]

1. The paper should discuss briefly the quality control methods used to ensure that the data are complete and accurate. A reliable procedure should be cited for ensuring that all patients entered in the study are actually reported upon. If no such procedures are in place, their absence should be noted. Any procedures employed to ensure that assessment of major endpoints is reliable should be mentioned (e.g., second-party review of response) or their absence noted.

2. All patients registered in the study should be accounted for. The report should specify for each treatment the number of patients who were not eligible, died, or withdrew before treatment began. The distribution of follow-up times should be described for each treatment, and the number of patients lost to follow-up should be given.

3. The study should not have an inevaluability rate greater than 15% for major endpoints from early death, protocol violation, and missing information. Not more than 15% of eligible patients should be lost to follow-up.

4. In randomized studies, the report should include a comparison of survival and/or other major endpoints for all eligible patients as randomized, that is, with no exclusions other than those not meeting eligibility criteria.

5. The sample size should be sufficient to either establish or conclusively rule out the existence of effects of clinically meaningful magnitude. For "negative" results in therapeutic comparisons, the adequacy of sample size should be demonstrated by either presenting a confidence interval for the true treatment difference or calculating the statistical power for detecting differences. For uncontrolled Phase II studies, a procedure should be in place to prevent the accrual of an inappropriately large number of patients when the study has shown the agent to be inactive.

6. Authors should state whether there was an initial target sample size and, if so, what it was. They should specify how frequently interim analyses were performed and how the decisions to stop accrual and report results were arrived at.

7. All claims of therapeutic efficacy should be based upon explicit comparisons with a specific control group, except in the special circumstances where each patient is his/her own control. If nonrandomized controls are used, the characteristics of the patients should be presented in detail and compared with those of the experimental group. Potential sources of bias should be adequately discussed. Comparison of survival between responders and non-responders does not establish efficacy and should not be included. Reports of Phase II trials that draw conclusions about antitumor activity but not therapeutic efficacy do not require a control group.

8. The patients studied should be adequately described. Applicability of conclusions to other patients should be carefully dealt with. Claims of subset-specific treatment differences must be carefully documented statistically as more than the random results of multiple-subset analyses.

9. The methods of statistical analysis should be described in sufficient detail that a knowledgeable reader could reproduce the analysis if the data were available.

ACKNOWLEDGMENTS

The author would like to thank Drs. Edward L. Korn and K.K. Gordon Lan for their comments and suggestions.

REFERENCES

1. Ries, L.A., Hankey, B.F., Edwards, B.K., eds., *Cancer Statistics Review 1973-87, NIH Publication No. 90-2789*, National Institutes of Health, Bethesda, MD, 1990.
2. Bailar, J.C. III and Smith, E.M., Progress against cancer? *N. Engl. J. Med.*, 314, 1226–1232, 1986, correspondence on progress against cancer, *N. Engl. J. Med.*, 315, 963–968.
3. Doll, R., Are we winning the fight against cancer? An epidemiological assessment, *Eur. J. Cancer*, 26, 500–508, 1990.
4. Extramural Committee to Assess Measures of Progress Against Cancer, Measures of progress against cancer, *J. Natl. Cancer Inst.*, 82, 825–835, 1990.
5. Kessler, D.A., The regulation of investigational drugs, *N. Engl. J. Med.*, 320, 281–288, 1989.
6. O'Shaughnessy, J.A., Wittes, R.E., Burke, G. et al., Commentary concerning demonstration of safety and efficacy of investigational anticancer agents in clinical trials, *J. Clin. Oncol.*, 9, 2225–2232, 1991.
7. Byar, D.P., Schoenfeld, D.A., Green, S.B. et al., Design considerations for AIDS trials, *N. Engl. J. Med.*, 323, 1343–1348, 1990.
8. Pocock, S.J., A perspective on the role of quality-of-life assessment in clinical trials, *Controlled Clin. Trials*, 12, 257S–265S, 1991.
9. Aaronson, N.K., Quality of life: what is it? How should it be measured? *Oncology*, 2, 69–74, 1988.
10. National Cancer Institute. *Investigator's Handbook. A Manual for Participants in Clinical Trials of Investigational Agents Sponsored by the Division of Cancer Treatment National Cancer Institute*, National Cancer Institute, Bethesda, MD, 1986.
11. Edler, L., Statistical Requirements of Phase I Studies, *Onkologie*, 13, 90–95, 1990.
12. Collins, J.M., Grieshaber, C.K., and Chabner, B.A., Pharmacologically guided Phase I clinical trials based upon preclinical drug development, *J. Natl. Cancer Inst.*, 82, 1321–1326, 1990.
13. Storer, B.E., Design and analysis of phase I clinical trials, *Biometrics*, 45, 925–937, 1989.
14. Scheiner, L.B. and Beal, S.L., Bayesian individualization of pharmacokinetics: simple implementation and comparison with non-Bayesian methods, *J. Pharm. Sci.*, 71, 1344–1348, 1982.
15. Moore, T.D. and Korn, E.L., Phase II trial design considerations for small-cell lung cancer, *J. Natl. Cancer Inst.*, 84, 150–154, 1992.
16. Cheson, B.D., Cassileth, P.A., Head, D.A. et al., Report of the National Cancer Institute-sponsored workshop on definitions of diagnosis and response in acute myeloid leukemia, *J. Clin. Oncol.*, 8, 813–819, 1990.
17. Simon, R., Optimal two-stage designs for Phase II clinical trials, *Controlled Clin. Trials*, 10, 1–10, 1989.
18. Fleming, T.R., One sample multiple testing procedure for Phase II clinical trials, *Biometrics*, 38, 143–151, 1982.
19. Schultz, J.R., Nichol, F.R., Elfring, G.L., and Weed, S.D., Multiple-stage procedures for drug screening, *Biometrics*, 29, 293–300, 1973.
20. Cox, D.R. and McCullagh, P., Some aspects of analysis of covariance, *Biometrics*, 38, 541–561, 1982.

21. Byar, D.P., Simon, R.M., Friedewald, W.T. et al., Randomized clinical trials: perspectives on some recent ideas, *N. Engl. J. Med.*, 295, 74–80, 1976.

22. Durrleman, S. and Simon, R., When to randomize? *J. Clin. Oncol.*, 9, 116–122, 1991.

23. Peto, R., Pike, M.C., Armitage, P. et al., Design and analysis of randomized clinical trails requiring prolonged observation of each patient. I. Introduction and design, *Br. J. Cancer*, 34, 585–612, 1976.

24. Pocock, S.J. and Simon, R., Sequential treatment assignment with balancing for prognostic factors in the controlled clinical trial, *Biometrics*, 31, 103–115, 1975.

25. Simon, R., Restricted randomization designs in clinical trials, *Biometrics*, 35, 503–512, 1979.

26. Casagrande, J.T., Pike, M.C., and Smith, P.G., An improved formula for calculating sample sizes for comparing two binomial distributions, *Biometrics*, 34, 483–486, 1978.

27. Bernstein, D. and Lagakos, S.W., Sample size and power determination for stratified clinical trials, *J. Stat. Comput. Simul.*, 8, 65–73, 1978.

28. Rubinstein, L.V., Gail, M.H., and Santner, T.J., Planning the duration of a comparative clinical trial with loss to follow-up and a period of continued observation, *J. Chronic Dis.*, 34, 469–479, 1981.

29. Dunnett, C.W. and Gent, M., Significance testing to establish equivalence between treatments, with special reference to data in the form of 2×2 tables, *Biometrics*, 33, 593–602, 1977.

30. Gail, M.H., Applicability of sample size calculation based on a comparison of proportions for use with the logrank test, *Controlled Clin. Trials*, 6, 112–119, 1985.

31. Lachin, J.M. and Foulkes, M.A., Evaluation of sample size and power for analyses of survival with allowance for nonuniform patient entry, losses to follow-up, noncompliance, and stratifaction, *Biometrics*, 42, 507–519, 1986.

32. Lakatos, E., Sample size based on the log-rank statistics in complex clinical trials, *Biometrics*, 44, 229–241, 1988.

33. Halpern, J. and Brown, B.W. Jr., Cure rate models: power of the logrank and generalized Wilcoxon tests, *Stat. Med.*, 6, 483–489, 1987.

34. Kaplan, E.L. and Meier, P., Nonparametric estimation from incomplete observations, *J. Am. Stat. Assoc.*, 53, 457–481, 1958.

35. Berkson, J. and Gage, R.P., Calculation of survival rates for cancer, *Proc. Staff Meet. Mayo Clin.*, 25, 270–286, 1950.

36. Cutler, S.J. and Ederer, F., Maximum utilization of the life table method in analyzing survival, *J. Chronic Dis.*, 8, 699–712, 1958.

37. Gehan, E.A., A generalized Wilcoxon test for comparing arbitrarily singly-censored samples, *Biometrika*, 52, 203–223, 1965.

38. Prentice, R.L., Linear rank tests with right censored data, *Biometrika*, 65, 167–179, 1978.

39. Mantel, N. and Haenszel, W., Statistical aspects of the analysis of data from retrospective studies of disease, *J. Natl. Cancer Inst.*, 22, 719–748, 1959.

40. Mantel, N., Evaluation of survival data and two new rank order statistics arising in its consideration, *Cancer Chemother. Rep.*, 50, 163–170, 1966.

41. Tarone, R. and Ware, J., On distribution-free tests for equality of survival distributions, *Biometrika*, 64, 156–160, 1977.

42. Harrington, D.P. and Fleming, T.R., A class of rank test procedures for censored survival data, *Biometrika*, 69, 553–566, 1982.
43. Early Breast Cancer Trialists' Collaborative Group, Systemic treatment of early breast cancer by hormonal, cytotoxic, or immune therapy: 133 randomized trials involving 31,000 recurrences and 24,000 deaths among 75,000 women, *Lancet*, 1–15, 71–85, 1992.
44. Early Breast Cancer Trialists' Collaborative Group, Effects of adjuvant tamoxifen and of cytotoxic therapy on mortality in early breast cancer: an overview of 61 randomized trials among 28,896 women, *N. Engl. J. Med.*, 319, 1681–1692, 1988.
45. Cochran, W.G., Some methods of strengthening the common χ^2 tests, *Biometrics*, 10, 417–451, 1954.
46. Cox, D.R., The regression analysis of binary sequences, *J. R. Stat. Soc.*, B20, 215–242, 1958.
47. Cox, D.R., Regression models and life tables (with discussion), *J. R. Stat. Soc.*, B74, 187–220, 1972.
48. Kalbfleisch, J.D. and Prentice, R.L., *The Statistical Analysis of Failure Time Data*, Wiley, New York, 1980.
49. Gail, M. and Simon, R., Testing for qualitative interactions between treatment effects and patient subsets, *Biometrics*, 41, 361–372, 1985.
50. Meier, P., Statistical analysis of clinical trials, In *Clinical Trials: Issues and Approaches*, Shapiro, S.H. and Louis, T.A., eds., Marcel Dekker, New York, pp. 155–189, 1983.
51. Anderson, J.R., Cain, K.C., and Gelber, R.D., Analysis of survival by tumor response, *J. Clin. Oncol.*, 1, 710–719, 1983.
52. Armitage, P., McPherson, C.K., and Rowe, B.C., Repeated significance tests on accumulating data, *J. R. Stat. Soc.*, A132, 235–244, 1969.
53. Lan, K.K.G. and DeMets, D.L., Discrete sequential boundaries for clinical trials, *Biometrika*, 70, 659–663, 1983.
54. Pocock, S.J., Group sequential methods in the design and analysis of clinical trials, *Biometrika*, 64, 191–199, 1977.
55. O'Brien, P.C. and Fleming, T.R., A multiple testing procedure for clinical trials, *Biometrics*, 35, 549–556, 1979.
56. DeMets, D.L. and Gail, M.H., Use of logrank tests and group sequential methods at fixed calendar times, *Biometrics*, 41, 1039–1044, 1985.
57. Pocock, S.J., Interim analyses for randomized clinical trials: the group sequential approach, *Biometrics*, 38, 153–162, 1982.
58. Jennison, C. and Turnbull, B.W., Interim analyses: the repeated confidence interval approach (with discussion), *J. R. Stat. Soc.*, B51, 305–361, 1989.
59. Lan, K.K.G., Simon, R., and Halperin, M., Stochastically curtailed tests in long-term clinical trials, *Commun. Stat. Sequential Anal.*, 1, 207–219, 1982.
60. Zelen, M., Guidelines for publishing papers on cancer clinical trials: responsibilities of editors and authors, *J. Clin. Oncol.*, 1, 164–169, 1983.
61. Simon, R. and Wittes, R.E., Methodologic guidelines for reports of clinical trials, *Cancer Treat. Rep.*, 69, 1–3, 1985.

7 Recent Statistical Issues and Developments in Cancer Clinical Trials

Weichung Joe Shih

CONTENTS

I. INTRODUCTION

Chen (in Chapter 6) and many others (e.g., Ref. 1) have given excellent general overviews of clinical trial in cancers. This chapter will deal with a review of some statistical methods and issues focusing on recent developments pertinent to the pharmaceutical industry. It will follow the traditional drug development process to organize the review in terms of phase I to phase III trials and will also discuss about a recent major challenge to seamlessly link these kinds of traditional phased-designs.

II. PHASE I CLINICAL TRIALS

Many general design considerations for clinical trial of cancer are similar to that for other categories of diseases. However, a major difference starts from the so-called phase I clinical trial. In most drug testing in diseases other than cancer, healthy (normal) volunteers (subjects) are recruited for phase I trials in order to study the clinical pharmacology and toxicity of the drug. Using healthy subjects reduces the risk of serious toxicity problems and avoids confounding pharmacologic and disease effects. Once comfort against acute toxicity is established, dose-ranging studies to determine tolerable doses typically follow, again with healthy subjects. This is not the case for cancer phase I trials.

Phase I cancer clinical trials usually involve patients who have been heavily treated and, in most cases, have failed to respond to previous treatments (but still have good organ function to receive potential benefit from the investigational therapy). The types and grade levels of toxicity are specifically defined. In the U.S.A., the National Cancer Institute (NCI) *Common Toxicity Criteria* are used. The main goals of a phase I cancer clinical trial with cytotoxic drugs are to find the maximum tolerated dose (MTD) of the drug for a specific mode of administration and to characterize the most frequent dose-limiting toxicities (DLT).[2] Sequential dose-finding strategies are always used for ethical reasons.

Two types of sequential strategies are used: algorithm-based designs and model-based designs. The so called "3 + 3" design is the typical algorithm-based design (see Chen in Chapter 6) and has been referred to as *the standard method* by Korn et al.[3] and *a conventional method* by Simon et al.[4] Because of its practical simplicity, many clinical investigators favor this conventional design. The algorithm does not have to be limited to "3 + 3", and many variants in fact have also frequently been used in practice. Lin and Shih[5] presented examples and derived in rigorous details the statistical properties of the generalized "A + B" designs, with or without dose de-escalation schemes. The statistical properties include:

- the probability of a dose chosen as MTD
- the expected number of patients at each dose level
- the target toxicity level (TTL), i.e., the expected DLT incidences at MTD
- the expected DLT incidences at each dose level
- the expected overall DLT incidences.

All these statistical properties are derived based on the assumed toxicity rate at each dose level selected for the trial. Though the exact dose–toxicity rates are not known in advance, the clinicians should have some knowledge or rough idea of the drug–toxicity based on similar trials or other source of information; otherwise, it would be very difficult for the investigator to justify the dose levels selected for testing. Usually several different scenarios, including the best and worst possible cases, may be considered back and forth during the planning stage. By considering these properties, statisticians also help the clinical investigators to gain insights on selecting the dose levels to be tested in the trial. It is clear from Ref. 5 that the algorithm-based "A + B" designs do not really have a fixed TTL; in particular, they showed that the TTL of 33% for the "3 + 3" design is a misconception. One should understand that the algorithm-based designs are to identify a dose-level that does not exhibit too much toxicity on a very small group of patients so as not to produce accurate estimates of a target quantile. The S-plus program used in Ref. 5 is available at http://www2.umdnj.edu/~linyo.

In model-based sequential designs, the MTD is a quantile corresponding to the desired TTL of the assumed dose–toxicity distribution model. Methods for estimating the MTD based on parametric models are also used in industry-sponsored trials. These include the "continual reassessment method" (CRM),[6,7] modified CRM,[8–10] extended CRM,[11] and "escalation with overdose control" (EWOC).[12] The main feature of the CRM and EWOC methods is using an initial monotonic dose–toxicity working model with prior distributions on the model parameters and accruing data to update the current estimate of the MTD. The modifications and extension of CRM for practical concerns include the following:

- Always start with lowest dose.
- Never skip a dose level (in the discrete case).
- Never increase by more than twice the previous dose.
- Use the conventional "3 + 3" algorithm for the first two or three dose levels until the first toxicity is observed and then engage in the CRM mode.

O'Quigley and Shen[13] noted that CRM could be developed according to the likelihood without Bayes theorem, similar to sequential maximum likelihood techniques. It is clear that the likelihood approach requires at least one toxicity case for parameter estimation and restriction of the dose–toxicity model to only one parameter. The modified or extended CRM procedure is always used in practice instead of the CRM. Shen and O'Quigley[14] and Cheung and Chappell[15] discussed sufficient conditions under which the procedure is consistent (i.e., converging to the correct MTD). Proper stopping-rules need to be set to allow early termination, such as rules based on confidence intervals,[16] binary outcome trees,[17] and allocation limits.[18] Some of these rules are based on precise probabilistic calculations and are not easy to implement. In practice, a maximum number of patients to be treated in the trial (usually under 30) is imposed as the stopping-rule and may undermine the dose convergence.

EWOC is also a Bayesian method based on a location-scale family of models. The scheme introduces over-dose control such that the predicted probability of the next dose assigned to a new patient exceeding MTD is fixed at a given level. Zacks et al.[19] studied the consistency of this procedure. Evaluation of the predicted probability requires intensive computations, but with recent developments of the Markov Chain Monte Carlo method and the widely available computer software "BUGS" (Bayesian inference Using Gibbs Sampling), the task of computation has been easier.

A major concern for model-based methods is model misspecification. The sufficient conditions given in Refs. 14 and 15 for consistency of CRM relate to the true dose–toxicity curve. Because the true dose–toxicity curve is unknown, the conditions are not verifiable. For a given working dose–toxicity model, Cheung and Chappell[15] suggested a reasonable approach to determine an interval of probabilities in which the toxicity of the converged recommended dose will fall. The shorter the range, the less sensitive the working model is to the underlying true model and *vice versa*. Similar to studying the "A + B" properties by Lin and Shih[5] using these sufficient conditions and simulations, statisticians are able to evaluate the operating characteristics of CRM in advance and can help in selecting doses for experimentation; see examples in Ref. 20.

Storer[21] investigated several "up and down" designs that target TTL at 33%. Random walk rules (RWRs) generalize these rules to any quantile of interest.[22] Up and down and RWRs are nonparametrics having no concerns in possible model misspecification. A RWR creates a unimodal distribution around the target quantile. The estimate of MTD can then be obtained from the empirical mode of frequency distribution, and it is consistent but is highly variable with a small number of patients. Also, as in CRM, some patients will be assigned above the MTD. Properties of RWRs have been developed and a simple software in MATLAB is also available.[22]

More reviews on phase I designs can be found in Ref. 23 including other methods such as decision–theoretic approaches.[24] Leung and Wang[25] also used a decision theory approach to optimize the number of patients treated at the MTD. Because the phase I trial has to define the MTD, with due consideration to efficacy, strategies based on efficacy and toxicity responses in combination phase I/II trials by Thall and Russell[26] have great potential to expedite drug development in the industry. Phase I/II trial designs first use one of the above strategies to find the MTD or RPTD (recommended phase II dose), then with the same protocol continue the same study to treat patients with the RPTD and examine the tumor response rate. Such seamless switching from phase I to phase II within the same protocol is practical only when the study does not require different patient populations, defined by the inclusion and exclusion criteria, for phase I and II parts of the protocol.

III. PHASE II CLINICAL TRIALS

The main objective of a phase II cancer trial is to determine whether a new therapy has sufficient activity against a specific type of tumor to warrant its further (phase III) development.[27] A major difference between cancer phase II trials and those of many other diseases is that the former are usually conducted single-arm without a parallel control. Historical control is often referred to for comparison.[28] In the industry, these are often referred to as phase IIA studies and extensive epidemiological data and literature review and meta-analysis are crucial to the interpretation of a phase IIA cancer trial using historical controls. The primary endpoint for cancer phase IIA trials is usually the tumor response rate defined clinically based on a combination of reduction in tumor size and changes in biochemical markers. Complete and partial responses are usually pooled together when a single (overall) response rate is calculated. Sometimes investigators also collect data on survival, but confidence intervals are usually wide because of small samples. Since there is no randomization in these Phase IIA studies, the starting time of survival is rather arbitrary.

A hypothesis testing approach is carried out in a phase IIA trial based on response rates because one has to decide whether or not to proceed to a phase IIB/III trial. The therapy will be deemed uninteresting if the true response rate (p) is no more than a certain level, and accepted for further investigation in larger groups of patients (i.e., phase IIB/III studies) if the true response is greater than some target level. The "uninteresting level" of response rate (p_0) may be obtained from the literature regarding the standard therapy. The target level of response rate (i.e., the alternative hypothesis, p_*) is usually set based on the investigator's expectation of the new therapy. Typically, for ethical and practical considerations a two- or three-stage design is used for these phase IIA trials so that an ineffective treatment can be dismissed early at the end of the first stage.

In the early 1960s, when the anticancer agents had low activity, Gehan's two-stage design was used widely, in which p_0 was set to be zero.[29] Later, Simon generalized p_0 and introduced "optimal" and "minimax" designs.[30] Simon's "optimal" design minimizes the expected sample size under the null hypothesis, and "minimax" design first minimizes the maximum of the total sample size and then chooses the "optimal" one among these solutions. In Simon's design, no early termination is allowed even when there is a long run of failures at the start. To overcome this difficulty, Ensign et al.[31] introduced an optimal three-stage design, in which the first stage is to allow early stopping when a moderately long sequence of initial failures occur and the remaining two stages are the same as in Simon's design.

While Simon's two-stage design has been the most popular method for phase IIA cancer trials, another recent development is an adaptive two-stage design, which copes with the uncertainty in setting the alternative hypothesis associated with power at the planning stage. To illustrate, consider a study to investigate the weekly administration of vinorelbine, bleomycin, and gemcitabine combination therapy for treating patients with recurrent or refractory Hodgkin's disease. Because each of the single agents has been known to be active against Hodgkin's disease when given alone, p_0 was set at .40 to distinguish the combination from the single agents. The principal investigator targeted the response rate of the combination therapy at $p_* = .60$ based on his expectation. The testing of H_0: $p \leq .40$ vs. H_A: $p \geq .60$ is considered. With the type I error $\alpha \leq 5\%$ and type II error $\beta \leq 20\%$, using Simon's two-stage optimal design, 16 patients will be recruited to the first stage of the study. The therapy will not be interesting (i.e., H_0 accepted) if there are no more than seven responses out of the 16 patients, otherwise an additional 30 patients will be recruited to the second stage of the study. The combination therapy will not be interesting if there are no more than 23 responses out of the total of 46 patients.

When the true response rate is actually 55% (i.e., 15% above p_0), the probability of accepting H_0 (rejecting the therapy) will be 40%, twice as large as the chosen type II error. If the true response rate is 50% (i.e., 10% above p_0), the probability of rejecting the drug will be 64%, more than triple the type II error. The problem is even more pronounced when one chooses $\beta \leq 10\%$. If the true response rate is 55%, the probability of rejecting the therapy will be 26.9%, almost triple the chosen type II error. If the true response rate is 50%, the probability of rejecting the therapy will be 54.2%, more than five times the type II error.

It is conceivable that in many situations the response rates of 55 or 50% are still worth pursuing, even though 60% is initially targeted based on the investigator's expectation of the new therapy. In general, using Simon's design, there is a high probability of rejecting a promising new therapy if the initial expectation is set optimistically.

From the above illustration, we can see that it is crucial to choose the right p_* when planning a phase IIA study. Unfortunately, we usually have very little information about p_* at the planning stage of studying a new cancer therapy, and are often concerned with the uncertainty in setting a value for it. A natural way to resolve this dilemma is to choose p_* with some flexibility. Lin and Shih[32] proposed an adaptive two-stage design, which enables the investigator to set a higher target (p_2) in the beginning but to switch to a lower rate (p_1) for testing if necessary, or *vice versa*, depending on the observed number of responses after the first stage of the study, and then determine the number of patients needed for the second stage accordingly. The procedure is briefly described as follows. Let x be the number of the observed responses out of n_1 patients in the first stage:

- If $x \leq s_1$, reject the therapy and stop the trial (i.e., accept H_0).
- If $s_1 < x \leq r_1$, power the study of $(1 - \beta_1)$ at $p_* = p_1$ and enter $m_2 = m - n_1$ additional patients into the study.

Reject the therapy if later the total number of responses is $\leq s$ out of m patients.

- If $x > r_1$, power the study of $(1 - \beta_2)$ at $p_* = p_2$ and enter $n_2 = n - n_1$ additional patients into the study.

Reject the therapy if later the total number of responses is $< r$ out of n patients.

The adaptive two-stage design parameters are $(s_1, r_1, n_1, s, m, r, n)$. These have to satisfy the requirement of type I error $\leq \alpha$. It is reasonable to choose $\beta_1 \geq \beta_2$ in practice, although not required, because we would like to have higher power for detecting more improvement of the new therapy (p_2 vs. p_0), and, from the feasibility aspect, we need to lower the power for less improvement (p_1 vs. p_0) because the sample size could not be too big for a phase IIA study. This capping sample size for less effect (compromising the power somewhat) has also been used in the sample size re-estimation methods (see, e.g., Ref. 33). In addition, four optimality criteria for $(s_1, r_1, n_1, s, m, r, n)$ are considered:

- Optimality Type (O1): EN_0 is smallest
- Optimality Type (O2): $\max\{EN_i | i = 0, 1, 2\}$ is smallest

- Optimality Type (O3): $\max(n, m)$ is smallest among all solutions and EN_0 is smallest among such solutions
- Optimality Type (O4): $\max(n, m)$ is smallest among all solutions and $\max\{EN_i | i = 0,1,2\}$ is smallest among such solutions

where $EN_i = E(N|p_i)$ for $i = 0, 1, 2$.

O1 and O3 are similar to Simon's "optimal design" and "minimax design" criteria, respectively. As in Ref. 30, O1 design achieves reduction in EN_0 by having a smaller sample size at the first stage. This is desirable for ethical considerations in the case of inactive therapy. On the other hand, O3 design has a smaller maximum sample size. O2 and O4 designs are natural extensions of O1 and O3, respectively. In O2 and O4, the smallest expected number of patients is considered under the null hypothesis and also under the alternative as well. For O2 and O4, compared with O1 and O3, respectively, a larger sample size is needed at the first stage, but large savings in the total sample size are achieved. A larger sample size needed at the first stage is reasonable for O2 and O4 to ensure a sound decision based on the interim data for adaptive designs. Lin and Shih[32] provided theoretical proof of the existence of $(s_1, r_1, n_1, s, m, r, n)$ and algorithm to find the optimal solutions. Table 7.1 gives the designs for $\alpha = 0.05$, $\beta_1 = 0.20$, $\beta_2 = 0.10$, $p_1 - p_0 = .20$, and $p_2 - p_0 = .30$. More tables for other scenarios of $(\alpha, \beta_1, \beta_2, p_0, p_1, p_2)$ and the computer program used to generate these tables are available at the web site http://www2.umdnj.edu/~linyo.

Other various designs that extend Simon's design can be found in Refs. 34–36. All these designs and testing procedures are considered as some sort of optimal early stopping for futility or efficacy. Bayesian designs have also been proposed by, for example, Ref. 37. An earlier review of statistical designs of phase IIA cancer trials can be found in Ref. 38.

Recently, because of the pressure of getting medicines on the market for needy patients faster, more phase IIB studies are designed with a randomized active control group using time-to-progression or progression-free-survival as the primary endpoint and quality of life as the key secondary endpoint. This strategy is related to the use of seamless phase IIB/III design and the "Fast Track Drug Development Program," as discussed in the next section.

IV. PHASE III CLINICAL TRIALS

Key design considerations for phase III cancer trials, such as randomization, control agent, endpoints, sample size, study duration, interim analyses, Data Safety Monitoring Committee, etc., are similar to those for other life-threatening diseases, and have been discussed by many authors (e.g., Ref. 1). Some issues, those are specifically pertinent to the pharmaceutical industry sponsored cancer trials, are worth highlighting. These include the 1998 FDA's "Guidance for Industry: the Fast Track Drug Development Programs" (FTDDP) and the recent trend in filing equivalence or noninferiority for new cancer treatments. We discuss these two topics in the following.

TABLE 7.1

Designs for $\alpha = 0.05$, $\beta_1 = 0.20$, $\beta_2 = 0.10$, $p_1 - p_0 = .20$, and $p_2 - p_0 = .30$

p_0	p_1	p_2	Design Parameters			True			Expected Sizes			Optimal Type
			$s_1/r_1/n_1$	s/m	r/n	α	β_1	β_2	EN_0	EN_1	EN_2	
.05	.25	.35	0/1/7	2/19	3/24	0.041	0.200	0.059	10.84	20.17	22.24	1
			0/1/9	2/18	2/15	0.046	0.196	0.049	12.11	15.23	15.18	2
			0/1/9	2/17	2/16	0.044	0.198	0.048	11.89	15.70	15.96	3 & 4
.10	.30	.40	1/2/11	4/22	5/28	0.047	0.200	0.043	14.87	24.88	26.95	1
			0/2/9	5/25	3/16	0.050	0.198	0.038	18.32	19.52	17.92	2
			1/3/17	5/23	4/22	0.050	0.197	0.035	20.03	22.09	22.03	3 & 4
.15	.35	.45	2/5/12	8/35	7/24	0.050	0.199	0.047	18.03	29.18	28.83	1
			2/4/15	9/36	5/18	0.050	0.196	0.040	22.20	23.04	19.94	2
			2/3/15	6/25	7/28	0.050	0.199	0.031	19.49	26.86	27.77	3
			1/5/15	7/28	6/20	0.048	0.200	0.033	23.72	24.33	22.06	4
.20	.40	.50	3/7/13	12/43	8/24	0.050	0.200	0.048	20.56	36.09	36.10	1
			3/6/17	11/36	7/20	0.049	0.199	0.035	24.97	26.28	22.54	2
			3/6/17	10/32	9/31	0.047	0.200	0.026	23.73	30.75	31.07	3
			1/5/13	10/32	7/23	0.050	0.200	0.026	27.29	27.93	25.58	4
.25	.45	.55	4/7/15	14/40	9/24	0.049	0.200	0.032	22.56	31.45	28.91	1
			5/8/20	15/42	9/22	0.049	0.200	0.036	27.60	29.07	24.47	2
			3/6/16	12/34	13/35	0.050	0.196	0.022	26.79	34.13	34.81	3
			7/10/26	13/35	11/32	0.050	0.200	0.022	28.71	32.54	32.17	4
.30	.50	.60	5/9/15	18/46	14/32	0.050	0.199	0.036	23.58	39.21	39.31	1
			5/8/17	19/45	9/21	0.050	0.198	0.022	27.32	30.99	25.48	2

.35	.55	.65	6/11/22	15/36	13/34	0.050	0.200	0.020	29.05	34.80	34.43	3
			5/11/22	15/36	12/28	0.050	0.200	0.020	31.50	32.55	29.82	4
			6/9/16	20/44	15/33	0.050	0.199	0.027	24.48	36.50	35.79	1
			8/11/21	21/45	12/24	0.048	0.198	0.022	27.40	32.08	27.15	2
.40	.60	.70	7/11/23	18/38	17/37	0.049	0.199	0.017	31.73	37.08	37.06	3
			9/14/28	18/38	16/36	0.050	0.200	0.017	33.33	36.60	36.14	4
			7/11/16	23/46	14/26	0.050	0.200	0.028	24.42	38.40	36.23	1
			8/12/21	23/44	13/23	0.049	0.199	0.022	31.21	32.19	26.04	2
.45	.65	.75	6/10/17	20/39	20/37	0.050	0.199	0.016	29.08	37.34	37.38	3
			15/19/31	20/39	20/35	0.050	0.198	0.016	32.01	36.47	35.69	4
			7/11/15	24/43	14/23	0.050	0.198	0.021	24.58	36.38	33.29	1
			10/13/21	27/47	14/23	0.048	0.200	0.018	28.44	32.12	25.95	2
.50	.70	.80	12/16/24	22/39	21/35	0.050	0.199	0.014	27.59	36.16	35.83	3
			16/19/30	22/39	20/33	0.050	0.199	0.014	31.14	34.82	33.56	4
			8/12/15	26/43	20/30	0.050	0.200	0.021	23.45	37.68	37.32	1
			12/15/22	26/42	16/24	0.049	0.198	0.015	26.76	31.27	26.27	2
.55	.75	.85	8/13/17	23/37	15/23	0.050	0.200	0.011	26.91	33.37	29.26	3
			13/17/24	23/37	18/29	0.050	0.200	0.011	27.43	32.93	30.46	4
			9/13/15	28/43	14/17	0.050	0.199	0.023	22.26	36.76	34.25	1
			11/14/19	27/40	15/21	0.048	0.199	0.011	25.12	29.53	23.66	2
.60	.80	.90	15/19/24	24/36	20/28	0.050	0.199	0.009	26.05	32.57	30.22	3 & 4
			7/10/11	30/43	14/18	0.050	0.200	0.019	20.39	35.70	34.56	1
			13/15/20	30/41	17/23	0.050	0.196	0.006	24.33	27.85	23.73	2
			10/14/17	24/33	15/20	0.048	0.200	0.005	24.01	28.37	23.08	3 & 4
.65	.85	.95	6/8/9	28/37	17/22	0.049	0.197	0.009	18.13	29.58	27.31	1
			11/13/16	31/40	14/17	0.049	0.190	0.008	21.90	25.19	17.97	2
			13/16/18	23/30	20/24	0.050	0.199	0.003	20.24	27.21	25.34	3
			13/16/18	23/30	20/24	0.050	0.199	0.003	20.24	27.21	25.34	4

A. FAST TRACK DRUG DEVELOPMENT PROGRAMS

The FTDDP is a great opportunity for industry to bring effective treatment on the market faster to benefit patients. The issues involve endpoints switching and controlling different type I errors for conditional and final approvals of the drug. In general, overall survival benefit is the ultimate endpoint that a phase III cancer trial needs to show on the test treatment over the control in order to obtain the final approval of marketing authorization from the Food and Drug Administration. Time-to-progression, disease-free survival, tumor response rate, and quality of life scores can all serve as secondary endpoints for supportive evidence, but the primary endpoint is the overall survival. (Aside: Because it may well take a huge sample size and long time to show the benefit of overall survival, issues regarding interim analyses and trial monitoring arise. See Hwang and Lan in Chapter 14 for discussions of group sequential designs, which are almost always used for phase III cancer trials.)

In the past, the Oncology Drug Advisory Committee (ODAC) of the FDA has recommended conditional approval of new treatments based on well-conducted studies using secondary endpoints, such as disease progression and tumor response rate. The legal base of the conditional approval is the Food and Drug Administration Modernization Act of 1997 Section No. 112 entitled "Expediting Study and Approval of Fast Track Drugs."[53] The FDA issued "Guidance for Industry: the Fast Track Drug Development Programs" in 1998 to set the requirements for the FTDD programs.[54] First, it states that the purpose of FTDD programs is to "*facilitate the development and expedite the review of new drugs that are intended to treat serious or life-threatening conditions and that demonstrate the potential to address unmet medical needs.*" For cancer, this requires the investigation of the new treatment to be at a tumor site for which there is currently no effective medication. Second, it states that an application for approval of a fast track product may be granted if it is determined that "*the product has an effect on a clinical endpoint or on a surrogate endpoint that is reasonably likely to predict clinical benefit.*" For cancer treatments, the "clinical benefit" refers to the overall survival, and "a clinical endpoint or a surrogate endpoint" may be time-to-progression, progression-free-survival, or tumor response rate, because these are generally accepted as reasonably predictive of the overall survival.

The FTDD Programs also put limitations on such accelerated approvals: the sponsor has to "conduct appropriate postapproval studies to validate the surrogate endpoint or otherwise confirm the effect on the clinical endpoint." The FDA also may withdraw approval of a fast track product using expedited procedures if, among other things such as safety issues, "the sponsor fails to conduct any required study" or "a postapproval study of the fast track product fails to verify clinical benefit of the product." Therefore, the accelerated approval is only a conditional approval for the drug. Some authors have labeled as "phase IIB" those randomized studies that use time-to-progression, progression-free-survival, or tumor response rate as endpoints[39] and "phase III" for the postconditional-approval study.

Shih et al.[40,52] discussed two related issues involved in the FTDD programs: the so-called "postconditional-approval study" concept, and the kind of type I errors involved in the approval process. For the issue of postconditional-approval study, Shih et al. proposed a "seamless phase IIB/III" design, i.e., the "postconditional-approval study" does not have to be a separate study, but can be a proper continuation or extension of the same study upon which the early submission for accelerated approval is based. An obvious advantage of such an approach is savings of time and resources. It is also conceivable that in certain situations of severe diseases (such as pancreatic cancer) continuation or extension of the same trial, often very large in sample size, is the only feasible way to study the effect of treatment under investigation.

Seamless studies have obvious advantages of efficiency. But there are design and conduct considerations to continue a study properly so as to ensure that the final submission of the product satisfies the usual requirements of the traditional approval. For example, special attention needs to be paid to how to keep enough patients in the control arm of the study after a clear benefit of the investigational drug has been shown on the surrogate endpoint (and the drug is available on the market). Because the objective and endpoint often change in the continuation according to the design, some interesting questions are raised. Do we view the fast track approval submission as an interim analysis of the whole study, or view the final analysis as for a "poststudy extension" (i.e., the fast track submission is the main study)? If the fast track (accelerated approval) submission is an interim analysis, how does this type of interim analysis differ from the usual ones? What is the implication of the type I error rate when the first accelerated approval is only a conditional one? How should the type I error rate(s) be calculated and controlled?

The usual sense of overall (or experiment-wise) type I error rate means the probability of falsely rejecting any true hypothesis. This concept is not useful for the current situation where the final hypothesis regarding the overall survival ultimately dominates the fast-track hypothesis regarding the intermediate endpoint (time-to-progression or progression-free-survival) at a later time point with more data. Denote the "final approval type I error rate" by α_F, the "early submission type I error rate" during the gap time before final approval by α_E, and the tentative, conditional "accelerated approval type I error rate" during the gap time by α_A. Shih et al.[40] suggested that we should instead consider the following possible scenarios:

(1) Control α_F at 0.05 level.
(2) Control α_F at 0.05 level and, in addition, control α_E also at 0.05 level.
(3) Control α_F at 0.05 level and, in addition, control α_A at 0.01 level.
(4) Control $\alpha_F + \alpha_A$ at 0.05 level, for example, $\alpha_F = 0.04$ and $\alpha_A = 0.01$.

Scenario (1) views that the ultimate approval is the final conclusion of the drug's efficacy, only α_F needs to be controlled at the conventional 5% level. Scenario (2) views that the continuation of the trial is an extension study.

Each section of the submission process is controlled at the 5% level. Scenario (3) controls the final submission at the conventional 5% and the tentative conditional type I error rate at 1% (implying the imposition of a stricter risk protection for the accelerated approval of a yet-to-be confirmed but promising drug.) Scenario (4) is the most conservative way of controlling the accelerated and final approvals together at the 5% rate. When planning for an accelerated submission, discussion with the regulatory agency with regard to an appropriate scenario for α_F, α_E and α_A should be an essential part of the application for the FTDD programs.

B. NONINFERIORITY OR SUPERIORITY TRIALS WITH ACTIVE CONTROL

Because of ethical reasons many randomized phase III cancer trials are conducted using an active control agent ("A") for testing an experimental treatment ("T"). The active control treatment should have been shown to be efficacious as compared with placebo or a reference drug ("R").[41] Note that, because many recent phase III cancer studies have involved combinations of therapies, a single therapy such as 5-fluorouracil (5-FU) is often the ultimate reference ("R") rather than the placebo. There are usually two types of study objectives in an active controlled clinical trial. One is a superiority hypothesis that the experimental treatment is more effective than the active control. The other is a noninferiority (or equivalence) hypothesis that the experimental treatment is therapeutically no worse than (or equivalent to) the active control within a defined margin or range.[42] The superiority objective is of course much more desirable if achieved. Because the effect size of a new treatment relative to the active control is often hard to predict, the noninferiority objective is also valuable to consider if the experimental treatment is shown to have a similar effect, yet is less costly, safer, and more convenient to administer than the active control. Thus, both objectives are often included in the study protocol in practice.

For the noninferiority objective, the issue of determining the noninferiority margin has been at the center stage. First, one has to assure that the active control ("A") would have been superior to a standard reference ("R") if a standard reference were included in the present trial. The use of past (historical) standard reference-controlled trials often accomplishes this, but one must evoke a very strong assumption (namely, the *constancy assumption*) that the historical difference between the active control and reference therapy remains the same if the reference therapy had been used in the present trial. Second, one has to take into account the variability of the historical data by meta-analysis. Third, one has to demonstrate that the new therapy ("T") is superior to the putative "R" preserving at least a certain amount of the superiority of the active control ("A") over the reference therapy. See Hwang in Chapter 12, Refs. 43 and 44 for detailed reviews of fundamental issues in noninferiority trials in general. The "indirect confidence interval comparison method",[45] or so-called "two CI procedure",[46] is the most commonly used method to address the above issues. Although often conservative, it controls the type I error probability robustly against failure of the constancy assumption.

For keeping both objectives of superiority and noninferiority comparisons in the same study, Morikawa and Yoshida[47] and Dunnett and Gent[48] proposed using stepwise procedures, testing superiority first then noninferiority next depending on the outcome of the first test. The stepwise procedures are based on the closed testing principle valid without adjustment for the multiple comparisons. Note that their procedures are conducted with the usual fixed sample size design. Group sequential trials for either superiority or noninferiority can also be conducted by using the repeated confidence interval approach. Note that the conventional group sequential procedure is also based on fixed maximal information.

An adaptive design, which utilizes in-trial information to direct the future course of a trial, is sequential in nature and provides a strategy for flexible sample size (or information in general), trial duration, and other study design specifications. Adaptive designs have gained increasing popularity in recent years in clinical trials; see, for example, Pledger and Liu in Chapter 13, Refs. 49 and 50 for recent overviews. Wang et al.[42] have proposed an adaptive group sequential closed test procedure (AGSC) for testing the superiority or noninferiority hypotheses. Wang et al.'s AGSC is an extension of that of Cui et al.[51] In their AGSC, sample size can be adjusted once, and the test statistic is reconstructed to control the type I error rates for both superiority and noninferiority, based on the interim data. This procedure has the advantage of an early stop for superiority and continuing with a larger sample size if only inferiority is shown at the interim analysis.

Another adaptive strategy for testing the superiority and noninferiority hypotheses in an active-controlled study is proposed in Ref. 40, which uses the conditional power at the first stage to determine the course of the second stage. Differing from AGSC, they include consideration of an early stop for futility as a part of the interim decision making, and keep the final test statistic in its original likelihood ratio test form but recalculate the critical value to control the overall type I error rate. As a result, the proposed procedure is more flexible and more powerful compared with Wang et al.'s AGSC. Future cancer phase III trials in the pharmaceutical industry will likely be shaped with these new developments. The SAS computer program of Ref. 40 is available at the author's web site at http://www2.umdnj.edu/~shihwj.

REFERENCES

1. Simon, R.M., Design and conduct of clinical trials, In *Cancer Principles and Practice of Oncology*, DeVita, V.T. Jr., Hellman, S., and Rosenberg, S.A., eds., Lippincott, Philadelphia, PA, 1982.
2. Carter, S.K., The phase I study, In *Fundamentals of Cancer Chemotherapy*, Hellmann, K.K. and Carter, S.K., eds., McGraw Hill, New York, pp. 285–300, 1987.
3. Korn, E.L., Midthune, D., Chen, T.T., Rubinstein, L.V., Christian, M.C., and Simon, R.M., A comparison of two phase I trial designs, *Stat. Med.*, 13, 1799–1806, 1994.

4. Simon, R., Freidlin, B., Rubinstein, L., Arbuck, S.G., Collins, J., and Christian, M.C., Accelerated titration designs for phase I clinical trials in oncology, *J. Natl Cancer Inst.*, 89, 1138–1147, 1997.

5. Lin, Y. and Shih, W.J., Statistical properties of the traditional algorithm-based designs for phase I cancer clinical trials, *Biostatistics*, 2, 203–215, 2001.

6. O'Quigley, J., Pepe, M., and Fisher, L., Continual reassessment method: a practical design for phase I clinical trials in cancer, *Biometrics*, 46, 33–48, 1990.

7. O'Quigley, J. and Chevret, S., Methods for dose finding studies of cancer clinical trials: a review and results of a Monte Carlo study, *Stat. Med.*, 10, 1647–1664, 1991.

8. Faries, D., Practical modification of the continual reassessment method for phase I clinical trials, *J. Biopharm. Stat.*, 4, 147–164, 1994.

9. Goodman, S.N., Zahurak, M.I., and Piantadosi, S., Some practical improvement in the continual reassessment method for phase I studies, *Stat. Med.*, 14, 1149–1161, 1995.

10. Ahn, C., An evaluation of phase I cancer clinical trial designs, *Stat. Med.*, 17, 1537–1549, 1998.

11. Moller, S., An extension of the continual reassessment methods using a preliminary up-and-down design in a dose finding study in cancer patients, in order to investigate a greater range of doses, *Stat. Med.*, 14, 911–922, 1995.

12. Babb, J., Bogatko, A., and Zacks, S., Cancer phase I clinical trials: efficient dose escalation with overdose control, *Stat. Med.*, 17, 1103–1120, 1998.

13. O'Quigley, J. and Shen, L.Z., Continual reassessment method: a likelihood approach, *Biometrics*, 52, 673–684, 1996.

14. Shen, L.Z. and O'Quigley, J., Consistency of the continual reassessment method under model misspecification, *Biometrika*, 83, 395–406, 1996.

15. Cheung, Y.K. and Chappell, R., A simple technique to evaluate model sensitivity in the continual reassessment method, *Biometrics*, 58, 671–674, 2002.

16. Heyd, J.M. and Carlin, B., Adaptive design improvements in the continual reassessment method for phase I studies, *Stat. Med.*, 18, 1307–1321, 1999.

17. O'Quigley, J. and Reiner, E., A stopping-rule for the continual reassessment method, *Biometrika*, 85, 741–748, 1998.

18. O'Quigley, J., Continual reassessment designs with early termination, *Biostatistics*, 3, 87–99, 2002.

19. Zacks, S., Rogatko, A., and Babb, J., Optimal Bayesian-feasible dose escalation for cancer phase I clinical trials, *Stat. Probabil. Lett.*, 38, 215–220, 1998.

20. Ishizuka, N. and Ohashi, Y., The continual reassessment method and its applications: a Bayesian methodology for phase I cancer clinical trials, *Stat. Med.*, 20, 2661–2682, 2001.

21. Storer, B.E., Design and analysis of phase I clinical trials, *Biometrics*, 45, 925–937, 1989.

22. Durham, S.D., Flournoy, N., and Rosenberger, W.F., A random walk rule for phase I clinical trials in cancer, *Biometrics*, 53, 745–760, 1997.

23. Rosenberger, W.F. and Haines, L.M., Competing designs for phase I clinical trials: a review, *Stat. Med.*, 21, 2757–2770, 2002.

24. Whitehead, J. and Brunier, H., Bayesian decision procedures for dose determining experiments, *Stat. Med.*, 14, 885–893, 1995.

25. Leung, D.H.Y. and Wang, Y.G., An extension of the continual reassessment method using decision theory, *Stat. Med.*, 21, 51–64, 2002.

26. Thall, P.F. and Russell, K.E., A strategy for dose-finding and safety monitoring based on efficacy and adverse outcomes in phase I/II clinical trials, *Biometrics*, 54, 251–264, 1998.

27. Leventhal, B.G. and Wittes, R.E., *Research Methods in Oncology*, Raven Press, New York, 1988.

28. Thall, P.F. and Simon, R., Incorporating historical control data in planning phase II clinical trials, *Stat. Med.*, 9, 215–228, 1990.

29. Gehan, E.A., The determination of the number of patients required in a preliminary and a follow-up of a new chemotherapeutic agent, *J. Chronic Dis.*, 13, 346–353, 1961.

30. Simon, R.M., Optimal two-stage designs for Phase II clinical trials, *Control. Clin. Trials*, 10, 1–10, 1989.

31. Ensign, L.G., Gehan, E.A., Kamen, D.S., and Thall, P.F., An optimal three-stage design for phase II clinical trials, *Stat. Med.*, 13, 1727–1736, 1994.

32. Lin, Y. and Shih, W.J., Adaptive two-stage designs for single-arm phase IIA cancer clinical trials, *Biometrics*, 60, 482–490, 2004.

33. Gould, L.J. and Shih, W.J., Modifying the design of ongoing trials without unblinding, *Stat. Med.*, 17, 89–100, 1998.

34. Green, S.J. and Dahlberg, S., Planned versus attained designs in phase II clinical trials, *Stat. Med.*, 11, 853–862, 1992.

35. Chen, T.T., Optimal three-stage designs for phase II cancer clinical trials, *Stat. Med.*, 16, 2701–2711, 1997.

36. Shuster, J., Optimal two-stage designs for single arm phase II cancer trials, *J. Pharm. Stat.*, 12, 39–51, 2002.

37. Tan, S.B. and Machin, D., Bayesian two-stage designs for phase II clinical trials, *Stat. Med.*, 21, 1991–2012, 2002.

38. Mariani, L. and Marubini, E., Design and analysis of phase II cancer trials: a review of statistical methods and guidelines for medical researchers, *Int. Stat. Rev.*, 64, 61–88, 1996.

39. Simon, R., Wittes, R., and Ellenberg, S., Randomized phase II clinical trials, *Cancer Treat. Rep.*, 69, 1375–1381, 1985.

40. Shih, W.J., Quan, H., and Li, G., Two-stage adaptive strategy for superiority and noninferiority hypotheses in active controlled clinical trials, *Stat. Med.*, 23, 2781–2798, 2004.

41. Temple, R. and Ellenberg, S.S., Placebo-controlled trials and active-controlled trials in the evaluation of new treatments: Part 1: Ethical and scientific issues, *Ann. Intern. Med.*, 133, 455–463, 2000.

42. Wang, S.J., Hung, H.M.J., Tsong, Y., and Cui, L., Group sequential test strategies for superiority and noninferiority hypotheses in active controlled clinical trials, *Stat. Med.*, 20, 1903–1912, 2001.

43. D'Agostino, R.B., Massaro, J.M., and Sullivan, L.M., Noninferiority trials: design concepts and issues — the encounters of academic consultants in statistics, *Stat. Med.*, 22, 169–186, 2003.

44. Hung, H.M.J., Wang, S.J., Tsong, Y., Lawrence, J., and O'Neil, R.T., Some fundamental issues with noninferiority testing in active controlled trials, *Stat. Med.*, 22, 213–226, 2003.

45. Wang, S.J., Hung, H.M.J., and Tsong, Y., Utility and pitfalls of some statistical methods in active controlled clinical trials, *Control. Clin. Trials*, 23, 15–28, 2002.

46. Rothmann, M., Li, N., Chen, G., Chi, G.Y.H., Temple, R., and Tsou, H.H., Design and analysis of noninferiority mortality trials in oncology, *Stat. Med.*, 22, 239–264, 2003.

47. Morikawa, T. and Yoshida, M., A useful testing strategy in phase III trials: combined test of superiority and test of equivalence, *J. Biopharm. Stat.*, 5, 297–306, 1995.

48. Dunnett, C.W. and Gent, M., Significance testing to establish equivalence between treatments, with special reference to data in the form of 2×2 tables, *Biometrics*, 33, 593–602, 1996.

49. Shih, W.J., Sample size reestimation — Journey for a decade, *Stat. Med.*, 20, 515–518, 2001.

50. Wittes, J., On changing a long-term clinical trial midstream, *Stat. Med.*, 27, 2789–2795, 2002.

51. Cui, L., Hung, H.M.J., and Wang, S.J., Modification of sample size in group sequential trials, *Biometrics*, 55, 853–857, 1999.

52. Shih, W.J., Ouyang, P., Quan, H., Lin, Y., Michiels, B., and Bijnens, L., Controlling type I error rate for fast track drug development programmes, *Stat. Med.*, 22, 665–675, 2003.

53. U.S. Department of Health and Human Services, *Section 112 of the Food and Drug Administration Modernization Act of 1997: Expediting Study and Approval of Fast Track Drugs*. http://www.fda.gov/cder/guidance/index.htm, 1997.

54. U.S. Department of Health and Human Services, *Guidance for Industry: Fast Track Drug Development Programs — Designation, Development, and Application Review*, http://www.fda.gov/cder/guidance/index.htm, 1998.

8 Design and Analysis of Testosterone Replacement Therapy Trials

Ted M. Smith

CONTENTS

I. INTRODUCTION

Testosterone (abbreviated as T in this chapter) in the male is associated with sexual function and fertility, intellectual capacity, depression, fatigue, body composition (muscle and fat mass), muscle strength, bone mineral density (BMD), and red blood cell production.[1] Deficiency in testosterone has been associated with sexual dysfunction of low libido, poor sexual performance, lack of spontaneous erections, poor erectile quality,[2] reduced muscle mass, increased body fat (visceral fat), increased risk of osteoporosis, negative mood and/or depression, and decreased red blood cell production.

Primary hypogonadism is defined as a testicular failure to produce T and can be caused by Klinefelter's Syndrome, cryptorchidism, vanishing testis syndrome, bilateral torsion, orchitis, orchiectomy, chemotherapy or toxic damage from radiation, alcohol, or heavy metals. Secondary hypogonadism is defined as hypothalamic–pituitary failure to simulate testicular testosterone production and can be caused by idiopathic gonadotropin or luteinizing hormone releasing hormone (LHRH) deficiency or pituitary–hypothalamic injury from tumors, trauma, radiation, or Kallmann's Syndrome. Age-dependent decline in testosterone levels is with associated decreases in muscle mass and strength, BMD, libido and sexual desire, or increases in body fat.[3] Testosterone levels have been reported to decrease in males over 40 years of age at a rate of approximately 1% a year.[4] As a result, 12% of men in the age bracket of 50 to 59 years are estimated to have a deficiency in testosterone, 19% of men between 60 and 69 years, 28% of men between 70 and 79 years, and 49% of men over 80 years.

A. PHYSIOLOGY

Testosterone is approximately 98% bound to the sex hormone-binding globulin (SHBG) in the blood and albumin. Approximately 2% of T in circulation is unbound (free T). Because of the high affinity between T and SHBG, the T bound to SHBG is not available to most tissues for androgenic action, whereas the free T and the T bound to albumin is bioavailable to most tissues for androgenic action (bioavailable T = 70% of circulating T). SHBG levels increase with age and as a result, many older men will have total T levels in the low-to-normal range but will have free or bioavailable T levels that are below the normal range for young men.[5]

The active metabolites of T are estradiol (E2) and 5 alpha-dihydrotesto-sterone (DHT). These metabolites, in part, may mediate many of the actions of T. DHT is a more potent androgen than T.

B. GOALS OF TESTOSTERONE REPLACEMENT

Goals of testosterone replacement therapy (TRT) are to restore libido and regain sexual function, improve energy and restore positive mood, improve mental acuity, reduce body fat, restore muscle mass and strength, and improve BMD.[1]

Current options for testosterone replacement are oral testosterone, injectable testosterone esters, transdermal patches, and transdermal gels. Oral formulations suffer from inconsistent serum T levels and possible hepatotoxicity. Injectables provide more infrequent dosing options, but suffer from supraphysiological serum T levels that return to subtherapeutic levels before the next injection. Transdermal patches maintain serum T levels in a normal range, but suffer from high dermal reactions that often result in discontinuation. Transdermal gels maintain serum T levels in a normal range with long-term therapy with a convenient once a day dosing but have a potential for transfer to a partner or child.

II. GENERAL DESIGN CONSIDERATIONS OF TRT TRIALS

Goals of TRT trials should be two-fold:

1. Establish that serum T levels are increased into the normal range.
2. Establish that clinical endpoints such as sexual functions, body composition, mood, and BMD improved through the increase in serum T levels.

The first goal is essentially pharmacokinetic and should be established relative to an active comparator, e.g., transdermal patches or transdermal gels. Because of the large intersubject variation in response to TRT, the trial should include a component with titration of the dosage of T in the treatment regimen to provide useful information for prescribing physicians. The titration decision should be based on the steady state T levels obtained after an initial dosing period. The titration decision can be part of a double-blind trial or part of an open label extension.

The second is a clinical goal and must be established relative to a placebo comparator to achieve clinical objectivity. Depending on the choice of active comparator and experimental treatment regimen, it may not be possible to have a completely blinded clinical trial with placebo and active comparator. A new drug application (NDA) approved by the FDA included an open label active comparator of a transdermal patch and blinded treatment arms of two doses of a transdermal gel and a matching placebo gel. Both TRT goals were achieved with this design.[6]

A. SERUM TESTOSTERONE LEVELS

Testosterone levels follow a daily circadian variation in untreated healthy young men with the maximum levels observed in the morning (8 to 9 a.m.) and minimum levels observed in the afternoon.[9] A 24 h pharmacokinetic (PK) profile on specific days throughout the study is required to establish the first goal with the number of serum sample collection time points depending on the pharmacokinetics of the specific TRT. Typically, serum collection time points of 0 h (predose), 2, 4, 8, 12, and 24 h (postdose) will often suffice. A collection time between 12 and 24 h postdose is only required if a significant maximum concentration is expected during that time period. Otherwise, this additional collection time does not add much to the establishment of the first goal and adds a tremendous burden for the clinical trial centers and their subjects.

In contrast to many other areas of clinical trial research, there are endogenous levels of T circulating in the body naturally, even in most men with testosterone deficiency. Testosterone supplementation adds exogenous T to this circulating system. The body's natural biofeedback system will alter the level of endogenous T levels in response to the addition of exogenous T. After TRT, the T levels are a combination of both naturally occurring endogenous T and supplemented exogenous T. Consequently, to measure the effect of the TRT, a baseline 24 h PK profile is required before treatment begins, which measures the naturally occurring endogenous T levels.

Serum profiles should be collected at baseline and once a month for the duration of the study for T, free T, and DHT. Serum E2 levels should be collected at a single collection time during each 24 h PK profile. This is usually during the predose 0 h collection time point. Serum T, DHT, and free T levels should be measured by a central laboratory because of large interlaboratory variations in the assays available. It is critical that the appropriate assay method be used to measure each of the serum parameters, particularly for free T.

B. Clinical Endpoints

Three potential clinical endpoints are presented, which address very different clinical questions. Sexual function is a question of lifestyle and quality of life. Body composition is a question of ability to carry out daily activities easily and efficiently and may also be related to diabetes.[7] BMD is really a surrogate for osteoporosis and risk of fractures. Although older men may have a lower risk of fractures compared with women, the mortality from these fractures may be higher.[8]

The time of response to TRT for these three endpoints varies significantly. Sexual function parameters may respond within the first 30 days of treatment, body compositions will respond within 90 days of treatment, whereas BMD will take 12 to 18 months before a measurable effect will be seen. In contrast, the impact on fracture rates has yet to be studied and may require a trial duration of 5 years or more to see an effect. Consequently, the duration of the clinical trial depends on which clinical endpoints are required for the indication sought.

Other clinical endpoints may be used, depending on the indication and population of interest. A comprehensive summary of other clinical endpoints, especially for older men, is presented in Ref. 5.

1. Sexual Functions

Sexual function can be measured using several methods. A number of questionnaires have been developed for different aspects of sexual function. The questionnaire selected for the clinical trial should measure to some degree erectile dysfunction, spontaneous erections, sexual performance in general, sexual motivation, and libido/desire. Some methods or questions are required to accommodate sexual activity with and without a partner.

Most questionnaires are administered periodically and are based on either the recall method for the last 2 to 4 weeks or on diaries kept daily for 1 week prior to the office visit. One daily diary questionnaire was adapted for use with an interactive voice response system (IVRS) using the telephone. This system required the subject to call each day with the response to several questions. The advantage of this system was that responses were captured in "real time" as opposed to the recall method or to paper diaries, which may be completed on the same day for all days. Thus, both the recall method and paper diaries can be very inaccurate. These questionnaires could be modified for use with other electronic diary techniques such as hand-held personal digital assistants (PDA).

2. Bone Mineral Density

Lumbar spine BMD is the primary endpoint for determining the impact of TRT on BMD. The gold standard for measuring BMD is dual x-ray absorptiometry (DXA). This technique allows the use of intercenter calibration, if needed, when pooling across centers. Data can be analyzed by a central reader, to increase consistency. If possible, a machine produced by the same manufacturer should be used at all centers.

3. Body Composition

Recent advances in DXA technology has made this technique a viable way to also measure whole body composition of lean mass and fat mass. Percent fat is derived from the total mass and fat mass. As with BMD measurements, a central reader reads these measurements. If required, specific body areas (such as abdominal fat) can be targeted for special consideration and measurement.

Because muscle mass can also change as a result of muscle/strength training, subjects should either be instructed to not be involved in any muscle training activities or be kept on a constant level of training for the duration of the clinical trial. In the latter case, there may be need of some adjustment either at the time of randomization or at the time of analysis to account for possible differences in level of muscle training.

III. INCLUSION/EXCLUSION CRITERIA

Inclusion/exclusion criteria should reflect the population that will eventually receive the TRT. Listed below are criteria from Phase III TRT trials submitted to the FDA.

A. INCLUSION CRITERIA

The two primary inclusion criteria are the serum T levels and symptoms of testosterone deficiency presented during screening. Two serum T levels should be obtained 1 week apart, and both should be below 300 ng/dl (nanograms per deciliter). Intrasubject variability is high enough so that approximately 15% of men with normal serum T levels will have a single morning serum T level below 300 ng/dl.[9] The serum levels must be taken during the morning (8 to 9 a.m.) because of the diurnal variation observed in T levels. Also, levels of luteinizing hormone (LH) and follicle-stimulating hormone (FSH) should be measured to provide a complete gonadotropic picture at baseline. In addition, a subject should present with one or more symptoms of low testosterone (i.e., fatigue, decreased muscle mass, reduced libido, or reduced sexual functioning of a nonmechanical nature).

Other inclusion criteria are as follows. Subject should be judged to be in otherwise good health, based upon the results of a medical history, physical examination, and laboratory profile. Subject's body mass index (kg/m^2) should be between 18 and 31. It should be noted that subjects who are extremely obese may have difficulty having BMD or body composition measured by DXA. Subjects receiving lipid-lowering agents, anxiolytics, lithium, antidepressants, hypnotics, or antipsychotics must have been on a stable dose for at least 3 months prior to entering the study. Subjects who have benign prostatic hypertrophy (BPH) can be allowed into the study if they have normal prostate specific antigen (PSA) levels and, in the investigators' opinion, are not at risk for urinary obstruction. Subjects receiving treatment α_1 blockers or herbal treatment for BPH must have been on a stable dose for at least 3 months prior to entering the study.

B. EXCLUSION CRITERIA

The two primary sets of exclusion criteria are concerned with subjects taking medications that may interfere with or enhance androgen metabolism and with subjects who have undiagnosed prostate cancer.

The following relate to prohibitive medications. Subject is using medications that may interfere with androgen metabolism (i.e., spironolactone, finasteride, or ketoconazole). Subject has received any estrogen therapy, a lutenizing hormone releasing hormone (LHRH) antagonist, or human growth hormone therapy within the last 12 months prior to the screening visit. Subject was treated with either a testosterone ester injection within the last 8 weeks, or with an oral or transdermal patch or gel androgen within the last 6 weeks prior to start of dosing. Subject is receiving supplements that are supposed to be anabolic such as dehydroepian-drosterone (DHEA) and creatine.

A patient who has diagnosed prostatic cancer or a history thereof, palpable prostatic masses or serum levels of PSA > 4 ng/ml is excluded.

Other diseased populations to exclude are: subject currently has uncontrolled diabetes, subject has clinically significant anemia or renal dysfunction, subject has any evidence of hepatic dysfunction, and subject has hyperparathyroidism. In later trials these men may be studied. Subjects receiving Viagra® or other treatments for erectile dysfunction should be excluded if sexual function is a clinical endpoint.

IV. EFFICACY

A. Serum T, Free T, DHT Levels

The following PK parameters should be computed for each 24 h PK profile for serum T, free T, and DHT:

- C_{avg} = area under the 24 h concentration curve using the linear trapezoidal rule divided by the length of the 24 h sampling time period. This parameter can also be viewed as a time-dependent weighted average of the serum levels from the 24 h sampling period.
- C_{min} = minimum measured postdose serum concentration.
- C_{max} = maximum measured postdose serum concentration.

1. Normalization of Serum T Levels

Normalization of T levels has not been a simple concept to quantify because of the history of the various types of testosterone replacement therapies currently on the market. The initial and very intuitive definition is based on C_{avg} alone, namely:

- Definition 1: Serum T levels are normalized if C_{avg} is within the normal range of young healthy men, usually 300 to 1000 ng/dl.

Typically, many of the current TRT will result in approximately 60 to 80% of all subjects showing normalization of T levels, depending on the dose level. However, the different TRTs achieve this degree of normalization in many different ways, often with large fluctuations over the dosing period including T levels that approximated pretreatment T-deficient levels. In light of large fluctuations over a dosing period, the FDA proposed a more restrictive definition of normalization:

- Definition 2: Serum T levels are normalized if both C_{avg} and C_{min} are within the normal range (300 to 1000 ng/dl).

This definition will separate injectable forms of TRTs and transdermal patch TRTs from transdermal gel TRTs. Typically, transdermal patches will have a smaller normalization rate than those achieved with transdermal gels.

2. Analysis of T Levels

The primary analysis should be based on the comparison of the normalization rate of the experimental TRT with an active comparator TRT. The analysis could be used to show equivalence/superiority of one dose of the experimental TRT to a comparable dose of the active comparator, as well as to show a dose response between two doses of the experimental TRT.

Further characterization of the response profile can be obtained with an Analysis of Covariance (ANCOVA) of the change from baseline for the individual PK parameters with the appropriate baseline parameter as a covariate. The change from baseline is the appropriate parameter that adjusts for the existence of endogenous T levels occurring naturally before T supplementation. The addition of the baseline values to the analysis of covariance will adjust the comparison for any potential differences at baseline that may occur. In addition, if only one screening T level was obtained instead of the recommended two screening levels, the baseline C_{avg} could be used to stratify those subjects with baseline C_{avg} below 300 ng/dl from those with baseline C_{avg} above 300 ng/dl. Then this stratification variable could be used in the final analysis. However, the inclusion of this stratification typically does not affect any of the conclusions.

3. Analysis of Free T and DHT

There are no acceptable definitions of normalization of free T or DHT in T-deficient men. Therefore, the ANCOVA analysis should be used for changes from baseline in the three PK parameters for free T and DHT. In a short-term study it is expected that free T will follow the same pattern as T levels.

The response for DHT will depend on the type of experimental TRT being studied. The metabolism of T to DHT can occur internally as well at various locations on the skin and genital areas. For example, the DHT response is different between transdermal patches and transdermal gels, probably because of the conversion of T to DHT taking place at the skin and the difference in skin area exposed to the exogenous T between the gel and the patch. This difference in conversion sites is also reflected in the ratio of DHT/T, once converted to the same unit. Serum T levels are typically measured in ng/dl and serum DHT levels in picograms per milliliter (pg/ml). Hence, an additional characterization of the DHT response is provided by an ANCOVA for the change from baseline in this ratio.

B. Serum E2

The same ANCOVA analysis for the change from baseline, as used with serum T, should be used for serum E2. A similar pattern as seen with serum T is expected because the primary source of E2 is from conversion of serum T.

C. Clinical Endpoints

Each of the proposed clinical endpoints should be analyzed also with an ANCOVA for the actual value or the change from baseline with the appropriate baseline parameter as covariate. In addition, there may be several other baseline parameters, which may help explain the degree of clinical effect that could be used in multivariate exploratory and/or confirmatory analyses.

There are still open questions about potential threshold levels for serum T above which no additional clinical benefit may be seen. These threshold levels will vary for the different clinical endpoints. There are enough data to explore pharmacokinetic/pharmacodynamic relationships between clinical endpoints and serum T, free T, and/or DHT levels.

D. Sample Size Considerations

Typically for a phase III trial 80 to 90 subjects per treatment arm will be sufficient to establish equivalence/superiority of treatment regimens with respect to normalization of serum T levels based on Definition 2. Sample sizes will increase when the different clinical endpoints are considered. The largest studies will be those based on fracture rates, in which several thousand subjects per treatment regimen will be required to show clinical benefit.

Approximately one of every three men who present with some symptom of T deficiency will also have a serum T level below 300 ng/dl. Consequently, one would expect to need to screen approximately three men who may have symptoms of low T to randomize one man for a clinical trial.

V. SAFETY

Potential risks for TRT include polycythemia (increased red blood cell mass [RBC]), increased hemoglobin (Hgb), increased hematocrit (Hct), changes in PSA levels, gynecomastia, and sleep apnea. Unknown at this time is the effect of TRT on BPH or prostate cancer. Therefore, in addition to standard safety surveillance for any clinical trial, special considerations must be given to monitoring RBC, Hgb, Hct, and PSA levels, symptoms of BPH, and prostate cancer.

A. PROSTATE

Periodic assessment for BPH symptoms using the International Prostate Symptom Score (I-PSS) should be obtained throughout the clinical trial. In addition, at minimum a pre- and end-study examination of the prostate, including a digital rectal exam (DRE) and PSA level, should be performed for all subjects.

VI. CONCLUSION

TRT trials in men with testosterone deficiency have increased in number over the last decade. Short-term trials have clearly indicated that various techniques are available for delivery of exogenous testosterone to men, which will increase circulating T levels into the normal range for healthy young men. In addition some placebo-controlled trials have shown the clinical benefit of TRT for some clinical parameters. The FDA is exploring guidelines for such trials. At the same time, there is a need to conduct longer term trials in larger numbers of subjects to see the actual long-term benefits and long-term risks for TRT in men with testosterone deficiency.

REFERENCES

1. Morales, A., Heaton, J.P.W., and Carson, C.C. III, Andropause: a Misnomer for a true clinical entity, *J. Urol.*, 163, 705–712, 2000.
2. Morales, A. and Lunenfeld, B., Replacement therapy in aging men with secondary hypogonadism, *Aging Male*, 4, 151–162, 2001.
3. Vermeulen, A., Commentary: androgen replacement therapy in the aging male-A critical evaluation, *J. Clin. Endocrinol. Metab.*, 86, 2380–2390, 2001.
4. Harman, S.M., Metter, E.J., Tobin, J.D., Pearson, J., and Blackman, M.R., Longitudinal effects of aging on serum total and free testosterone levels in healthy men. Baltimore longitudinal study of aging, *J. Clin. Endocrinol. Metab.*, 86, 724–731, 2001.
5. Matsumoto, A.M., Andropause: clinical implications of the decline in serum testosterone levels with aging men, *J. Gerontol. Med. Sci.*, 57A, M76–M99, 2002.
6. Testim™ North American Study Group, Steidle, C., Schwartz, S., Jacoby, K., Sebree, T., Smith, T., and Bachand, R., AA2500 testosterone gel normalizes androgen levels in aging males with improvements in body composition and sexual function, *J. Clin. Endocrinol. Metab.*, 88, 2673–2681, 2003.
7. Abate, N., Haffner, S.M., Garg, A., Peshook, R.M., and Grundy, S.M., Sex steroid hormones, upper body obesity, and insulin resistance, *J. Clin. Endocrinol. Metab.*, 87, 4522–4527, 2002.
8. Center, J.R., Nguygen, T.V., Schneider, D., Sambrook, P.N., and Eisman, J.A., Mortality after all major types of osteoporotic fracture in men and women: an observational study, *Lancet*, 353, 878–882, 1999.
9. Spratt, D.I., O'Dea, L.S.L., Schoenfeld, D., Butler, J., Rao, P.N., and Crowley, W.F. Jr., Neuroendocrine–gonadal axis in men: frequent sampling of LH, FSH, and testosterone, *Am. J. Physiol.*, 254, E658 1988.

9 Clinical Trials of Analgesic Drugs

Cynthia G. McCormick

CONTENTS

I. INTRODUCTION

Tremendous groundwork has been laid over the last half century by pioneer researchers in analgesic drug evaluation. Early analgesic trials to evaluate the properties of opioid drug products brought out critically important insights through *in vivo* human assays, the single-dose relative potency studies. These trials were designed to answer the basic question, whether a test intervention had any analgesic effect. These early trials attempted to accurately and reliably measure pain, the subjective outcome, in the context of a clinical experiment. The clinical pharmacology experiments performed by these early researchers have had a lasting effect on the field. Their legacy was the modern randomized controlled clinical trial in analgesic drug evaluation.

Approval of many of the early analgesic drug products were based on evidence from randomized controlled trials in single-dose studies. As drugs came under regulatory scrutiny, the limitations of these studies became evident without the benefit of basic experiments to define efficacy in the conditions and settings for which approval was sought. As new modified release formulations were developed to address dosing needs for patients suffering from chronic painful conditions, the single-dose pain models were shown to be inadequate to define effectiveness. With this observation it became clear that pain management in the chronic disease setting would require a different approach.

Advances in basic research have led to consideration that studies should be performed to evaluate the effect of drugs on the basic underlying mechanisms of pain, which could be many in the acute or chronic painful condition. This led to the conclusion that for many conditions, one agent may not be sufficient to control pain elicited by a variety of mechanisms, unless a final common pathway could be defined. This approach of polypharmacy-targeting-specific underlying mechanisms has scientific appeal but has not yet gained sufficient practical application.

The innovative beginning of analgesic trials has given way to more traditional approaches, recognizing that the one-size-fits-all trial may not be adequate to characterize the potential drug product for its ultimate usefulness. With the development of agents with unique pharmaco-kinetic properties the clinical trial methodology has matured. Discoveries in basic science have enhanced our understanding of the mechanisms underlying pain so that we can pose more sophisticated questions in the context of clinical trial. Nevertheless, current approaches to the challenge of defining a drug's efficacy as a pain reliever still focus on basic clinical questions, exploring a spectrum of the drug's utility in trials designed to replicate the target conditions. Central questions to the design of these trials include the target population, duration of trial, appropriate dose, outcome measures, high-placebo effects and high-drop-out rates. This chapter focuses on the key elements of studies, which will define the efficacy of an intervention for pain.

II. DESIGN OF ANALGESIC DRUG TRIALS

A. SELECTING THE TARGET PATIENT POPULATION

From the early studies in analgesic development evolved the popular concept of the "pain models," the workhorses of the latter part of the 20th century. These studies were often small, single-dose assays, performed in standard settings, such as the postoperative setting, third molar extraction, or other acute painful conditions. The studies were popular because these were economic and relatively easy to conduct. Despite the usefulness, these studies had limitations. In one sense these were not always true "models" for all of the representative conditions, but rather were founded on the somewhat naive assumption that if the test drug was successful in an analgesic model of pain the results could be generalized to the vast spectrum of painful conditions regardless of etiology or chronicity. While often successful in demonstrating an effect in the acute setting, these models left questions about the dose, duration, and regimen.

It is necessary to evaluate the effectiveness of analgesic interventions in the representative population intended to be used. The likely target population for an analgesic under development may depend on a number of factors including the purported mechanism of action, likely biochemical or physiological target determined from nonclinical studies, past performance of drugs in a similar class, pharmaco-kinetic properties of the drug in human, and manner in which the drug is formulated to achieve that pharmaco-kinetic profile. It is not feasible or necessary to test a drug in all potentially relevant clinical settings; it is important to try to define the most representative of these in which to perform the key clinical trials.

B. THE CHOICE OF CONTROL GROUP

The selection of the control group is one of the most challenging and important decisions in designing a clinical trial for analgesic drug products. The particularly high placebo response rate characteristic of analgesic trials, the frequent occurrence of variable and even negative performance of known analgesics across studies, and the subjective nature of the outcome being measured all argue for the use of a solid anchor to establish the sensitivity of the analgesic trial.[1] The placebo control is by far the highest standard for the analgesic trial.

Ethical and practical concerns are often raised about performing studies with an untreated or placebo control group in painful conditions particularly for studies of 3 or 6 months' duration. These concerns can be overcome by applying a variety of strategies or trial designs to minimize the untreated state. One of these includes the use of rescue medication.

In the setting of clinical analgesic trials, rescue is a strategy by which a known analgesic treatment is introduced to alleviate painful symptoms that arise during any phase of the clinical trial. Rescue medication may be administered to patients in the placebo group or even to the experimental treatment group, depending on the study design and conditions of blinding. The rescue medication is administered after the primary outcome measurement is obtained. The use of rescue medication may be helpful in preventing symptom-related attrition from clinical trials; however, caution is warranted, as the use of this strategy may dilute the difference in effect size between the placebo and treated groups. Whenever rescue medication is used, provisions should be made to analyze the influence of the rescue medication on the outcome of the trial.

It may be appropriate in some instances to design a study using more than one type of concurrent control. Whereas U.S. regulatory standards for drug approval do not require the demonstration of superiority to an existing marketed product, from the perspective of patient care, it is often useful to know how agents compare with each other in certain clinical settings. Therefore, use of an active control in addition to a placebo can provide a useful clinical internal gauge of the sensitivity of the trial to assay analgesic effect and may be useful when considering international marketing.

Active control trials that do not make use of a concurrent internal placebo comparator are often subject to misinterpretation and may lead to erroneous conclusions. The comparison of the test drug against a standard analgesic drug may yield useful information if the test drug is shown to be statistically and significantly superior to the standard analgesic or *vice versa*. If the drugs perform in a similar manner, and no significant difference can be demonstrated, such a finding may simply reflect inadequate sensitivity of the assay to distinguish between the treatments and does not establish the effectiveness of either drug. To avoid such an ambiguous outcome, the use of an internal placebo anchor can be incorporated into the study design. In this way, the assay should be able to distinguish the placebo from the standard control defining its level of activity in this population, setting and trial as conducted. This design will allow for the optimal comparison of the test drug with a commonly used analgesic.

The dose-controlled study is a variation on the placebo-controlled trial. In such a study, two or more doses of the test drug are compared with each other with or without a placebo group. In selecting doses one should explore the entire dose-response curve of the test drug. Data should be collected on doses that are expected to be above and below the recommended doses. When this trial design is used it is important to take into account the pharmaco-kinetic profile of the drug, avoiding any overlap in plasma concentrations or area under the plasma concentration curve (AUC). These dose-ranging studies are conducted as fixed-dose trials in which patients are randomized to one of several doses of the treatment drug that remains constant throughout the duration of the study. Such designs are of tremendous usefulness in evaluating the minimum effective dose in a population that is being initiated on therapy. However, for chronic dosing studies, particularly in the case of the opioid drug products with a wide therapeutic window, where dose individualization and escalation have occurred, fixed dose studies may not be meaningful or feasible. In this latter setting, other more flexible dosing strategies may be required.

Regardless of the control group or groups chosen, the success of the analgesic trial is determined by having some internal measure of assay sensitivity. In general, the performance of a test analgesic in a clinical trial varies across the population studied. In most of the studies the relief of painful symptoms is partial and quite variable. The demonstration of efficacy in one study may not predict a similar performance of the drug in another study, even when the methodology is ostensibly similar. A study that does not contain some measure of assay sensitivity is not considered capable of providing substantial evidence for the effectiveness of a new analgesic.

C. Outcome Measures

Pain is a purely subjective and patient-based symptom, but it is clearly of interest in analgesic trials and the evaluation of an analgesic drug should measure pain as the primary outcome. There are a number of parameters that could be considered in this evaluation, including pain intensity (PI) and pain relief (PR), temporal aspects of pain, pain quality, and distribution. It is not necessary for a given clinical trial to encompass all of these types of outcomes, and one is selected as the principal outcome of interest—most frequently it is PI.

While it can be argued that pain is an inherently subjective symptom complex modulated by a host of physiological and psychological factors, there are a number of metrics that define and quantify this symptom complex. In selecting a measurement tool to assess this outcome in analgesic trials, one should consider how reliable a measurement is in assessing the patient's self-report of symptoms. The measurement's reliability partly depends on the patient's ability to understand and apply the scales.

An abundance of scales exists but by far the most widely used are the single item ratings of PI such as the Visual Analog Scales (VAS), the Numerical Rating Scales (NRS), and the Verbal Rating Scales (VRS). The VAS is constructed to allow the patient to choose from an entire spectrum of possible levels of pain, showing no pain on one end of a line (usually the left of a horizontal line) and extreme pain on the other end, usually the right in a scale of zero to 100. The patient places a mark on the line, which corresponds to the degree of pain experienced at the time of assessment. The VAS pain score is the distance from zero (no pain). The scale is accepted as sensitive because there is a wide range of choice available to reflect the interpretation of symptoms. One of the shortcomings of the VAS is the patient's subjectivity required to arrive at an appropriate numeral and in some cases it may be more difficult for patients to correctly understand and interpret the pain in terms of the scale even with assistance. Nevertheless, this scale is reliable with high correlation within studies of other measures of PI.

Use of NRS in measuring PI is another approach to quantify subjective symptoms of pain. The NRS consists of a spectrum of numbers, usually between zero and ten as in the case of the Likert scale, ranging from no pain to extreme pain or "the worst pain that you can imagine." Patients are asked to respond, most often verbally, with their assessment about where their pain falls within this spectrum. The properties of this rating scale are similar to those of the VAS. One notable shortcoming is the tendency of patients to be conservative about their assessment of numerals anticipating that pain may indeed worsen with time. Most of these scales are simple, quick and easy to administer, and are relatively easy to understand.

Another form of a pain assessment is the VRS in which the patient chooses among a variety of categories describing the intensity of pain or degree of PR. For example, in the traditional four-point categorical scale of PI, the patient must choose among four categories described as *none*, *slight*, *moderate*, and *severe*, with numbers assigned to the categories for purposes of calculation and analysis. These scores are reported as continuous variables. The advantage to this type of scale is that the descriptors are easy to interpret; the disadvantage is that there may not be sufficient degrees of gradation to adequately characterize the patient's pain. These measures provide a relatively intuitive means to assess outcome, both for the patient and for the person interpreting the results.

The scales can be used to measure PI or PR. There are advantages and disadvantages to these approaches. The direct measurement of PI has the advantage of measuring contemporaneous pain and does not rely upon memory of past symptoms. It assumes that other factors that may influence the patient's interpretation of pain are stable or at least random, which will reduce power. The measurement of PR, on the other hand, allows the patient to incorporate some degree of interpretation of symptoms as better, worse or the same. Littman et al.[2] compare visual pain analog, verbal PI and verbal PR and conclude that these scales are highly correlated with minimal difference in sensitivity. These analgesic rating scales provide a simple means for patients to rate PI in a unidimensional scale.

In many clinical trials that use rescue medication, a quantification of rescue medication is used as a confirmation or a cross-check against the results of the pain rating assessment. It is quite clear that the results of the VAS may be influenced by the amount, timing, and characteristics of the rescue medication. It is common for the use of rescue medication to dilute the effect of an active treatment by providing response in the placebo arm of a trial. In the case of a less effective active medication, if the trial is found to be successful because of the excessive use of rescue in the treatment arm, the results can be misleading.

Some trials are specifically designed to study the effect of rescue medication directly as a primary outcome. In these trials the use of active rescue compared with placebo rescue can be used to assess the effect of an intervention on the treatment of breakthrough pain.

Studies that focus only on indirect outcomes such as analgesic sparing effect or time to rescue medication, have been proposed. These studies, while they provide some useful information, do not necessarily capture the essential features of the effect of the drug on the outcome of interest, that is, their primary performance as an analgesic.

D. DURATION OF STUDY

The duration of the analgesic trial should be determined by the characteristics of the condition being evaluated. For example, studies in acute pain should not last longer than the expected duration of the pain. Postoperative pain studies should be designed duly considering the fact that the intensity of pain can be expected to be maximal once the effect of anesthetics has subsided and the pain will gradually attenuate with time following the surgery. Ideally the duration of the study should last no longer than the period of maximal pain, unless the goal of the study is to evaluate tapering strategies.

In the case of chronic pain, there may be day-to-day or even week-to-week fluctuations in the intensity of pain, and in some cases because of underlying disease factors, symptoms may even intensify over time. Clinical trials evaluating the effect of a drug in chronic pain should be of sufficient length to allow for a trend in the response to treatment rather than the natural fluctuations to be measured. In general, chronic pain studies should be conducted for a duration of no less than 3 months.

In the case of the opioid drug products, the phenomenon of tolerance may be expected to occur after the first few weeks to a month. Tolerance can be suspected if there are increasing symptoms of pain associated with an increasing requirement for medication. Trials of several months duration allow for this phenomenon to be identified and studied in a controlled setting. In some instances, it may be desirable to specifically design a trial to study the development of tolerance as it may have important clinical and safety implications.

E. DESIGN

There is a multitude of study designs that have been and can be used in the evaluation of analgesic drugs, but by far the three most widely used include *prospective randomized parallel-group design, placebo-controlled add-on trial*, and *crossover design*. These will be discussed in order of importance and regulatory stature.[3]

1. Parallel-Group Design

The simplest, commonest and most straightforward design is the prospective parallel-design trial in which randomized groups are treated simultaneously for a set period of time. The controls are concurrent and treated identically. Any changes to protocol are applied contemporaneously to all groups.

The parallel-group design is quite flexible and may allow for the addition of a number of features to improve the quality of information gained from the trial. For example, some investigations allow for stratification into subgroups for specific analysis, such as baseline pain, anticipating an analysis of the results as a function of disease severity. Other examples of stratification allow for analysis by gender, previous treatment, or etiology of pain.

Parallel design trials may incorporate titration paradigms to allow for gradual acclimation onto treatment regimens, and fixed vs. flexible dosing. This feature is of particular value for treatments for which there is an anticipated high attrition because of adverse events. Titration may considerably reduce the intolerance to side effects, risk of unblinding and burden of imputing results caused by drop-outs related to adverse events.

Parallel design trials may be conducted as fixed dose trials or may employ strategies such as individualization of dose. The latter is a particularly common strategy for chronic pain trials of opioids, where tolerance and disease severity have resulted in considerable variability in baseline opioid medication dosage in patients entering the trials. The trial includes a period prior to randomization during which the patient is stabilized on a formulation and dose of the active intervention (test drug), which is predicted to be comparable with the patient's existing therapy. This is done in an effort to reduce the possibility of withdrawal effects or rebound pain. While properties of opioids may vary from one another, and doses cannot be predicted with complete accuracy, this strategy is found to be helpful in reducing the early drop-outs.

Fixed dose parallel-group studies are the preferred design for acute pain studies. This design, when combined with the dose comparator and placebo control, has the clear advantage of accurately determining the minimum effective dose for treatment of pain and may lend itself to strategies of measuring time to onset of effective treatment.

2. Add-on Design

A study design, which has not been commonly used in the evaluation of therapies for chronic pain, is the add-on study where the intervention is studied against a background of existing analgesic therapy. The placebo-controlled add-on trial is the most basic design in this class. This trial design has the clear advantage of being able to evaluate a new medication in a relevant clinical context while maintaining a stable regimen. It also allows for the comparison to proceed over several months and virtually eliminates the need for the usual heavy reliance upon rescue medication, resulting in a cleaner comparison of the two study arms. The clearest advantage of this design is that it will allow for a clean straightforward placebo-controlled comparison to take place without the:

- concern about deterioration over the course of several months
- risk of disproportionate drop-outs in the control group
- necessity to use rescue medication

This design also offers a closer approximation of actual clinical practice than the alternatives, providing valuable information about safety, tolerance, and effectiveness in the context of existing concomitant treatments. Some of the apparent lack of popularity of this design results from the expectation that such a trial would likely lead to an adjunctive therapy indication.

3. Crossover-Design

The crossover-design is one in which each patient receives both or all treatments in the study, but in a randomized prespecified sequence. The design has the advantage of being able to increase the sensitivity by allowing within-patient comparisons, rather than between-patient comparisons.

There are many disadvantages to this study design and it is rarely used for regulatory decisions. The studies have been criticized because of carryover effects from one analgesic treatment period to the next because of inadequate time between treatments, even when pharmaco-kinetics would have predicted that no residual plasma blood levels are measurable. This is of particular concern in chronic pain studies.

In acute pain studies, such as postoperative or dental pain, the intensity of the pain will likely have changed from one period to the next based solely on natural history, rendering the within-patient comparison invalid and the results impossible to interpret. This study design is not really feasible for short duration pain.

III. INTERPRETATION OF RESULTS

The efficacy of a particular dose of a test drug is most commonly established by demonstrating a statistically significant difference in analgesic effect on the selected analgesic measure between the treatment and placebo groups by comparing group means of a given outcome.[4] Alternatively, one could, based on an *a priori* definition of response, demonstrate a statistically significant difference between the percentage of patients who meet the definition of responders in the treatment and the responders in the placebo group. How one defines a responder in this setting is a matter of debate.

Assessing the clinical meaningfulness of a change, whether measured by patient report of PR or a difference in the PI values recorded on a scale, is a challenge. Attempts to define a clinically meaningful outcome have relied largely on either an arbitrary definition set by the investigator, or by the use of global rating scales that may be influenced by a number of factors, some unrelated to the intervention's ability to control pain. One approach that has considerable promise is the correlation of the change in VAS with a categorical measurement of patient improvement.[5] Such an approach allows the correlation of a percentage of improvement with a patient's own assessment of clinically meaningful improvement. Additional objectivity can be gained by measuring the effect of an intervention on other dimensions such as pain quality, temporal aspects of pain, and pain distribution.

IV. UNIQUE CHALLENGES IN THE ANALGESIC TRIAL

One of the most significant challenges to the success of an analgesic trial for drugs that are centrally acting is the effect of the profile of central nervous system (CNS) adverse events. These effects may result in unblinding of the study, influencing the validity of pain measurements, or leading to an unacceptably high level of drop-outs.

Blinding is an important tool in reducing bias in a controlled trial. In the cases where a treatment with a very prominent or bothersome adverse event profile is compared with placebo, successful blinding may be a significant challenge. This is of particular concern with CNS adverse effects. Strategies that reduce the CNS effects such as slow induction may serve to attenuate the difference between treatment and placebo groups.

Another significant challenge of analgesic trials is the recognized problem of differential drop-out rates. This problem arises when in the course of a chronic dosing study, the patients receiving placebo withdraw because of a lack of perceived effectiveness, while patients in the treatment arm may have an early but significant attrition because of intolerable adverse events. This differential drop-out rate may tend to amplify the effectiveness of the drug when prescribed in the manner studied, when indeed the patient may never realize adequate PR at the tolerated doses.

The use of rescue medication has been alluded to as a means to reduce the excessive attrition from placebo-controlled trials because of a lack of perceived effectiveness in the placebo arm. This practice can have the unwanted result of diluting the differences in treatment between the two arms, resulting in a very small effect size or no separation between the treatments. Timing of the measurement of outcomes relative to rescue medication is as essential as the comparison of the quantity of rescue medication between the treatment and control arms of the study.

A unique feature of analgesic trials of opioid medications is the phenomenon of tolerance. Tolerance can be described as the increase in the dosage requirement for medication over time, combined with the reduction in effectiveness of a previous dose. The result of tolerance to opioids is the increase in doses over time in individuals who require chronic treatment. The phenomenon is accompanied by acclimatization to many of the adverse effects of these medications, such as respiratory depression and somnolence, such that higher doses can be tolerated without serious risk to the patient. The challenge that tolerance presents in the evaluation of clinical trials is that the effectiveness of the drug may appear to be lost at the end of the evaluation period, if this effect is not anticipated and analysis is planned.

V. CONCLUSION

Tremendous progress has been made in the design and interpretation of clinical trials for analgesic drug products over the last half century. It is expected that as further progress is made in the basic understanding of pain mechanisms, more sophisticated outcome measures will be developed and validated allowing for greater precision and predictability of response to analgesic drugs.

REFERENCES

1. ICH topic E10. *Choice of a Control Group in Clinical Trials (CPMC/ICH/364/ 96)*, 27 July, 2000 (http://www.emea.eu.int/pdfs/human/ich/036496en.pdf).
2. Littman, G.S., Walker, B.R., and Schneider, B.E., Reassessment of verbal and visual analog ratings in analgesic studies, *Clin. Pharmacol. Ther.*, 38, 16–23, 1985.
3. Guideline for the Clinical Evaluation of Analgesic Trials. US Department of Health and Human Services, Public Health Service, FDA, December 1992.

4. Green, J.W., Design and analysis of clinical trials of analgesic drugs, In *Statistics in the Pharmaceutical Industry, Revised and Expanded*, 2nd ed., Buncher, C.R. and Tsay, J.Y., eds., Marcel Dekker, New York, pp. 181–191, 1994.
5. Farrar, J.T., Young, J.P. Jr., La Moreaux, L., Werth, J.L., and Poole, R.M., Clinical importance of changes in chronic PI measured on an 11-point numerical pain rating scale, *Pain*, 94, 149–158, 2001.

10 Statistical Issues in HIV/AIDS Research

Ronald J. Bosch and C. Ralph Buncher

CONTENTS

I. INTRODUCTION

In the last decade, the field of HIV/AIDS research has changed dramatically. The introduction of potent antiretroviral combination therapy ("cocktail" therapy) in the mid 1990s has led to significant decreases in HIV/AIDS morbidity and mortality in those countries where patients can afford these regimens.[1] These regimens are difficult to tolerate, though, and drug toxicities may require additional treatment. However, the spread of the world HIV/AIDS pandemic continues, especially in southern Africa, where antiretroviral treatment is still only minimally available. An HIV vaccine is urgently needed to alter the devastating course of this disease that infects 38 million people worldwide, of whom only a fraction in need are receiving antiretroviral treatment.[2]

This review chapter highlights various statistical issues relevant to HIV/AIDS research. Statisticians in this field have created or improved many statistical methods of design and analysis. Awareness of these issues and the cited references should aid statisticians working in this field. Many of these issues, especially relating to the use of surrogate markers in clinical trials, are relevant to statisticians and clinicians investigating other diseases where clinical disease may take years to develop.

II. CHARACTERISTICS OF HIV/AIDS TRIALS VS. OTHER PHARMACEUTICAL RESEARCH

– Chronic disease, many years to clinical disease — use of surrogate markers as study endpoints.
– Multidrug combination therapy. Studies examine the optimal use of different manufacturers' drugs used in combination. Sequential strategies of drug combinations are impacted by the development of drug resistance, especially multidrug resistance.
– HIV vaccine research. With potentially minimal return on investment in developing countries for preventive vaccines, public/nonprofit/private funding mechanisms are used to support HIV vaccine development (e.g., International AIDS Vaccine Initiative/AlphaVax, NIH/VaxGen).

III. DESIGN AND ANALYSIS OF HIV CLINICAL TRIALS

A. THERAPEUTICS

Corresponding to the changes in treatment and improved outcomes, the design of clinical trials to evaluate anti-HIV therapeutics has changed substantially in the last 10 years. Early trials were powered to detect differences in clinical endpoint rates, such as progression to AIDS and death.[3–6] However, as potent antiretroviral regimens including protease inhibitors became available and clinical progression rates were thereby reduced, the necessary sample size and duration for comparative trials with clinical endpoints became very large. Also, in the mid 1990s, viral load assays were developed to measure the concentration of HIV virions in blood plasma.[7] These HIV RNA-based measures of viral load were shown to be prognostic of HIV disease progression,[8–12] and were more quantitative and sensitive than earlier assays.[13,14]

These developments led to new antiretroviral drugs becoming FDA-approved based on their ability to suppress viral load levels after 16 to 24 weeks of treatment. Moreover, short-term viral endpoint studies could be conducted more quickly, and with fewer subjects, than clinical endpoint studies. The FDA continues to view viral load as a key surrogate marker for evaluating antiretroviral agents.[15,16] In addition to predicting clinical outcome, viral load is a natural marker of the biological activity of an antiviral agent. But to be a surrogate marker of therapeutic efficacy, a marker needs to fully account for the clinical efficacy of the therapeutic agent.[17] Yet an important surrogacy issue remains, where studies frequently have not presented purely viral load-based endpoints.[18] Rather, a composite endpoint is constructed so that a subject is considered a success only if viral load is suppressed and the subject also remained on the study-prescribed regimen.[19] Follow-up for viral load and other measurements is often discontinued after stopping or switching the randomized treatment, so that true intent-to-treat virologic suppression rates, without consideration of whether the randomized treatment was still being taken, cannot be determined. This adversely affects the conclusions one can draw from such a study. Continued follow up of all subjects — even after treatment discontinuation — is urged.

Clinical endpoint studies, however, are still being conducted. In particular, the immune-based therapy interleukin-2 (IL-2) is being evaluated in two large, multi-year clinical endpoint studies.[20] While IL-2 plus antiretroviral therapy has been shown to produce a sustainable rise in CD4 counts (decline in CD4 cell counts is a marker of the progress of the disease), exceeding what can be achieved using antiretroviral therapy alone, the clinical benefit of these greater CD4 counts has not yet been established.

For immune-based interventions, such as therapeutic HIV vaccines, there are a large number of immunologic assays to evaluate the effects of the interventions. However, none of these assays is considered the "gold standard" for assessing improved host immune control of HIV. For this reason, many immune-based intervention studies have viral setpoint as the primary endpoint. In such a study, the randomized immune-based intervention, or placebo, is given while subjects are on combination antiretroviral therapy. Then subjects have their antiretroviral treatment withdrawn, and the viral setpoint is determined by the viral load level obtained a certain number of weeks after treatment withdrawal or after the dynamic viral load rebound has stabilized. An intervention can then be evaluated relative to the placebo arm in terms of its ability to substantively lower the viral load level in the absence of antiretroviral treatment. This endpoint, however, has some anticipated statistical challenges, most importantly because of the fact that withdrawal of antiretroviral treatment has safety concerns and some subjects may have treatment reinitiated because of high viral load levels or declining CD4 counts. Therefore, not all randomized subjects will have an observed viral setpoint, leading to statistical approaches such as worst-rank imputation analyses using rank-based analysis methods and planned sensitivity analyses to incorporate information on the reasons for unavailable viral setpoints.

In terms of study design, factorial designs continue to be used to evaluate anti-HIV drugs and strategies. A 2 × 3 factorial design was used in AIDS Clinical Trials Group (ACTG) 384,[21] where the two factors represented two components of the combination antiretroviral regimen. This factorial structure permitted six different initial antiretroviral combinations to be evaluated in an efficient design. The results of this study revealed statistically significant interactions,[22] highlighting the challenging task of defining optimal multi-drug combination regimens when the efficacy of one drug vs. another may depend on the other drugs in the regimen. Because an antiretroviral combination regimen with too few drugs may be clinically inappropriate, factorial designs having factors representing the use or nonuse of specific drugs are not directly applicable to evaluate combinations of antiretroviral drugs. ACTG 398[23] was a four-arm study of protease-inhibitor-based regimens in subjects previously failing a regimen containing a protease inhibitor. The randomization in this study was stratified and restricted to prevent, to the extent possible, subjects from being randomized to protease inhibitors to which they had prior exposure. Thus, for the main comparison of the efficacy of single vs. dual protease inhibitor regimens, a stratified analysis was required, because not every subject was eligible for randomization to every arm. This planned stratified analysis was key to the design of this study.

B. PREVENTIVE VACCINES

A variety of HIV vaccine products and strategies are in the early stages of testing, in animals and in Phase I and Phase II trials.[24,25] The first Phase III clinical trials of a preventive HIV vaccine have been concluded. Though the overall analyses were negative, subgroup analyses were highlighted that showed a vaccine effect. However, concern about the statistical issues of multiple testing and subset analyses have led to criticism of the reporting of these results from this high-profile study.[26] A subsequent, thorough statistical evaluation, corrected for multiple comparisons, failed to identify a vaccine effect in any of the subgroups.[27]

A review article discussed statistical issues inherent to HIV vaccine studies.[28] One challenging issue derives from the expectation that available HIV vaccines may have only a modest effect on blocking infection, but may be able to confer protection against high levels of HIV replication and also may slow HIV disease progression. Thus, an important co-primary or secondary endpoint in preventive HIV vaccine trials will be to compare viral load levels and disease course between placebo-recipient vs. vaccine-recipient infecteds. As these comparison groups are selected post-randomization (i.e., when these subjects become HIV infected), a standard statistical test that compares viral load distributions does not assess a causal effect of the vaccine. To address this problem, a class of logistic selection bias models has been developed, which can be used to quantify how the inferred causal effect of vaccination varies with the presumed magnitude of selection bias.[29] This framework to assess randomized comparisons in post-randomization-selected subgroups is an illustrating example of recent statistical research in causal inference.[30]

IV. ANALYSIS ISSUES RELATED TO ASSAY CHARACTERISTICS

A. VIRAL LOAD

As outlined above, viral load as measured by HIV RNA in blood plasma is a key surrogate marker in HIV/AIDS, and a major goal of antiretroviral treatment is to suppress HIV RNA levels below the lower limit of the assay. Combination antiretroviral therapy, especially in antiretroviral-naïve populations, can lead to reductions in viral load of more than 3 $\log_{10}$ (99.9% reduction), resulting in a majority of subjects with viral load measurements below the lower limit of the assay. This in turn has led to statistical research in methods for analyzing such left-censored data. One approach has been to create study endpoints that are not affected by this assay limitation. For example, virologic failure can be defined as failure to suppress HIV RNA by 24 weeks or a subsequent confirmed rise in viral load above a threshold. This virologic failure definition has clinical interpretation and also can be analyzed using standard time-to-event statistical methods.[31]

Because of clinical interest in estimating the magnitude (in $\log_{10}$ units) of viral load reduction induced by antiretroviral regimens, statistical methods have been developed, for example, by modifying standard right-censored data analysis approaches.[32] However, bias in these estimates of change in viral load remains an issue and it is recommended to use an analysis of covariance (ANCOVA) approach, with adjustment for baseline viral load. Longitudinal mixed effects models have also been generalized, using the EM algorithm, to allow for repeated measurements that may be left-censored below assay limits.[33]

B. Timing of HIV Infection

One of the greatest successes in HIV treatment has been the ability to reduce mother-to-child transmission of HIV. However, identification of the timing of HIV transmission is challenging. For this reason, HIV transmission rates in mother-to-child studies are based on Kaplan–Meier estimates.[34] Statistical methods have also been developed to account for possible false-positive and false-negative test results in estimating the timing of infection,[35] for example, in order to estimate the probability of HIV transmission during delivery vs. subsequently via breast-feeding.

C. Viral Genotype and Resistance

Drug resistance can now be evaluated by genotyping the circulating virus in an individual. Statistical and bioinformatical approaches to examine HIV genotypic resistance data are rapidly developing areas of research. We refer the reader to several papers that highlight the multidimensional nature of genotype data[36,37] and a framework for relating resistance information to viral load responses.[38] One challenge to conducting research in HIV resistance is that diagnostic companies have developed proprietary algorithms for assessing drug resistance, which are not made publicly available.

D. Phenotypic Susceptibility

In addition to sequencing the viral genotype, there are phenotypic assays that evaluate the *in vitro* growth of the virus in the presence of antiretroviral drugs. The result of a phenotype assay is a fold-change for each antiretroviral drug evaluated, representing the amount of drug required to suppress the growth of the patient's virus by 50%, relative to a control virus. Identifying the optimal clinical utility of the phenotype assay is also an important and timely area of research, because the choice of a new antiretroviral drug regimen should be guided by the anticipated resistance to the new regimen. We have recently analyzed baseline phenotypic susceptibility data and related these to virologic outcome in terms of both dichotomous (threshold-based) and continuous scoring systems.[39] In particular, the continuous scoring system was developed because drug resistance/susceptibility is likely to be truly a continuous phenomenon, with drugs having partial activity against mutant viruses and patients having variability in drug exposure, metabolism, and distribution to sites of virus replication. We also found evidence for hypersusceptibility to the antiretroviral drug efavirenz,[40] in which viruses that have become highly resistant to the earliest class of antiretrovirals show increased susceptibility to efavirenz.[41] These findings provide a rationale to consider interactions between multiple drugs with respect to resistance profiles, a task that will require substantial research given the thousands of possible drug combinations using the more than 15 approved antiretroviral HIV drugs.

E. ACTIVATION AND FUTURE SURROGATE MARKERS

While CD4 and viral load remain the main surrogate markers in HIV disease, it should be noted that these commonly used biomarkers do not directly reflect many of the toxicities associated with antiretroviral drugs. As numerous assays continue to be developed and evaluated, appropriate statistical analysis approaches will be needed to identify the value of these markers.[17] Of particular interest are markers of immune activation,[42–44] which may become increasingly important as new and improved antiretroviral regimens are successful in maintaining long-term viral load suppression.

ACKNOWLEDGMENTS

The authors thank Donna Mildvan and John Spritzler for valuable discussions. This work was supported in part by NIH grant AI-38855.

REFERENCES

1. Palella, F.J.J., Delaney, K.M., Moorman, A.C. et al., Declining morbidity and mortality among patients with advanced human immunodeficiency virus infection, *N. Engl. J. Med.*, 338, 853–860, 1998.
2. UNAIDS, *Report on the global AIDS epidemic*, 2004, http://www.unaids.org/bangkok2004/report.html
3. Volberding, P.A., Lagakos, S.W., Koch, M.A. et al., Zidovudine in asymptomatic human immunodeficiency virus infection: a controlled trial in persons with fewer than 500 CD4-positive cells per cubic millimeter, *N. Engl. J. Med.*, 322, 941–949, 1990.

4. Hammer, S.M., Katzenstein, D.A., Hughes, M.D. et al., A trial comparing nucleoside monotherapy with combination therapy in HIV-infected adults with CD4 cell counts from 200 to 500 per cubic millimeter, *N. Engl. J. Med.*, 335, 1081–1090, 1996.

5. Aber, V., Aboulker, J.P., Babiker, A.G. et al., Delta: a randomized double-blind controlled trial comparing combinations of zidovudine plus didanosine or zalcitabine with zidovudine alone in HIV-infected individuals, *Lancet*, 348, 283–291, 1996.

6. Hammer, S.M., Squires, K.E., Hughes, M.D. et al., A controlled trial of two nucleoside analogues plus indinavir in persons with human immunodeficiency virus infection and CD4 cell counts of 200 per cubic millimeter or less, *N. Engl. J. Med.*, 337, 725–733, 1997.

7. Fessel, W.J., Human immunodeficiency virus (HIV) RNA in plasma as the preferred target for therapy in patients with HIV infection: a critique, *Clin. Infect. Dis.*, 24, 116–122, 1997.

8. O'Brien, W.A., Hartigan, P.M., Martin, D. et al., Changes in plasma HIV-1 and CD4 + lymphocyte counts and the risk of progression to AIDS, *N. Engl. J. Med.*, 334, 426–431, 1996.

9. Katzenstein, D.A., Hammer, S.M., Hughes, M.D. et al., The relation of virologic and immunologic markers to clinical outcomes after nucleoside therapy in HIV-infected adults with 200 to 500 CD4 cells per cubic millimeter, *N. Engl. J. Med.*, 335, 1091–1098, 1996.

10. Babiker, A., Bartlett, J., Breckenridge, A. et al., Human immunodeficiency virus type 1 RNA level and CD4 count as prognostic markers and surrogate end points: a meta-analysis, *AIDS Res. Hum. Retroviruses*, 16, 1123–1133, 2000.

11. Kim, S., Hughes, M.D., Hammer, S.M. et al., Both serum HIV type 1 RNA levels and CD4 + lymphocyte counts predict clinical outcome in HIV type 1-infected subjects with 200 to 500 CD4 + cells per cubic millimeter, *AIDS Res. Hum. Retroviruses*, 16, 645–653, 2000.

12. Demeter, L.M., Hughes, M.D., Coombs, R.W. et al., Predictors of virologic and clinical outcomes in HIV-1-infected patients receiving concurrent treatment with indinavir, zidovudine, and lamivudine, *Ann. Intern. Med.*, 135, 954–964, 2001.

13. Spector, S.A., Kennedy, C., McCutchan, J.A. et al., The antiviral effect of zidovudine and ribavirin in clinical trials and the use of p24 antigen levels as a virologic marker, *J. Infect. Dis.*, 159, 822–828, 1989.

14. Fiscus, S.A., DeGruttola, V., Gupta, P. et al., Human immunodeficiency virus type 1 quantitative cell microculture as a measure of antiviral efficacy in a multicenter clinical trial, *J. Infect. Dis.*, 171, 305–311, 1995.

15. Murray, J.S., Elashoff, M.R., Iacono-Connors, L.C., Cvetkovich, T.A., and Struble, K.A., The use of plasma HIV RNA as a study endpoint in efficacy trials of antiretroviral drugs, *AIDS*, 13, 797–804, 1999.

16. FDA. Guidance for industry, Antiretroviral Drugs Using Plasma HIV RNA Measurements — Clinical Considerations for Accelerated and Traditional Approval, FDA Center for Drug Evaluation and Research, 2002, http://www.fda.gov/cder/guidance/index.htm

17. Mildvan, D., Landay, A., DeGruttola, V., Machado, S.G., and Kagan, J., An approach to the validation of markers for use in AIDS clinical trials, *Clin. Infect. Dis.*, 24, 764–774, 1997.

18. Kirk, O., Pedersen, C., Law, M. et al., Analysis of virologic efficacy in trials of antiretroviral regimens: drawbacks of not including viral load measurements after premature discontinuation of therapy, *Antivir. Ther.*, 7, 271–281, 2002.
19. Gilbert, P.B., DeGruttola, V., Hammer, S.M., and Kuritzkes, D.R.,Virologic and regimen termination surrogate end points in AIDS clinical trials, *J. Am. Med. Assoc.*, 285, 777–784, 2001.
20. Pett, S.L. and Emery, S., Immunomodulators as adjunctive therapy for HIV-1 infection, *J. Clin. Virol.*, 22(3 Special Issue SI), 289–295, 2001.
21. Smeaton, L.M., DeGruttola, V., Robbins, G.K., and Shafer, R.W., ACTG (AIDS Clinical Trials Group) 384: a strategy trial comparing consecutive treatments for HIV-1, *Control. Clin. Trials*, 22, 142–159, 2001.
22. Robbins, G.K., De Gruttola, V., Shafer, R.W. et al., Comparison of sequential three-drug regimens as initial therapy for HIV-1 infection, *N. Engl. J. Med.*, 349, 2293–2303, 2003.
23. Hammer, S.M., Vaida, F., Bennett, K.K. et al., Dual vs. single protease inhibitor therapy following antiretroviral treatment failure — A randomized trial, *JAMA*, 288, 169–180, 2002.
24. Letvin, N.L., Strategies for an HIV vaccine, *J. Clin. Invest.*, 110, 15–20, 2002.
25. Mwau, M. and McMichael, A.J., A review of vaccines for HIV prevention, *J. Gene Med.*, 5, 3–10, 2003.
26. McCarthy, M., HIV vaccine fails in phase 3 trial — Sceptics question subset analysis that suggests HIV vaccine could be protective in non-white people, *Lancet*, 361, 755–756, 2003.
27. Follmann, D., Gilbert, P., Self, S. et al., An independent analysis of the effect of race in VAX004, 11th Conference on Retroviruses and Opportunistic Infections, 2004, Abstract #106.
28. Gilbert, P.B., Some statistical issues in the design of HIV-1 vaccine and treatment trials, *Stat. Methods Med. Res.*, 9, 207–229, 2000.
29. Gilbert, P.B., Bosch, R.J., and Hudgens, M.G., Sensitivity analysis for the assessment of causal vaccine effects on viral load in HIV vaccine trials, *Biometrics*, 59, 531–541, 2003.
30. Frangakis, C.E. and Rubin, D.B., Principal stratification in causal inference, *Biometrics*, 58, 21–29, 2002.
31. Gilbert, P.B., Ribaudo, H.J., Greenberg, L. et al., Considerations in choosing a primary endpoint that measures durability of virologic suppression in an antiretroviral trial, *AIDS*, 14, 1961–1972, 2000.
32. Hughes, M.D., Analysis and design issues for studies using censored biomarker measurements with an example of viral load measurements in HIV clinical trials, *Stat. Med.*, 19, 3171–3191, 2000.
33. Hughes, J.P., Mixed effects models with censored data with application to HIV RNA levels, *Biometrics*, 55, 625–629, 1999.
34. Connor, E.M., Sperling, R.S., Gelber, R. et al., Reduction of maternal–infant transmission of human immunodeficiency virus type 1 with zidovudine treatment, *N. Engl. J. Med.*, 331, 1173–1180, 1994.
35. Balasubramanian, R. and Lagakos, S.W., Estimation of a failure time distribution based on imperfect diagnostic tests, *Biometrika*, 90, 171–182, 2003.
36. Kowalski, J., Pagano, M., and DeGruttola, V., A nonparametric test of gene region heterogeneity associated with phenotype, *J. Am. Stat. Assoc.*, 97, 398–408, 2002.

37. Moore, C.B., John, M., James, I.R. et al., Evidence of HIV-1 adaptation to HLA-restricted immune responses at a population level, *Science*, 296, 1439–1443, 2002.
38. DeGruttola, V., Dix, L., D'Aquila, R. et al., The relation between baseline drug resistance and response to antiretroviral therapy: reanalysis of retrospective and prospective studies using a standardized data analysis plan, *Antivir. Ther.*, 5, 41–48, 2000.
39. Katzenstein, D.A., Bosch, R.J., Hellmann, N. et al., Phenotypic susceptibility and virologic outcome in nucleoside-experienced patients receiving three or four antiretroviral drugs, *AIDS*, 17, 821–830, 2003.
40. Bosch, R.J., Downey, G.F., Katzenstein, D.A., Hellmann, N., Bacheler, L., and Albrecht, M.A., Evaluation of cutpoints for phenotypic hypersusceptibility to efavirenz, *AIDS*, 17, 2395–2396, 2003.
41. Shulman, N., Zolopa, A.R., Passaro, D. et al., Phenotypic hypersusceptibility to non-nucleoside reverse transcriptase inhibitors in treatment-experienced HIV-infected patients: impact on virological response to efavirenz-based therapy, *AIDS*, 15, 1125–1132, 2001.
42. Giorgi, J.V., Hultin, L.E., McKeating, J.A. et al., Shorter survival in advanced human immunodeficiency virus type 1 infection is more closely associated with T lymphocyte activation than with plasma virus burden or virus chemokine coreceptor usage, *J. Infect. Dis.*, 179, 859–870, 1999.
43. Grossman, Z., Meier-Schellersheim, M., Sousa, A.E., Victorino, R.M., and Paul, W.E., CD4 + T-cell depletion in HIV infection: are we closer to understanding the cause? *Nat. Med.*, 8, 319–323, 2002.
44. Sousa, A.E., Carneiro, J., Meier-Schellersheim, M. Grossman, Z., and Victorino, R.M., CD4 T cell depletion is linked directly to immune activation in the pathogenesis of HIV-1 and HIV-2 but only indirectly to the viral load, *J. Immunol.*, 169, 3400–3406, 2002.

11 The Wonders of Placebo

C. Ralph Buncher

CONTENTS

I. INTRODUCTION

After a fall, a small child cries in pain. The parent picks up the child, kisses the source of pain, and says that now it will feel better. Remarkably, the child shows less pain and stops crying.

It is well known that in studies of pharmaceutical preparations, the subjects who receive a pill or capsule without any of the pharmacological properties of the "active" medication will also show some signs of efficacy and some side effects. This preparation is called "placebo" from the Latin for "I shall please" (*placebo Domino in regione vivorum* — I shall please the Lord in the land of the living). The name is very old and was often used as a derogatory term recognizing the fact that almost all medications used more than a century ago were without proven therapeutic efficacy. Still these medications were used because the recipients found relief from their complaints. They are also frequently called "sugar pills" since they are usually made up from noncaloric sugar with again the overtone that, it is only their sweetness which makes one feel better.

There are many definitions of placebo, which depend on the point of view and emphasis of the writer. An excellent and comprehensive definition was given by Shapiro[1]:

> A placebo is any therapy (or component of therapy) that is deliberately or knowingly used for its nonspecific, psychologic, or psychophysiologic effect, or that is used unknowingly for its presumed or believed effect on a patient, symptom, or illness, but which, unknown to patient and therapist, is without specific activity for the condition being treated.

In more modern times when drugs were being tested for efficacy, it soon became clear that a concurrent control preparation was essential if one needed to prove to others the difference between pharmacologic efficacy and perceived efficacy. Anyone working in this field needs to have read some of the older literature including the classic paper of Beecher[2] and others who studied placebos before the advent of Informed Consent and Institutional Review Boards in the early 1970s. In those days one could deceive subjects and therefore discover physiologic effects while controlling the thoughts of the subjects. One problem is that many conditions, such as pain, will decrease over time and thus a no-treatment group will also "improve" over the course of a clinical trial. The belief system of the patient is an important element of the placebo effect. For example, Comstock[3] reported that customers who in a past day believed that pasteurization spoiled the flavor of their milk complained of the awful pasteurized milk delivered to them. It seems the label was recently changed to note the pasteurization, although the milk was unchanged from what they had been receiving. When the label was changed back, the complaints ceased.

One interesting example was a study of the effect of iron pills on women.[4] In this study, three groups of subjects were established. In one, the women were given iron pills and were told that they were taking iron pills. A second group received the placebo for the iron pills and was told that they were receiving the placebo. A third group also received the placebo for the iron pills but they were told that they were receiving the iron pills. The outcome was that, both groups who thought they were taking iron pills reported many more side effects than the group who thought they were taking placebo. Because the two groups who thought they were taking iron pills reported the same results and the two groups who were on placebo had different results, the conclusion is that the side effects were caused by what the women thought and not by the physiologic effects. "Virtually no toxic effects were reported from 'known' control pills containing lactose, but the exactly similar 'unknown' control pills, which were thought by the subjects to contain iron, produced as many side effects as the pills that did, in fact, contain it."[4]

Another study, this time with second year medical students, is also illustrative.[5] This study, though not original in concept, is classic because the results were so predictable to illustrate this field. In fact we placed the predicted results in a sealed envelope prior to the study to emphasize that we were pretty sure we knew what would happen. The students were studying stimulants and sedatives in their pharmacology classes, and were asked to participate in a blindfold experiment on the psychological and physiological effects of stimulant and sedative drugs. At baseline and one hour later, after attending a lecture, the students who volunteered measured each other's pulse, blood pressure, and pupil size. They reported on twelve possible desirable and undesirable psychological effects. Students received their medication dose as one or two blue or pink capsules.

Only three students did not report any change and 27% of the class reported at least seven of the 12 responses. A statistically significant but small change was observed in pulse rate and systolic blood pressure. Subjects in a comment section reported headaches, difficulty in concentrating, and dizzy feelings. Additional effects were noted by single individuals. Later in the day, two subjects were sufficiently concerned that they sought reassurance from the faculty and one had to be driven home. Those who took two capsules demonstrated more pronounced but not more frequent changes than those who took only one, a typical dose response. Blue capsules produced more sedative effects than pink capsules.

These results were presented to the students two weeks later when they were also told that all students consumed only placebo. After a pause, presumably to process this information and to reevaluate, the students burst out laughing. Almost all of the responses to a questionnaire on the impact of the experiment rated the experience in a favorable light. This included five students who felt humiliated but still rated the learning-experience as good or excellent.

Most physicians and patients have not had the experience of taking and reacting to something that is later revealed to be a placebo especially in the last decades when Informed Consent and Institutional Review Boards constrict researchers on what can be told to the recipients. The literature suggests that almost everyone will respond to a placebo if put into a conducive situation. It is also clear that a reaction today does not do a good job of predicting what will happen tomorrow in a slightly different situation. In fact, researchers have tried the approach of a run in period to find and eliminate those who respond to placebo. This approach has not been successful because placebo effects are still observed during the study even after putative placebo responders have been eliminated from starting the study.

It should also be emphasized that in spite of its name, placebo effects include both the positive and negative when compared with a standard of no treatment. Thus Buncher[6] reported as follows:

> Placebo is well known to be a good analgesic. It cures or reduces the pain from headaches, backaches, postoperative pain, rheumatoid arthritis, angina pectoris, and cardiac pain. It has cured motion sickness, gastric hyperacidity, the symptoms of common cold, and clinical cough. It can tranquilize or stimulate. One tenth of women proven to be anovulatory then ovulated following administration of a placebo under study conditions.[7] Moreover, side effects from placebo therapy are even more extensive than the list of conditions that are aided by placebo. Headaches, nausea, vomiting, dizziness, diarrhea, pain, dermatitis, drowsiness, anxiety-nervousness, weakness-fatigue, dry mouth, abdominal pain, insomnia, urinary frequency, urticaria, loss of libido, tinnitus, and so forth, have all been caused by the administration of placebos.

Also, the results sometimes indicate that placebo is the better treatment. Occasionally people fall into the trap of believing that either the active treatment is better or the same as placebo. One example is the cardiac arrhythmia suppression trial discovering that the placebo group had fewer deaths from arrhythmia or shock after acute recurrent myocardial infarction. This study was stopped by the

Data and Safety Monitoring Board when they observed more deaths in the encainide and flecainide treatment groups than in the placebo group.[8]

In pharmaceutical trials, the purpose of a placebo is to provide a comparison such that one can tell what would have happened if the new "active treatment" had no pharmacologic effect. One should not think that the results in the placebo group are necessarily causal. Some effects are causal but some are caused by changes over time in the disease or the patient, regression towards the mean, other human factors, and so forth. One illuminating example appeared in a news account of AIDS testing.[9] "Four weeks after enrolling in a trial, John G. saw his CD4 cells (a marker for the progress of the disease) rise from 300 to 649. Thrilled, he called up other infected friends to urge them to get the drug. He started to take better care of himself — he ate three meals a day, he exercised — seeing a future for himself again. Then he found out he was on a placebo. …'I was totally shocked,' John G., a 31 year old circulation manager for a magazine in Manhattan, said. 'I thought it was the miracle drug'."

We have to note that thinking you are doing better can be autocorrelated with actions that make you healthier. This anecdote also raises the complicated issue of how to tell a patient at the end of a trial that you have been taking a placebo.[10]

One particularly important study should be understood by all who work in pharmaceutical statistics. This is part of the Coronary Drug Project that evaluated several lipid-influencing drugs.[11] The five-year mortality rate was 20.9% in the placebo group and 20.0% in the clofibrate group — a nonsignificant difference. Further analysis showed that good adherers, defined as those who took 80% or more of the assigned medication had a 15.0% mortality rate compared with 24.6% in those who took less of the medication — a highly significant difference. Then the same analysis was done for the placebo group with the same results — 15.1% mortality for those who took at least 80% of their placebo and 28.3% for those who took less of the placebo, again a highly significant difference. The usual interpretation is that those who took at least 80% of their medication, whether clofibrate or placebo, were "better patients" who also followed other advice to keep them as healthy as possible, such as exercising and using a more healthy diet. As an aside, this study put a bright spotlight on the danger of evaluating treatment efficacy in subgroups determined by patient responses and lead to the much greater use of the "intent-to-treat" analysis.

Explanations of the placebo effect have been sought and include factors such as a cascade of events resulting in the release of endorphins in the brain. Thus we understand how a chemical drug can fit into a receptor site on a cell of an organ and then trigger a series of events resulting in the positive effects of the drug or even the side effects if a receptor on a different organ is triggered. Then how does a placebo work if we cannot point to a chemical pathway? In spite of a great quantity of results and better understanding, the process is still being studied. I do object to an advertisement that stated "No placebos. What we do for you really works" since that statement misses the point that, the "really works" and the placebo effect are indistinguishable in any individual.

I think of it this way. We know that the brain, in response to a stimulus such as a sight, a sound, a smell, a touch, or a taste, can trigger thoughts that in turn will turn on or off parts of the genetic system. That is a gene can be turned on by the brain to produce a protein or turned off to stop producing a protein. Thus there is a parallel system with the brain as intermediary to the system of drug induced molecular changes. One can imagine an ancient ancestor walking and seeing or hearing a lion. Molecular changes to start the fight or flight reaction would be induced by the sensing of this potential problem. We also know that sometimes that ancestor might be mistaken in the identification but would still trigger the reaction. Alpha and beta errors suggest that it was probably better for us if our ancestors overreacted to potential danger. Thus we have this biologic system that translates sense organ signals into chemical reactions, which in the experimental setting of pharmacological research we would designate as a placebo reaction.

A fascinating example of the role of placebo in research was given by Roy L. Sanford in the second edition of this book,[12] and it is repeated here.

II. A CASE STUDY OF A CLINICAL TRIAL OF THE DRUG CHYMOPAPAIN

Published results of studies with chymopapain serve to illustrate the revealing nature of placebo-controlled, double-blind trials and the importance of not underestimating the magnitude of the placebo effect. A brief historical review is in order. Chymopapain is an enzyme that dissolves the protein in injured vertebral discs. According to Smith, the dissolution of this protein may alleviate the pain experienced by slipped-disc sufferers. In 1963 Smith[13] injected the enzyme intradiscally into patients with symptomatic lumbar disc disease and termed his new treatment, chemonucleolysis. Prior to 1975, almost 17,000 patients had undergone chemonucleolysis by neurosurgeons and orthopedists. These studies were uncontrolled, and success rates ranged from 50% to 80% from investigator to investigator. FDA approval of chemonucleolysis seemed a formality. In 1974 the American Academy of Orthopedic Surgeons endorsed chymopapain as "safe" and "effective." However, prior to approval, it was determined that a placebo-controlled, double-blind study was necessary in the United States. Based on the successful uncontrolled clinical experience since 1963, this study was considered by many to be unethical. Unfortunately, the only therapy available other than chemonucleolysis was surgery and could not be accommodated in a double-blind format.

This situation prompted the election of a placebo-controlled study. Four hospitals were selected to participate in a double-blind clinical study that was conducted for approximately one year and was completed on December 31, 1975. A total of 106 patients were admitted with 56 patients receiving a placebo injection and 50 receiving chymopapain. The placebo injection consisted of the vehicle without the enzyme but with an inert substance for bulk. The vehicle consisted of cysteine hydrochloride and ethylenediamine tetraacetic acid with sodium iothalamate, and was considered to be pharmacologically inert when included as part of the injection procedure. All other aspects of the treatment program were identical for both the control and treatment groups. At the end of one year, out of 50 patients receiving chymopapain, 20 patients were determined to be treatment failures, and out of 56 treated in the control group, 28 were determined to be treatment failures. Determination of treatment failure was made jointly by the physician and patient. The overall success rates were not found to be significantly different between control and treatment groups, nor did any additional evaluation of all the data collected demonstrate a significant benefit in favor of chymopapain compared with the placebo control. Long-term followup did not alter this situation. Further details and results were reported by Schwetschenau et al.[14] and Martins et al.[15]

This one chymopapain study raised numerous questions. Was the placebo response rate caused by true pharmacological activity on the part of the vehicle, or was the true placebo response rate under these circumstances comparable with those of chemonucleolysis and surgery? Should measurement of patient improvement and the reduction of pain from lower back problems have been carried out differently to result in a more efficient estimate of the contrast in success rates between chymopapain and placebo? How long should patients be followed before success or failure is determined? Should a larger sample size have been used? Lower back problems tend to reverse themselves and then recur. Should different patient entry criteria be used? Based on the findings of this study, the new drug application (NDA) was not approved and further use of chymopapain in the United States was discontinued. Several articles appeared in the press[16,17] questioning the nonapproval of the NDA and the conduct of the study, two congressional investigations were launched, documentaries appeared on television, and scientific papers were published in different journals discussing chemonucleolysis.

McCulloch[18] published results of a seven-year, unblinded, single-treatment study of 480 patients who underwent enzymatic dissolution of the nucleus pulposus with chymopapain. He reported that 70% of patients with the clinical criteria for a disc herniation had a favorable response to chemonucleolysis. Those patients with spinal stenosis or psychogenic components or those having had a previous operation were found to have poor results. In 1976 Smith, the discoverer of chemonucleolysis, indicated, "In comparison with usage of the drug over 12 years, this one study (referring to the double-blind study) is relatively insignificant." The controversy continued for years. Final approval of chymopapain was received from the FDA in 1982 after two additional placebo-controlled studies were completed. One was conducted in Australia and is reported by Fraser.[19] The other was conducted by Smith Laboratories and is reported by Haines[20] in a review of the three published randomized clinical trials of chymopapain. The three published studies were double-blind placebo-controlled studies utilizing a total of 234 patients. Haines[20] pooled the results of these studies on the basis that study design, selection criteria, technique, and outcome assessment were very similar. He concluded that the odds of successful outcome were 2.6 times as great with chymopapain as with placebo, or that chemonucleolysis provided a 23% increase in the number of successfully treated patients compared with placebo. The pooled success rate for chymopapain was 70% and for placebo was 47%. Haines demonstrated that in these three studies the estimated powers for finding a 50% increase in success rate for chymopapain relative to placebo ranged from 0.51 to 0.61, and he concluded that "the failure of the original double-blind study … probably resulted from small sample size." Two recent reports provide an update on the situation. Wittenberg[21] reported on a later clinical trial and Kim[22] reviewed 3000 cases.

In conclusion, we can reflect on the example just given and our understanding of the placebo effect. As we continue to make progress in pharmacologic treatment, there are more and more active medications that can be used to treat disease conditions. While patients may be willing to forgo a medicine to relieve pain in an experiment or to reduce itching or the symptoms of allergy, we do not think that a study should use a placebo to treat a debilitating disease or for birth control or cancer treatment, in most situations. Vickers and deCraen[23] discuss some of the alternatives. Some condemn the use of placebo in any study when a proven treatment exists. The country of Brazil instituted this as a requirement.[24] Thus more and more studies will use an active control and not include a placebo. This raises a whole range of statistical issues because statistically "significantly better than placebo" as the goal can be replaced by "as good as the usual treatment." Even when comparing active treatments, the investigators must keep in mind that some of the effects are caused by the placebo effect. As background, consider a study that shows a placebo effect such that 30% of patients on placebo have their pain relieved compared with 60% on the active treatment. The conclusion is that the active treatment is effective. However, we should keep in mind that, based on these results, we must conclude that half of the patients on the active treatment are being cured by placebo effects.

Finally, there are always doubters and those who come up with new conclusions. One example is an article that appeared in the New England Journal of Medicine and was given publicity to the effect that the placebo effect was not real.[25] The news reports stated things like the placebo effect is nothing more than a myth. The authors searched for articles with well done studies that involved both a placebo and a no-treatment group so that they could measure the difference caused by the placebo effect. Their conclusion was that only for an effect on pain was there a statistically significant effect. If one looks at their data in Table 2, you can see a fundamental fallacy in this report. The table shows that the effect size is about the same for pain as for obesity, asthma, hypertension, and insomnia, although none of the latter is statistically significant. Then one notes that the sample size of patients fulfilling the authors' criteria was large for pain relief ($n = 1602$) and small for the other characteristics ($n =$ from 81 to 129). The authors then concluded that because the effect was not found at a statistically significant level, it did not exist. This is the classic fallacy of "accepting" the null hypothesis rather than concluding that the data are consistent with the null hypothesis as well as an array of alternative hypotheses.

In summary, few who have experienced the contingencies of life or carried out pharmacologic research will doubt the importance of the concept of the placebo effect. Eventually, after you have proven your medication effective, you still have to choose a color for it and if a blue color has more sedative effects, then...

REFERENCES

1. Shapiro, A.K., Placebo effects in psychotherapy and psychoanalysis, *J. Clin. Pharmacol.*, 73–78, 1970, Mar/Apr.
2. Beecher, H.K., The Powerful Placebo, *JAMA*, 159, 1602–1606, 1955.
3. Comstock, G.W., Snippets from the past: 70 years ago in the Journal, *Am. J. Epidemiol.*, 157, 183–184, 2003.
4. Kerr, D.N.S. and Davidson, S., Gastrointestinal intolerance to oral iron preparations, *The Lancet*, 2, 489–492, 1958.
5. Blackwell, B., Bloomfield, S.S., and Buncher, C.R., Demonstration to medical students of placebo responses and non-drug factors, *The Lancet*, 1, 1279–1282, 1972.
6. Buncher, C.R., Principles of experimental design for clinical drug studies, In *Perspectives in Clinical Pharmacy*, Francke, D.E. and Whitney, H.A.K. Jr., eds., Drug Intelligence, Hamilton, IL, pp. 504–525, 1972.
7. Johnson, J.E. Jr., Cohen, M.R., Goldfarb, A.F. et al. The efficacy of clomiphene citrate for induction of ovulation. A controlled study, *Intern. J. Fert.*, 11, 265–270, 1966.
8. Echt, D.S., Liebson, P.R., Mitchell, L.B. et al. Mortality and morbidity in patients receiving encainide, flecainide, or placebo. The Cardiac Arrhythmia Suppression Trial, *New Engl. J. Med.*, 324, 781–788, 1991.
9. Navarro, M., *Into the unknown: AIDS patients test drugs*, New York Times, New York, 1992, pp. 1, 10, February 29.
10. DiBlasi, Z., Kaptchuk, T.J., Weinman, J., and Kleijnen, J., Informing participants of allocation to placebo at trial closure: postal survey, *Br. Med. J.*, 325, 1329–1331, 2002.
11. Coronary Drug Project, Influence of adherence to treatment and response of cholesterol on mortality in the coronary drug project, *New Engl. J. Med.*, 303, 1038–1041, 1980.
12. Sanford, R.L., The wonders of placebo, In *Statistics in the Pharmaceutical Industry*, 2nd ed., Revised and Expanded, Buncher, C.R. and Tsay, J.Y., eds., Marcel Dekker Inc., New York, pp. 247–266, 1994, Chapter 13.
13. Smith, L., Enzyme dissolution of the nucleus pulposus in humans, *J. Amer. Med. Assoc.*, 187, 137–140, 1964.
14. Schwetschenau, P.R., Ramirez, A., Johnston, J., Barnes, E., Wiggs, C., and Martins, A.N., Double-blind evaluation of intradiscal chymopapain for herniated lumbar discs, *J. Neurosurg.*, 45, 622–627, 1976.
15. Martins, A.N., Ramirez, A., Johnston, J., and Schwetschenau, P.R., Double-blind evaluation of chemonucleolysis for herniated lumbar discs, *J. Neurosurg.*, 49, 816–827, 1978.
16. Star, J., Bad times for the bad-back drug, *Chicago*, 168–174, 1978, November.
17. Steinmetz, J., Dr. Lyman Smith tangles with the FDA over his papaya enzyme to treat bad backs, *People*, 5, 58–59, 1976.

18. McCulloch, J.A., Chemonucleolysis, *J. Bone Joint Surg., Series B*, 59, 45–52, 1977.
19. Fraser, R.D., Chymopapain for the treatment of intervertebral disc herniation. A preliminary report of a double-blind study, *Spine*, 7(6), 608–612, 1982, November–December.
20. Haines, S.J., The chymopapain clinical trials, *Neurosurgery*, 17(1), 107–110, 1985.
21. Wittenberg, R.H., Oppel, S., Rubenthaler, F.A., and Steffen, R., Five-year results from chemonucleolysis with chymopapain or collegenase: a prospective randomized study, *Spine*, 26, 1835–1841, 2001.
22. Kim, Y.S., Chin, D.K., Yoon, D.H., Jin, B.H., and Cho, Y.E., Predictors of successful outcome for lumbar chemonucleolysis: analysis of 3000 cases during the past 14 years, *Neurosurgery*, 51(Suppl.), S123–S128, 2002.
23. Vickers, A.J. and deCraen, A.J.M., Why use placebos in clinical trials? A narrative review of the methodological literature, *J. Clin. Epidemiol.*, 53, 157–161, 2000.
24. Vieira, C.L., Tough placebo rules leave scientists out in the cold, *Science*, 295, 264, 2002.
25. Hrobjartsson, A. and Gotzsche, P.C., Is the placebo powerless? An analysis of clinical trials comparing placebo with no treatment, *New Engl. J. Med.*, 344, 1594–1602, 2001.

12 Active-Controlled Noninferiority/ Equivalence Trials: Methods and Practice

Irving K. Hwang

CONTENTS

I. INTRODUCTION

Substantial evidence from "adequate and well-controlled" randomized clinical trials (RCTs), as outlined in FDA CFR Title 21, Part 314.126, 2000,[1] is required for medicinal product (e.g., drug, therapy, vaccine, or medical device) approval by the Food and Drug Adminstration (FDA) of the US. The "control" serves as a comparator that allows for discrimination of patient outcomes (changes in symptoms, signs, morbidity, or mortality) caused by the test treatment from that caused by other factors, such as the natural progression of the disease, patient and investigator expectation, or other treatments. The comparative information gained on the control is crucial for the determination of test treatment efficacy and safety, provided that the "bias" is minimized via randomization and/or blinding. The choice of control is well discussed in ICH E10 Guidance[2] and others.[3,4] Control can be "historical" or "concurrent." A historical control is a control selected from a defined patient population in a similar group of patients studied in historical trials. The patient population in the current trial may no longer be the same because of changes in medical practice and patient life style. Due to a lack of randomization and patient comparability of the test and control groups and its inability to minimize bias, historical control is only used in exceptional cases. A concurrent control is one selected from the same patient population as the test treatment group and treated in the same trial concurrently in adherence to the study protocol. Concurrent control, as described in ICH E10, can be classified into four types: namely, no-treatment control, placebo control, active control, and dose–response control. An important extension is multiple controls, where placebo and active controls are included in the same trial.

Within the limits of technical and practical feasibility of using placebo, the placebo-controlled RCT has been the gold standard in drug development for many decades and it continues to be the primary means to demonstrate efficacy and safety of a new test treatment. As more proved effective treatments are available, the utilities of the placebo-controlled trials from ethical consideration become questionable.[5–7] Recently in 2000, the World Medical Association (WMA) Declaration of Helsinki[8] further challenged the use of placebo-controlled trials by declaring, "in any medical study, every patient — including those of a control group, if any — should be assured of the best proved diagnostic and therapeutic method." This strong wording is literally interpreted by many and they consider it unethical to conduct placebo-controlled trials, if there is an effective treatment available. Some FDA experts[9,10] countered the extreme viewpoint and rectify use of placebo under certain conditions (e.g., where diseases are symptom-driven, nonfatal, or morbidity is reversible) even when effective treatments are readily available.

Nonetheless, the active-controlled trials have gained popularity in recent years, especially in the European Union (EU) and Japan, where these trials are routinely conducted to demonstrate test treatment efficacy and assess comparative effectiveness of the test treatment against standard control treatments. An active-controlled trial is one in which a test treatment is compared with a standard effective treatment. Active-controlled trials have two distinct objectives with respect to demonstrating efficacy:

1) *superiority*: to demonstrate efficacy by showing superiority of the test treatment to the active control treatment
2) *noninferiority or equivalence*: to prove efficacy of the test treatment by showing it is noninferior or equivalent to a standard effective treatment.

Active control has been used in trials with or without placebo. For trials involving placebo and active controls, active control usually plays a secondary role with respect to demonstrating the effectiveness of a test treatment. It is primarily used as a reference intended for verifying the assay sensitivity (AS) of the trial.

In Section II the utilities of the placebo-controlled trials vs. the active-controlled trials are briefly reviewed. Section III discusses the definitions of superiority, noninferiority, and equivalence trials in hypothesis testing and interval estimation settings. Section IV provides some basic formulae for sample size and power calculations under various trial designs and data distributions. Section V details the issues of AS, historical evidence of sensitivity-to-drug-effects (HESDE), appropriate trial conduct (ATC), and constancy assumption (CA). Section VI further discusses active control effect size (Δ), noninferiority/equivalence margin (δ), and fraction of active control effect preservation (ϕ) determination. AS, HESDE, CA, Δ, δ, and ϕ are the essential elements required for the design of a positive noninferiority/equivalence trial. Section VII and Section VIII describe switching objectives and general analysis issues, respectively. Next, in Section IX some caveats are presented. In Section X a summary discussion on the active-controlled noninferiority trials is provided, closing with a short remark regarding the role of the statistician.

II. PLACEBO VS. ACTIVE-CONTROLLED TRIALS

The utilities of placebo-controlled trials are well established. The placebo-controlled trials, using randomization and blinding, generally minimize patient selection, investigator assessment, and trial conduct bias. In such trials, patients are randomly assigned to a test treatment (e.g., drug) or to an identical-appearing inactive drug (i.e., placebo). A placebo is a "dummy" substance that appears as identical as possible to the test treatment with respect to physical characteristics such as color, weight, taste, and smell, but it does not contain the test treatment or any other active ingredient of drugs. The treatments can be titrated or given at one or multiple fixed doses. The placebo concurrent control design controls for the so-called "placebo" effect (see Chapter 11, this volume). Therefore, use of placebo concurrent control is able to separate the true pharmacologic effect of the test treatment from other confounded effects (e.g., natural progression of the disease, regression to the mean, patient, and/or investigator expectation, the effect of being treated in a trial, and bias of diagnosis/assessment). Placebo-controlled trials also have the ability to distinguish adverse effects caused by a treatment from those resulting from underlying disease or concomitant illness. However, use of a placebo raises problems of ethics, acceptability, and feasibility when an effective treatment is available, in particular, for some severe disease conditions (e.g., mortality and irreversible morbidity) under study. Nonetheless, it is often possible to address the ethical or practical limitations of placebo-controlled trials by including multiple doses of the test drug, a pseudo-placebo (a low-dose active control drug), a known effective active-control drug, or adopting some design alternatives or modifications to be discussed in Section IX.

In an active-controlled trial, patients are randomly assigned to the test treatment or to an active control treatment. Such trials are usually double-blind via the use of double-dummies, but this is not always feasible. Many oncology trials, for example, are difficult or impossible to blind because of different regimens, schedules/cycles, routes of administration, and induced toxicities. Active-controlled trials are generally considered to pose fewer ethical and practical problems than placebo-controlled trials because all patients receive active treatment. Active-controlled trials also can, if properly designed, provide information about test treatment efficacy in addition to relative efficacy to an active control treatment. A crucial design question for an active-controlled trial is whether the primary objective of the trial is intended to show superiority of the test treatment to the active control or merely to show noninferiority/equivalence. When this design is used to show superiority of the test treatment to an active control treatment, the approach is straightforward like the placebo-controlled trials. When superiority (significant difference between the test and active control treatments) is shown, AS of the trial is established, and efficacy of the test treatment is demonstrated. However, when it is used to show noninferiority/equivalence of the test treatment to an active control treatment, AS will need special consideration; it cannot be demonstrated directly, but rather deduced via HESDE of the chosen active control, CA of the control effect size, and ATC of the current noninferiority trial including adequate sample size and power as well as high trial quality. Predefinition of a trial design as a superiority trial or a noninferiority trial is necessary for proper trial design and analysis (e.g., choice of control, doses, patient populations, endpoints, sample size and power, clinical relevant effect size, noninferiority margin, analysis plan, and assay sensitivity). In practice, an active-controlled trial may include switching objectives as *a priori* in the trial design.[3,11,12]. These important topics on properties of the noninferiority/equivalence trials and switching objectives will be discussed in Section IV and Section VII, respectively.

III. SUPERIORITY, NONINFERIORITY, AND EQUIVALENCE TRIALS

One should be clear about the primary objective of any clinical trial regardless of the control used. Should the objective be to demonstrate superiority of the test treatment to the control (either placebo or a standard effective active treatment), noninferiority to the active control treatment, equivalence to the active control, or simply effectiveness of the test treatment? Each of these objectives requires a different set of hypotheses. Now let us review the framework of the hypotheses in terms of null and alternative for superiority, noninferiority, and equivalence trials as follows. Blackwelder[13] and many authors,[3,14–19] to name just a few, have addressed the hypotheses using slightly different formats and symbols. In this manuscript primarily those of Hwang and Morikawa[3] are used. Let T = test treatment, S = standard active control treatment, P = placebo, δ = noninferiority/equivalence margin, Δ = active control effect size, and ε = effect size to be detected between the test and active control treatments. To simplify the presentation, the letters T, S, and P will be loosely used to represent treatment groups/arms or primary endpoint of interest in population means, proportions, and event rates, etc., as appropriate. Also, positive effects are considered favorable (i.e., $\Delta > 0$, $\delta > 0$, and $\varepsilon > 0$). In addition, we assume Δ, δ, and ε are known (i.e., readily available from prior research). In Section VI, the cases when Δ and δ are not known but may be estimated from historical placebo-controlled trials will be discussed. For other specific formulations of null and alternative hypotheses (e.g., relative risk in means or event rates, odds ratio, or hazard ratio), the reader may refer specifically to these articles.[20–24]

A. SUPERIORITY TRIAL

A superiority trial is designed to detect a difference (Δ or ε) between the test and control treatments. The control can be placebo or an effective standard active treatment. The form of null and alternative hypotheses remains the same. Namely

$H_0 : T - P \leq 0$ vs. $H_1 : T - P > 0$ when control is placebo and
$H_0 : T - S \leq 0$ vs. $H_1 : T - S > 0$ when control is a standard active
treatment

Note that in sample size estimation, the clinically meaningful effect size between the test treatment and placebo to be detected is Δ, while the effect size between the test and active control treatments is ε, where $\Delta > \varepsilon > 0$. Note also that we assume the test is one-sided instead of the traditional two-sided test that the FDA has favored. In fact, a one-sided test at $\alpha = 0.025$ gives the same significance level as the two-sided test at $\alpha = 0.05$.

The test statistics are,

$z = (T - P)/s_{(t-p)}$ when control is placebo, and
$z = (T - S)/s_{(t-s)}$ when control is a standard active treatment,

where $s_{(t-p)}$ and $s_{(t-s)}$ are the sample standard errors of $T - P$ and $T - S$, respectively. Again, to simplify presentation, we assume the data are from a large sample with a common distribution for which the variance is finite and outliers are rare. We reject H_0 and conclude superiority of T to P or S, if $z > z_{1-\alpha}$ (a one-sided α-level test), where $z_{1-\alpha}$ is the usual $100 \times (1 - \alpha)\%$ point of the standard normal distribution.

Equivalently, we can use the confidence interval (CI) approach. To declare superiority we need to show that the one-sided $100 \times (1 - \alpha)\%$ CI, $[C_L, \infty)$, for $T - P$ or $T - S$ is included in $[0, \infty)$ or simply $0 < C_L$ as shown in the following sketch, where C_L is the lower limit of the CI.

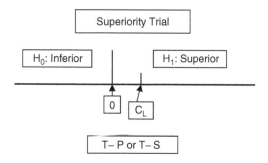

It should be noted that in a superiority trial involving a standard active control S, one cannot conclude the test treatment T is noninferior or equivalent to the active control S, when the trial failed to demonstrate superiority of T to S.

Many nonstatisticians often commit this kind of fallacy, simply because they do not understand that failing to reject the null hypothesis of inferiority (or no difference) for an active-controlled superiority trial does not imply that the null hypothesis is true. If one is interested in demonstrating T as noninferior or equivalent to S, then the corresponding hypotheses should reflect "noninferiority" or "equivalence" as follows.

B. NONINFERIORITY TRIAL

A noninferiority trial is to show that a test treatment is no less effective than an existing standard effective treatment by a small predefined noninferiority margin δ. In this context, "noninferiority" does not simply mean "not inferior," but rather "not inferior by as much as a predefined limit or margin, with respect to a particular endpoint under study." The control now is an effective standard active treatment. The null and alternative hypotheses are

$$H_0 : T - S \leq -\delta \text{ vs. } H_1 : T - S > -\delta,$$
where $\delta =$ predefined noninferiority margin

The test statistic is now $z = [(T - S) + \delta]/s_{(t-s)}$. We reject H_0 and conclude noninferiority of T to S if $z > z_{1-\alpha}$ (a one-sided α-level test).

To declare noninferiority of T to S using the CI approach, we need to show that the one-sided $100 \times (1 - \alpha)\%$ CI, $[C_L, \infty)$, for $T - S$ is included in $[-\delta, \infty)$ or simply $-\delta < C_L$ as shown in the graph below.

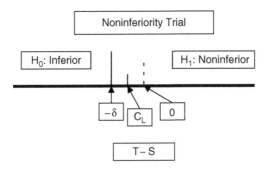

Note that we demonstrate noninferiority when $-\delta < C_L$. We may further claim superiority if $0 < C_L$. The discussion of switching objectives (i.e., superiority to noninferiority or *vice versa*) will be deferred to Section VII.

C. EQUIVALENCE TRIAL

An equivalence trial is designed to show either that the test treatment is not meaningfully different from an effective standard active treatment or that the test treatment is equivalent to the active control (i.e., bounded by a small predefined equivalence margin δ). Now the null and alternative hypotheses are two-sided:

$$H_0 : T - S \le -\delta \quad \text{or} \quad T - S \ge \delta \text{ vs. } H_1 : -\delta < T - S < \delta.$$

The two-sided hypotheses can also be expressed as paired (two) one-sided hypotheses[25,26]:

$$H_0 : T - S \le -\delta \text{ vs. } H_1 : T - S > -\delta \quad \text{and}$$
$$H_0' : T - S \ge \delta \text{ vs. } H_1' : T - S < \delta.$$

T and S are equivalent when the two-sided null hypothesis H_0 is rejected (or the paired null hypotheses H_0 and H_0' are simultaneously rejected). For testing equivalence, the test statistics for the paired one-sided α-level tests are:

$$z = [(T - S) + \delta]/s_{(t-s)} \quad \text{and} \quad z' = [(T - S) - \delta]/s_{(t-s)}.$$

Reject H_0 and H_0' to demonstrate equivalence of T and S. Chow and Shao[27] showed that the two one-sided tests procedure is a valid size α test.

To conclude equivalence of T and S in the CI approach (as shown in the following sketch), we need to show that the $100 \times (1 - 2\alpha)\%$ CI, $[C_L, C_U]$ is included in $[-\delta, \delta]$ or $-\delta < C_L < C_U < \delta$, where C_L and C_U are the lower and upper limits of the CI, respectively.

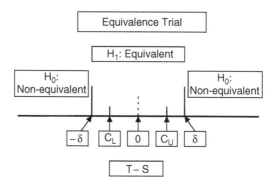

In fact, in late-phase drug development, noninferiority trials are more commonly used than equivalence trials. Sole assessment of therapeutic equivalence of two treatments (test vs. effective active control) may be inadequate in practice. The sponsor may want to demonstrate that the test treatment is no less effective than an effective active control treatment — it may have a similar effect or it may be even more effective than the active control. That is, it may involve an assessment of noninferiority and superiority in a stepwise fashion, not restricted to demonstrate equivalence. Because there is an incentive to demonstrate superior efficacy beyond noninferiority (unlike excess bioavailability in bioequivalence), the interest is fundamentally one-sided. As discussed in the next section, the formulae for sample size and power are also slightly different between the noninferiority and equivalence trials. The latter tends to need a larger sample size than the former. Therefore, the distinction between noninferiority and equivalence trials is important and needs to be clarified to avoid confusion, though this point has only been made clear recently.[11,12,28]

IV. SAMPLE SIZE AND POWER

Formulae for sample size estimates and their corresponding power can be derived via solving the following two simultaneous equations[29]:

$$\alpha = \Pr[z > z_c | H_0] \qquad \text{and} \qquad 1 - \beta = \Pr[z > z_c | H_1]$$

where z = the test statistic, z_c = the critical value, H_0 = the null hypothesis, and H_1 = the alternative hypothesis.

Some selected formulae for sample size estimates and their corresponding power under normal and binomial distributions[3,30] are provided as follows.

A. SUPERIORITY TRIAL

1. Normal Distribution

The formulae for sample size per group and its related power when control is placebo are

$$n = 2(s/\Delta)^2(z_{1-\alpha} + z_{1-\beta})^2 \qquad \text{and} \qquad 1 - \beta = \Phi[(\Delta/s)(n/2)^{1/2} - z_{1-\alpha}].$$

When control is an active treatment, one simply replaces Δ with ε as follows.

$$n = 2(s/\varepsilon)^2(z_{1-\alpha} + z_{1-\beta})^2 \qquad \text{and} \qquad 1 - \beta = \Phi[(\varepsilon/s)(n/2)^{1/2} - z_{1-\alpha}].$$

where n = sample size per group, $1 - \beta$ = power, δ = clinically meaningful mean difference of test vs. placebo (test treatment effect size), ε = mean difference between the test and active control treatments, which may not need to be clinically meaningful and in general $\Delta > \varepsilon$, s = pooled standard deviation, z_{1-x} remains the usual $100 \times (1 - x)\%$ point of the standard normal distribution, and $\Phi[x]$ denotes $\Pr[X \geq x]$ where X has the standard normal distribution.

2. Binomial Distribution

The formulae for sample size per group and its related power when control is placebo are:

$$n = 2[\pi(1 - \pi)/\Delta^2](z_{1-\alpha} + z_{1-\beta})^2 \qquad \text{and}$$

$$1 - \beta = \Phi[\{\Delta/[\pi(1 - \pi)]^{1/2}\}(n/2)^{1/2} - z_{1-\alpha}],$$

with $\Delta = T - P$, and $\pi = (T + P)/2$.

When control is an active treatment, one replaces Δ with ε:

$$n = 2[\pi(1 - \pi)/\varepsilon^2](z_{1-\alpha} + z_{1-\beta})^2 \quad \text{and}$$

$$1 - \beta = \Phi[\{\varepsilon/[\pi(1 - \pi)]^{1/2}\}(n/2)^{1/2} - z_{1-\alpha}],$$

with $\varepsilon = T - S$, and $\pi = (T + S)/2$.

B. NONINFERIORITY TRIAL

1. Normal Distribution

In the formulae for sample size per group and related power for a noninferiority trial, one needs to replace Δ or ε in a superiority trial with the noninferiority margin δ as follows:

$$n = 2(s/\delta)^2(z_{1-\alpha} + z_{1-\beta})^2 \quad \text{and} \quad 1 - \beta = \Phi[(\delta/s)(n/2)^{1/2} - z_{1-\alpha}],$$

when $T = S$.

2. Binomial Distribution

Again, we replace Δ or ε with δ; now the respective formulae become

$$n = 2[\pi(1 - \pi)/\delta^2](z_{1-\alpha} + z_{1-\beta})^2 \quad \text{and}$$
$$1 - \beta = \Phi[\{\delta/[\pi(1 - \pi)]^{1/2}\}(n/2)^{1/2} - z_{1-\alpha}],$$

at $T = S = \pi$.

C. EQUIVALENCE TRIAL

1. Normal Distribution

For an equivalence trial at $T = S$, the sample size formula for a noninferiority trial can be used, but with β replaced by $\beta/2$.[3,30,31] Here we assume that the equivalence margin δ is symmetric around 0

$$n = 2(s/\delta)^2[z_{1-\alpha} + z_{1-(\beta/2)}]^2 \quad \text{and}$$

$$1 - \beta = 2\Phi[(\delta/s)(n/2)^{1/2} - z_{1-\alpha}] - 1,$$

when $T = S$.

2. Binomial Distribution

Again, we replace β with $\beta/2$; now the respective formulae become

$$n = 2[\pi(1 - \pi)/\delta^2][z_{1-\alpha} + z_{1-(\beta/2)}]^2 \quad \text{and}$$
$$1 - \beta = 2\Phi[\{\delta/[\pi(1 - \pi)]^{1/2}\}(n/2)^{1/2} - z_{1-\alpha}] - 1,$$

at $T = S = \pi$.

Clearly in active-controlled trials whether the intention is to demonstrate superiority, noninferiority, or equivalence, the required sample size is usually much larger than a placebo-controlled superiority trial.

To take a closer view of this, let us arrange the sample size formulae of superiority, noninferiority, and equivalence on top of each other (e.g., under normal distribution) as follows:

$$n_{(\text{Sup: } T \text{ vs. } S)} = 2(s/\varepsilon)^2(z_{1-\alpha} + z_{1-\beta})^2,$$
$$n_{(\text{Sup: } T \text{ vs. } P)} = 2(s/\Delta)^2(z_{1-\alpha} + z_{1-\beta})^2,$$
$$n_{(\text{NI: } T \text{ vs. } S)} = 2(s/\delta)^2(z_{1-\alpha} + z_{1-\beta})^2, \quad \text{and}$$
$$n_{(\text{Eq: } T \text{ vs. } S)} = 2(s/\delta)^2[z_{1-\alpha} + z_{1-(\beta/2)}]^2,$$

where Sup = Superiority, NI = Noninferiority, and Eq = Equivalence.

Clearly, $n_{(\text{Eq: } T \text{ vs. } S)} > n_{(\text{NI: } T \text{ vs. } S)} > n_{(\text{Sup: } T \text{ vs. } P)}$, and $n_{(\text{Sup: } T \text{ vs. } S)} > n_{(\text{Sup: } T \text{ vs. } P)}$, because $\Delta > \delta > \varepsilon$ and $z_{1-(\beta/2)} > z_{1-\beta}$. In particular, if one chooses an equivalence margin to be less than one half of the active control effect size (i.e., let $\delta < \Delta/2$), then $n_{(\text{Eq: } T \text{ vs. } S)} > 4n_{(\text{Sup: } T \text{ vs. } P)}$. It should be emphasized again that $n_{(\text{Eq: } T \text{ vs. } S)} > n_{(\text{NI: } T \text{ vs. } S)}$ is caused by the fact that $z_{1-(\beta/2)} > z_{1-\beta}$. Therefore, one can generalize that an active-controlled trial needs larger sample size than a placebo-controlled trial.

Following are a couple of examples in sample size and power estimation in active-controlled noninferiority trials.

Example 1. Company X is developing a new antiarthritis (RA) disease drug X-111 — a selective COX-2 inhibitor. It has been proved in historical placebo-controlled trials that the standard drug, ibuprofen, is effective in treating RA, but might induce gastrointestinal (GI) side effects such as ulcer, which is usually confirmed by endoscopy. X-111 is also proved effective (vs. placebo) in Phase III placebo-controlled trials, but now the FDA wants Company X to conduct a study to ascertain that the possible GI side effects for X-111 is substantially better (lower) than ibuprofen, but not worse than placebo by much. You, the project statistician, are called upon to design this study to provide response to the FDA. The historical ulcer rates for ibuprofen and placebo are approximately 20 to 22% and 2 to 3%, respectively. The noninferiority margin is assumed readily known to be no greater than 5%.

Assignment. 1. What trial design would you suggest? How many treatment arms would you include? Which formula would you use to calculate the sample size as defined in this simple mythical example? (Assume that the sample size required for demonstrating noninferiority of X-111 to placebo is more than adequate for showing superiority of X-111 to ibuprofen in causing ulcer.) 2. What historical ulcer rates for ibuprofen and placebo would you use? What noninferiority margin to define? Give brief rationale. 3. Provide n, sample size per group (equal allocation) at $\alpha = 0.025$ (one-sided) and power $(1 - \beta) = 0.80$, 0.90, and 0.95, respectively. 4. Provide the power for $n = 100$, 200, and 300 per group, respectively.

Answer. 1. A mixture design with three treatment arms (i.e., X-111, ibuprofen, and placebo) to demonstrate superiority (X-111 to ibuprofen) and noninferiority (X-111 to placebo). In this hypothetical example, GI side effect (i.e., ulcer) is of safety concern. Therefore, the role of placebo is very different in assessing safety than efficacy and one needs to demonstrate that the ulcer rate of the test treatment X-111 is not much greater (i.e., the GI side effects were not much worse) than that of placebo (a standard control for safety). Because the sample size required for demonstrating noninferiority of X-111 to placebo is greater than for showing superiority of X-111 to ibuprofen in developing ulcer, the formula for a noninferiority trial under binomial distribution is used:

$$n_{(\text{NI: } T \text{ vs. } S)} = 2[\pi(1 - \pi)/\delta^2](z_{1-\alpha} + z_{1-\beta})^2$$

at $T = S = \pi$, where $T = $ X-111, $S = $ placebo, $T = S = \pi = 0.03$, $\delta = 0.05$, $z_{0.8} = 0.84$, $z_{0.9} = 1.282$, $z_{0.95} = 1.645$, and $z_{0.975} = 1.96$. 2. The ulcer rates used in sample size estimation are 20% for ibuprofen and 3% for placebo. The noninferiority margin used is 5%. The simple reason is that these rates provide a larger sample size to safeguard adequate power. 3. Sample sizes per group calculated and estimated:

Power (%)	n per Group (Calculated)	n per Group (Estimated)
80	183	185
90	245	245
95	303	305

Note: Sample size estimation is not an exact science. Usually in practice the calculated numbers are rounded up to some reasonable whole numbers. 4. The following table lists the calculated power for given $n = 100$, 200, and 300 per group:

n per Group Given	Power $= (1 - \beta)$ (%)
100	54
200	83
300	94

Example 2. The following example describes a complex case about a Phase III trial in oncology. The original trial design was to demonstrate that the test treatment (T) is noninferior in overall survival (OS) to an active standard treatment (S). The noninferiority margin for the hazard ratio of OS was assumed to be 0.70. Later, it was revised to 0.75 and eventually settled at $\delta = 0.80$ per insistence of the regulatory authority. In reviewing the draft protocol, the authority further requested the sponsor to include a co-primary endpoint — tumor response rate (RR) such that the test treatment (T) retains at least 75% of the active control response rate. The sample size section of the revised draft protocol is shown as follows (note that drug names are withheld and some wordings are also changed to preserve anonymity):

"The primary efficacy objective is to demonstrate that treatment with regimen T results in noninferior OS and RR as compared with treatment with the conventional regimen S. Statistically, it is to demonstrate noninferiority concurrently in both the co-primary endpoints such that:

1. The lower limit of the two-sided 95% CI or equivalently, the lower limit of the one-sided 97.5% CI of the hazard ratio on OS of T vs. S is greater than or equal to a noninferiority margin of 0.80.
2. The lower limit of the two-sided 95% CI or equivalently, the lower limit of the one-sided 97.5% CI on the difference of the RR between T and S excludes a noninferiority margin such that T retains at least 75% of the RR of S. Or, the lower limit of the one-sided 97.5% CI on the relative risk of the response rates between T and S is greater than or equal to a noninferiority margin of 0.75.

To design a noninferiority trial as suggested in ICH E10 Guidance, first it requires a determination that there exists HESDE of the chosen active control and then an estimation of the control effect size via appropriate statistical methodology (e.g., mixed-effects meta-analysis). Next, it needs to show that the test drug preserves appropriate fraction of the active control effect. Unfortunately, the HESDE of the active control S, was not well established and the control effect size for neither OS nor RR can be appropriately estimated. Alternatively, various estimates for the control effect size, based primarily on one positive trial were used. Tables 12.1 and 12.2 provide the sample size estimates for the co-primary endpoints of OS and RR under various assumptions, respectively.

Assume that the survival of this patient population follows an exponential distribution with a constant hazard and the time to median survival of the control group is approximately 18 months. For an average patient follow-up of 24 months (36 months maximum and 12 months minimum for a 24-month accrual period and an additional 12 months follow-up), the active control group mortality rate is estimated to be approximately 0.60. The total sample size required is approximately 780 patients (390 patients per group) at the significance level of $\alpha = 0.025$ (one-sided), power $(1 - \beta) = 90\%$, and the noninferiority margin

TABLE 12.1

The Sample Size Estimates for Demonstrating Noninferiority of T to S in OS Under Various Assumptions at $\alpha = 0.025$ (One-Sided), $1 - \beta$ (Power) = 90%, with a Noninferiority Margin $\delta = 0.80$ on Hazard Ratio of OS

$S_{0.5}$	λ_s	T	S_s	π_s	δ	n	N	N^*	D^*
21	0.0330	24	0.45	0.55	0.110	430	860	950	580
		30	0.37	0.63	0.126	310	620	690	480
20	0.0347	24	0.43	0.57	0.114	400	800	880	550
		30	0.35	0.65	0.130	280	560	620	450
18	*0.0385*	*24*	*0.40*	**0.60**	*0.120*	*350*	*700*	**780**	*520*
		30	0.32	0.68	0.136	250	500	550	410
16	0.0433	24	0.35	0.65	0.130	280	560	620	450
		30	0.27	0.73	0.146	195	390	430	350

$S_{0.5}$ = Time to median survival for the active control group in months; λ_s = Hazard rate for the active control group under exponential survival; T = Time of average patient follow-up (accrual time + follow-up time) in months; S_s = Active control group survival rate; π_s = Active control group mortality rate; δ = Noninferiority margin corresponding to the active control group mortality rate; n = Sample size per group; N = Total sample size; N^* = Total sample size adjusted for noncompliance (drop-out and lost-to-follow-up); D^* = Total information (total expected number of deaths) of the trial based on OS alone.

on hazard ratio of the OS at 0.80. The total information (total expected number of deaths) of the trial based on survival alone is estimated to be approximately 520 deaths.

The point and interval (95% CI) estimates for the active control RR in the single historical trial were, respectively, 0.44 and (0.35, 0.51). Assume that the active control (S) RR is approximately 0.45. To retain 75% of that effect, a noninferiority margin is estimated to be around 0.1125. To demonstrate that T retains at least 75% of the control response rate, the total sample size required is approximately 910 patients (455 patients per group) at the significance level of $\alpha = 0.025$ (one-sided) and power $(1 - \beta) = 90\%$. The total information (total expected number of responders) of the trial based on RR alone is estimated to be approximately 360 responders.

In summary, at $\alpha = 0.025$ (one-sided) and 90% power, it requires 780 patients (520 deaths) in OS and 910 patients (360 responders) in RR to show noninferiority, respectively. To assure that the overall power is at least 80% for demonstrating noninferiority in both the co-primary endpoints, it is imperative to maintain that the individual power for each endpoint is at least 90%. Therefore, the trial will randomize a total of 910 (the greater of 910 and 780) patients with a follow-up of 36 months or observe a total of 360 responders and a minimum of 520 deaths, whichever comes last."

TABLE 12.2
The Sample Size Estimates for Demonstrating Noninferiority of T to S in RR with the Active Control Rates Ranged from 0.40 to 0.50 at $\alpha = 0.025$ (One-Sided), $1 - \beta$ (Power) = 90%, and T Retains $\geq 75\%$ of the S Response Rate

π_s	π_t	δ	n	N	N^*	R^*
0.40	0.3000	0.1000	505	1010	1120	392
0.41	0.3075	0.1025	485	970	1080	388
0.42	0.3150	0.1050	465	930	1030	378
0.43	0.3225	0.1075	445	890	990	372
0.44	0.3300	0.1100	430	860	950	366
0.45	*0.3375*	*0.1125*	*410*	*820*	*910*	*360*
0.46	0.3450	0.1150	395	790	880	354
0.47	0.3525	0.1175	380	760	840	346
0.48	0.3600	0.1200	365	730	810	340
0.49	0.3675	0.1225	350	700	780	334
0.50	0.3750	0.1250	340	680	750	330

π_s = Active control group response rate; π_t = Test treatment group response rate; δ = Noninferiority margin corresponding to the active control group response rate; n = Sample size per group; N = Total sample size; N^* = Total sample size adjusted for noncompliance (drop-out and lost-to-follow-up); R^* = Total expected number of responders based on RR alone.

Comments. Working with moving targets in trial design was extremely frustrating. Because HESDE for the active control S was not well supported, the meta-analysis was not performed. Therefore, the approach of using "putative placebo" suggested by Hasselblad and Kong,[32] to estimate the fraction of active control effect S preserved by the test treatment T, was not attempted. The estimated sample size based on two co-primary endpoints was overly large for the sponsor to conduct. Because of the size and cost, the trial never got off the ground and was finally shelved by the management of the sponsor.

V. ASSAY SENSITIVITY (AS), HISTORICAL EVIDENCE OF SENSITIVITY-TO-DRUG-EFFECTS (HESDE), APPROPRIATE TRIAL CONDUCT (ATC), AND CONSTANCY ASSUMPTION (CA)

Now in this section we begin to provide in-depth discussions on the essence of active-controlled trials, in particular, the noninferiority trial. As noted earlier most active-controlled equivalence trials are practically noninferiority trials intended to establish the efficacy of a new treatment. The new treatment can be shown noninferior as well as superior to the active control treatment, not limited to equivalence. Hence, the term of equivalence will be dropped hereafter in most of this manuscript.

A. AS

As defined in ICH E10, AS is "a property of a clinical trial that has the ability to distinguish an effective treatment from a less effective or ineffective treatment." AS is crucial in any trial but has different implications for trials intended to demonstrate superiority vs. noninferiority. In the superiority trial setting whether the control is placebo or an active treatment, AS refers to the ability of a specific trial to detect a difference between treatments, if one exists. For active-controlled noninferiority trials, AS requires the presence of an active control treatment effect of a minimum size so that a specific trial, properly designed and conducted, has the ability not to falsely conclude an ineffective treatment noninferior. Because the effect size of the active control in the current noninferiority trial is not measured directly relative to placebo, AS must be deduced. When AS is not supported in a superiority trial whether the control is placebo or an active treatment, it will fail to show that the test treatment is superior and therefore will fail to demonstrate test treatment efficacy. In contrast, if a trial intended to demonstrate efficacy by showing a test treatment is noninferior to an active control lacks AS, the trial may find an ineffective treatment to be noninferior and could lead to an erroneous conclusion of efficacy. Therefore, when a finding of noninferiority is used as evidence of efficacy, AS of the trial is absolutely critical and the evidence of AS may be deduced from HESDE of the chosen active control treatment in historical placebo-controlled trials and an ATC of the current noninferiority trial. That is, in a noninferiority trial AS depends not only on the sample size and quality, but also on the effect of the active control (i.e., its effect size and constancy to the size observed in historical trials) in the current trial.

B. HESDE

ICH E10 defines HESDE as "similarly designed trials in the past regularly distinguish effective treatments from less effective or ineffective treatments". Superficially, AS and HESDE appear to be synonymous in terms of distinguishing effective treatments from less effective or ineffective treatments *per se*. There is indeed a difference between AS and HESDE. The former defines the ability of differentiating effective treatment from an ineffective one for any trial, historical or current, placebo or active-controlled trials, while the latter specifically emphasizes the historical placebo-controlled trials involving a chosen active control, which regularly demonstrated effectiveness over placebo. In fact, HESDE should be evaluated at the beginning of designing a noninferiority trial. That is, as described in ICH E10, "it should be determined in the specific therapeutic area under study, appropriately designed and conducted trials that used a well-defined dose of a specific active treatment, or other treatments with similar effects, reliably showed an effect of at least a minimum size." In plain language, HESDE means that the chosen active control for the current designed noninferiority trial should have shown efficacy with a clinically meaningful effect size over placebo regularly and consistently in the historical placebo-controlled trials in a specific therapeutic area of interest. The chosen active control with HESDE ensures that demonstrating noninferiority will not falsely conclude an ineffective treatment effective provided that a noninferiority margin is appropriately chosen and the current trial is conducted with high quality. It should be noted that in many therapeutic areas for symptomatic treatments such as depression, anxiety, seasonal allergic rhinitis, exercise tolerance in CHF, and symptomatic gastro-esophageal reflux, historical trials clearly did not have proved HESDE and AS for the test treatments vs. placebo. The effectiveness was not regularly and consistently demonstrated possibly because of high placebo response, small or marginal treatment effects, and excessive variability in trials. In these cases, it will be impossible to design and conduct noninferiority trials, because HESDE for those active control candidates cannot be supported.

C. ATC

ATC means that noninferiority trials currently conducted do not undermine the ability to distinguish effective treatments from less effective or ineffective treatments. For a planned noninferiority trial to be similarly sensitive to drug effects, it is essential that the trial design characteristics (e.g., the entry criteria, concomitant medications, the primary and secondary endpoints, and timing of assessments) should be similar to the historical trials in all aspects as possible, except that the current trial is intended to demonstrate noninferiority of the test treatment to the active control, while the historical trials were mostly placebo-controlled involving the selected active control treatment as the test treatment. Most importantly, the trial should be conducted with high quality not to undermine its AS.

Similarly designed and well-conducted trials may not ensure constancy in active control effect size. This brings about the next important issue in noninferiority trials.

D. CA

CA means that the historical active control effect size vs. placebo is holding unchanged in the setting of the current noninferiority trial. Therefore, demonstration of efficacy by showing noninferiority of the test treatment to an active control rests on some critical assumptions that the selected active control with proved HESDE does have an effect and that the CA of the control effect does hold. Unfortunately, as pointed out by many authors,[19,20,21,33] CA is a strong evoked assumption in noninferiority trials that may not be directly verifiable. Nonetheless, this may be accomplished via the so-called putative (imputed) placebo approach,[32] in which an imputed placebo P is compared with the test treatment T via comparing T vs. S in the current noninferiority trial in conjunction with S vs. P in historical placebo-controlled trials. When T is demonstrated to be superior to the imputed P, T is deduced to be effective.

Together with HESDE, ATC, and CA, it provides evidence of AS in the currently designed trial and a successful active-controlled noninferiority trial thus involves four critical steps[2]:

1. Determining that HESDE of the chosen active control exists. Without this determination, demonstration of efficacy from a showing of noninferiority is not possible and should not even be attempted. If HESDE exists for the chosen active control, one then needs to determine its effect size based on appropriate statistical methodology (refer to Section VI).
2. Designing a trial similar to the historical trials. The trial design (e.g., study population, concomitant therapy, endpoints, trial duration, and assessments) needs to adhere closely to the design of the trials for which HESDE has been determined.
3. Setting an appropriate margin provided that the CA holds. An acceptable noninferiority margin should be chosen taking into account the active control effect size based on the historical data and relevant clinical and statistical considerations (also see Section VI).
4. Conducting the trial with high quality. The trial conduct should also adhere closely to that of the historical trials and should be of high quality.

VI. ACTIVE CONTROL EFFECT SIZE (Δ) AND NONINFERIORITY MARGIN (δ)

A. ACTIVE CONTROL EFFECT SIZE (Δ)

When there exist no credible historical placebo-controlled trials or no HESDE involving the chosen active control, an active-controlled noninferiority trial should not be designed and conducted, or even attempted. However, in some therapeutic areas such as infectious disease and hypertension, historical active control effects are well documented and readily available. An active-controlled noninferiority trial should pose no major difficulty. Nonetheless, in most therapeutic areas the active control effects are not well known, but adequate and well-controlled (i.e., placebo-controlled) trials may be available; it may be possible to estimate the active control effect size Δ. Therefore, the difficulty in most noninferiority trials lies in the fact that the presumed active control effect is not measured directly in the current trial, but rather estimated indirectly via historical placebo-controlled trials. This means that most noninferiority trials inherited some strong assumptions with uncertain validity, if the active control effect is not readily known.

To estimate such an active control effect can be problematic. A meta-analysis of DerSimonian and Laird[33] on the data, if available, from the historical placebo-controlled trials involving the active control or other relevant treatments, may provide a reliable estimate of the control effect size Δ and the relevant within- and between-trial variability. Limitations and problems of an appropriate meta-analysis are well known.

First, trial selection bias may be of major concern in practice. Which trials to include — all placebo-controlled trials, trials showing positive results, or trials with similar design to the current noninferiority trial? If only favorable trials are included in the meta-analysis, the active control effect will be overestimated. On the other hand, if all trials are included indiscriminately, the control effect will be underestimated because of increased heterogeneity of trials, not to mention that some trials with negative or equivocal results have never been published because of publication bias.

Second, selection of estimates from a meta-analysis can be problematic. Which estimate to adopt, point estimate or interval estimate (e.g., the lower limit of the CI)? What level α or $100 \times (1 - \alpha)\%$ CI to use? One or two-sided? Some authors[34,22] have shown that use of a point estimate may overestimate the true control effect size, while use of the lower limit of a one-sided 95% CI may underestimate the true control effect for being over conservative in adopting the worst scenario.

Third, the trial data and critical information for meta-analysis may not be readily available. More often the historical placebo-controlled trial data are proprietary and owned by the funding sponsor(s). Gaining access to these trial data may be difficult in practice, though negotiation with the sponsor or use of Freedom of Information Act may help. Also, some trials may only report mean differences without standard errors or CIs or in mortality trials may only report median survival times, number of events (e.g., deaths) and logrank p values without giving hazard ratios and the corresponding standard error estimates or CIs. Though occasionally it may be possible to extract some of the necessary information,[35] the process may be difficult and sometimes implausible.

Fourth, correct model selection is important in meta-analysis. To obtain an overall active control effect one needs to choose between the fixed effect and random effect model, where appropriate. When historical trials are abundant, a random (mixed) effect model utilizes between-trial variation in estimation will be a logical choice. However, when available trials are scant (e.g., one or two), one cannot utilize the between-trial variability despite the fact that the within-trial variability estimate remains available.

Though the active control effect may be estimated via the data from historical placebo-controlled trials, the active control effect in the current noninferiority trial may still be different (usually smaller is the concern) because of changes in patient population, improved care, health awareness, and advanced medical practice. The current trial should be designed as similarly as possible to the historical placebo-controlled trials including important factors, which may influence the trial outcome. Most importantly, some adjustment (discounting by a fraction f) of the historical control effect may be necessary by introducing a reduced active control effect size Δ' as

$$\Delta' = f\Delta,$$

where $0 < f < 1$. The fraction f can be determined by clinical judgment, examining the within- and between-trial variability of the historical trials, and consulting with the experts in that particular therapeutic area, in the absence of regulatory guidance.

When the active control effect is readily available or estimated via historical trials, the next step will be choosing the noninferiority margin δ.

B. Noninferiority Margin (δ)

What is δ? δ is a term used to represent the noninferiority (or equivalence) margin. It states in ICH E10,[2] "This margin is the degree of inferiority of the test treatment to the control that the trial will attempt to exclude statistically. ...The margin chosen for a noninferiority trial cannot be greater than the smallest effect size that the active drug would be reliably expected to have compared with placebo in the setting of the planned trial, but may be smaller based on clinical judgment." ICH E9[36] states, "An equivalence margin should be specified in the protocol; this margin is the largest difference which can be judged as being clinically acceptable and should be smaller than differences observed in superiority trials of the active comparator. For the active control equivalence trial, both the upper and lower equivalence margins are needed, while only the lower margin is needed for the active control noninferiority trial. The choice of equivalence margins should be justified clinically." Blackwelder[13] states, "In a study designed to show equivalence of the therapies, the quantity δ is sufficiently small that the therapies are considered equivalent for practical purposes if the difference is smaller than δ." Hwang and Morikawa[3] defines, "The noninferiority/equivalence margin, δ, is the degree of acceptable inferiority between the test and active control drugs that a trial needs to predefine at the trial design stage. This margin chosen for a noninferiority trial should be smaller (usually a fraction) than the effect size, Δ, that the active control would be reliably expected to have compared with placebo in the setting of the given trial." The 2004 CPMP Points to Consider draft[37] articulates, "The selection of the noninferiority margin is based upon a combination of statistical reasoning and clinical judgment. An appropriate selection should be at the minimum provide assurance that the test drug has a clinically relevant effect greater than zero. ...The choice of margin should be independent of consideration of power. It should be based upon the clinical and statistical principles...not upon issues of sample size, as the size of the clinically important difference is not altered by the size of the study." For more definitions of δ, refer to Ng.[38] Before we discuss choosing an appropriate margin for a noninferiority trial, it can be asserted, in line with many authors, that δ should be based on the active control effect size Δ

derived from the historical placebo-controlled trials and more specifically, a small fraction of the control effect size Δ determined by good clinical judgment with sound statistical reasoning and it must be carefully stated in the trial protocol. In fact, the active control effect size, variability, and constancy as well as the trial objective are some of the major factors for determination of the noninferiority margin. In practice, the statistician and clinician, in consultation with the therapeutic area experts and regulatory authority (e.g., FDA), should define an appropriate margin at study design stage together for all active-controlled noninferiority trials intended for new drug registration. Wiens[18] suggested three strategies for choosing a margin, namely: the putative placebo strategy, the clinical importance strategy, and the statistical strategy. The first strategy appears to be one of the mainstream approaches in design and analysis of noninferiority trials.

In choosing an appropriate margin for a noninferiority trial, two inter-related objectives regarding the effectiveness of the test treatment arise. One objective is to demonstrate that the test treatment is not much less effective than the active control treatment by a prespecified margin. To attain this objective one must prespecify a fixed noninferiority margin. The other objective is simply to establish the effectiveness of the test treatment. In this case a prespecified margin is not necessary, but rather one needs to define a certain fraction of active control effect to be retained or preserved. Articles by Wang et al.,[34] Hung et al.,[20] Rothmann et al.,[21] and Chi et al.[22] have articulated the discussion of the above mentioned objectives and corresponding statistical methods for active-controlled noninferiority trials.

1.   Setting a Fixed Noninferiority Margin δ

The traditional framework for a noninferiority trial as shown in Section III requires a fixed noninferiority margin δ to be set in the null and alternative hypotheses. Whether it can be concluded that the test treatment T is effective in the absence of direct placebo comparison, if noninferiority to the active control S based on the predefined margin δ is demonstrated, remains a critical issue. When the active control effect size Δ or Δ' as defined earlier is readily known or estimated via historical placebo-controlled trials through a meta-analysis, one can simply set

$$\delta = \lambda\Delta \qquad \text{or} \qquad \delta \le \lambda\Delta'$$

where $0 < \lambda < 1$. The well known CBER/FDA "50% rule" defines $\lambda = 0.5$, when the control effect size Δ is set as the lower limit of the one-sided 95% CI on $S - P$ through a meta-analysis on the historical placebo-controlled trials involving the active control S. Some use $\lambda = 0.8$ to compensate for the over conservatism. Alternatively, one can set $0 < \lambda < 1/2$, if Δ is defined as the point estimate (equivalent to the lower limit of the 0% CI) of the active control effects from the meta-analysis. In principle, the lower CI limit or point estimate reflects the "least" effect of the active control can be used. This is to ensure that an ineffective test treatment should not be erroneously concluded as effective via a fallacious noninferiority demonstration.

Most determinations of δ through Δ and λ depend on clinical judgment, statistical reasoning, historical experience in a specific therapeutic area, and regulatory guidance (if available) on a case-by-case basis. A general one-size-fits-all rule which is available for bioequivalence (e.g., log mean AUC ratio between log 0.80 and log 1.25) does not appear to be feasible for assessing therapeutic noninferiority in various therapeutic areas. In infectious disease, the adaptive stepwise equivalence margins adopted by the FDA Points to Consider[39] are set to 10, 15, or 20 percentage points depending on the response cure rates of $>90\%$, 80 to 90%, or $<80\%$ in the study, respectively. These margins' determination appeared to be primarily based on clinical reasoning without statistical justification. Recently, responding to many years' criticism, the Agency adopted a further conservative "10 percentage point" margin across the board for all noninferiority trials in antiinfectives. In Europe, a new test that allows the noninferiority margin to vary with the response rates is proposed by Phillips.[40] In oncology, the Agency used to set the margin around 0.70 to 0.80 for hazard ratio of active control to test treatment in OS and disease-free survival (DFS), but recently has moved towards preservation of a certain fraction of active control effect approach.[21,22]

In the traditional approach with an appropriate margin prespecified, noninferiority is demonstrated when the lower limit of the CI excludes the margin and the effectiveness of the test treatment is deduced in the absence of placebo. Wang et al.[34] referred to it as the indirect CI comparison (ICIC), because there is no direct placebo comparison in the active-controlled noninferiority trials, while Rothmann et al.[21] and Chi et al.[22] termed it as the Two (95%) CI Testing Approach.

Is *post hoc* change in the margin allowed? This question occasionally arises regarding changing the prespecified noninferiority margin after the trial is completed. The answer is clearly negative. An appropriate margin is supposed to be chosen during the study design based on historical active control effect size. Regulatory authorities will not accept a *post hoc* change in the margin to accommodate the less favorable study results.

2. Preservation of a Certain Fraction of Active Control Effect

The notion of considering preservation of a certain fraction of active control effect has been discussed by many authors.[32,20–22] Simon[41] gave an equivalent Baysian formulation. When the noninferiority testing is defined in terms of a fraction of active control effect to be preserved, it provides some advantages. First, the fraction of control effect to be preserved is specified according to the trial objective. Second, one does not need to prespecify a noninferiority margin, though a fraction of active control effect to be preserved still needs to be defined. Because, in an active-controlled noninferiority trial, there is no concurrent placebo, one cannot estimate the active control effect directly from the current trial. However, one can impute a placebo, called "putative placebo," from historical placebo-controlled trials and compare the test treatment indirectly to this putative placebo. For this to be valid, one again has to assume that the current active control effect has not changed over time (i.e., CA to hold) or assume that the current control effect has only reduced slightly (i.e., a large fraction of the historical control effect is preserved). Such a comparison of the test treatment with the putative placebo seems to be natural, but the difficulty is that it involves cross historical trials inference, which may be highly sensitive to many conditions, in particular, the constancy assumption.

This putative placebo or "imputed placebo" approach has been best discussed by Hasselblad and Kong.[32] This putative placebo comparison approach works under three basic assumptions:

- At least one historical placebo-controlled trial is available that estimates the active control effect,
- the current noninferiority trial comparing the test treatment to the active control has the same endpoint of interest in historical trials, and
- at least some common patient subpopulations exist in the current and historical trials.

The above assumptions reiterate the requirements of HESDE and CA of the active control, as well as AS of the current noninferiority trials. When these assumptions are met, two measures: (1) estimated test treatment effect via putative placebo, and (2) estimated fraction of active control effect preserved by the test treatment can be obtained for point estimates and CIs, as well as for hypothesis testing. The concept of this putative placebo approach will now be described.

a. Estimating the Test Treatment Effect (Relative to Putative Placebo)

Formulae estimating the test treatment effect for different effect measures: risk difference in means or event rates, relative risk in means or event rates, odds ratio, and hazard ratio can be summarized as follows.

Let T = test treatment and S = standard active treatment in the current noninferiority trial; S' = standard active treatment and P = placebo in the historical trials. Again, the letters T, S, S', and P will be loosely used to represent treatment, estimate in mean, event rate, or hazard rate, as appropriate. Let β_{ab} = log relative risk, log odds ratio, or log hazard ratio of a to b; $\hat{E}[x]$ = expectation estimate of x and $\hat{U}[x]$ = variance estimate of x. Further, $\ln(x) = \log_e(x)$. It may be noted that since the meta-analysis on the historical trials and the current active-controlled noninferiority trial are independent, the variance estimate of the indirect comparison is simply the sum.

i.   Risk Difference in Means or Event Rates. The expectation and variance estimates for test treatment to placebo (imputed) comparison can be derived as

$$\hat{E}(T - P) = \hat{E}[(T - S) + (S' - P)] = \hat{E}(T - S) + \hat{E}(S' - P) \text{ and}$$
$$\hat{U}(T - P) = \hat{U}[(T - S) + (S' - P)] = \hat{U}(T - S) + \hat{U}(S' - P).$$

Here $S = S'$, if the CA holds. With estimates of expectation (mean) and variance on the effect of the test treatment relative to placebo $(T - P)$ available, one can construct CI and perform hypothesis testing, as appropriate.

ii.   Relative Risk. Now the expectation and variance estimates for the relative risk of test treatment to placebo are simply:

$$\hat{E}(\beta_{TP}) = \hat{E}(\beta_{TS}) + \hat{E}(\beta_{S'P}) = \hat{E}[\ln(T/S)] + \hat{E}[\ln(S'/P)] \text{ and}$$
$$\hat{U}(\beta_{TP}) = \hat{U}(\beta_{TS}) + \hat{U}(\beta_{S'P}) = \hat{U}[\ln(T/S)] + \hat{U}[\ln(S'/P)].$$

Here $\beta_{ab} = $ log relative risk of a to b. For example, $\beta_{TP} = \ln(T/P) = $ log relative risk of T to P. Similarly, estimates for odds ratio and hazard ratio can be derived.

iii.   Odds Ratio

$$\hat{E}(\beta_{TP}) = \hat{E}(\beta_{TS}) + \hat{E}(\beta_{S'P})$$
$$= \hat{E}(\ln\{[T/(1 - T)]/[S/(1 - S)]\}) + \hat{E}(\ln\{[S'/(1 - S')]/[P/(1 - P)]\})$$

and

$$\hat{U}(\beta_{TP}) = \hat{U}(\beta_{TS}) + \hat{U}(\beta_{S'P})$$
$$= \hat{U}(\ln\{[T/(1 - T)]/[S/(1 - S)]\}) + \hat{U}(\ln\{[S'/(1 - S')]/[P/(1 - P)]\})$$

Here $\beta_{ab} = $ log odds ratio of a to b. For example, $\beta_{TP} = \ln\{[T/(1 - T)]/[P/(1 - P)]\} = $ log odds ratio of T to P.

iv.   Hazard Ratio

$$\hat{E}(\beta_{TP}) = \hat{E}(\beta_{TS}) + \hat{E}(\beta_{S'P}) = \hat{E}[\ln(T/S)] + \hat{E}[\ln(S'/P)] \text{ and}$$
$$\hat{U}(\beta_{TP}) = \hat{U}(\beta_{TS}) + \hat{U}(\beta_{S'P}) = \hat{U}[\ln(T/S)] + \hat{U}[\ln(S'/P)]$$

Here $\beta_{ab} = $ log hazard ratio of a to b. For example, $\beta_{TP} = \ln(T/P) = $ log hazard ratio of T to P.

**b.   Estimation of the Fraction of Active Control Effect
        Preserved by the Test Treatment**

The preservation of active control effect is defined as a fraction ϕ $(0 < \phi < 1)$. It is a computed value of the effect of the test treatment vs. placebo (imputed) relative to the effect of active control vs. placebo (historical). If the active control is highly effective, then the test treatment should not be considered to be much inferior to this active control. One may set ϕ to be close to one. On the other hand, if the test treatment offers some important benefits such as better safety profile, then ϕ may be set to be somewhat smaller. In this case, it may only be concluded that the test treatment is effective, but not noninferior to the active control. Again, under CA the point and CI estimates can be obtained via expectation and variance estimates for different measures in risk difference in means or event rates, relative risk, odds ratio, and hazard ratio. Now, the expectation and variance estimates for the preservation fraction ϕ for risk difference are, respectively,

$$\hat{E}(\phi) \approx 1 + [(T - S)/(S' - P)] \quad \text{and}$$
$$\hat{U}(\phi) \approx [(T - S)/(S' - P)]^2 \{[\hat{U}(T - S)/(T - S)^2] + [\hat{U}(S' - P)/(S' - P)^2]\}$$

Similarly, for relative risk, odds ratio, or hazard ratio, the fraction ϕ of control effect preserved, can be estimated by

$$\hat{E}(\phi) \approx 1 + (\beta_{TS}/\beta_{S'P}) \quad \text{and}$$
$$\hat{U}(\phi) \approx [\beta_{TS}/\beta_{S'P}]^2 \{[\hat{U}(\beta_{TS})/\beta_{TS}^2] + [\hat{U}(\beta_{S'P})/\beta_{S'P}^2]\}$$

where $\beta_{ab} = \log$ relative risk, log odds ratio, or log hazard ratio of a to b, respectively, as previously defined. With estimates of expectation (mean) and variance available for the fraction effect preserved ϕ for the test treatment vs. placebo relative to the effect of active control vs. placebo, CI can easily be constructed and hypothesis testing be performed, as appropriate. It should be noted that preservation of a certain fraction of the active control effect on one measure (e.g., risk difference) does not necessarily translate to the same fraction of preservation on another measure (e.g., odds ratio). For formulae derivations and examples, see Refs. 21, 22, 32 and 34.

Wang et al.[34] referred to this preservation of fraction of control effect or the putative placebo approach as the virtual comparison (VC) method. The VC method compares the test treatment vs. a putative placebo by synthesizing the estimated effect of the test treatment vs. the active control and the estimated effect of the active control vs. the placebo from the historical trials. They compared the performance of the ICIC and VC methods in terms of Type I error rate — the probability of falsely concluding a test treatment is effective relative to a putative placebo and the test treatment preserves a certain fraction of the active control effect. By means of simulation studies, they showed that the ICIC method using the CBER 50% rule in defining the margin is naturally ultraconservative with respect to the Type I error rate. They also demonstrated that the VC method performed much worse in inflating the type I error rate than the ICIC method, which is a departure from the constancy assumption. In addition, they asserted that the risk ratio proposed by Hasselblad and Kong for estimating preservation of the active control effect is unreliable when sample size is small and historical data for active control are inadequate. Wang and Hung[42] further developed a two-stage active control testing (TACT) method. The TACT method consists of an examination phase and a two-stage testing phase. The first phase is for active control HESDE examination. The first stage of the next phase is for CA validation. The second stage then performs analysis using either the ICIC or VC method. On the contrary, Rothmann et al.[21] and Chi et al.[22] in their formulation of hazard ratio in survival data considered that hypotheses with any type of prespecified margin (i.e., the ICIC method) are in general problematic. They advocated that the hypothesis with a certain fraction of preservation of the active control effect (i.e., the VC method) is a preferred formulation for noninferiority trials. The contradictive assertions by these authors appear to be dependent on availability of historical trials, degree of CA deviation, and simulation studies used.

VII. SWITCHING OBJECTIVES

Predefinition of a trial design as a superiority trial or a noninferiority trial is necessary for proper trial design and analysis (e.g., choice of control, doses, patient populations, endpoints, sample size and power, clinical relevant effect size, noninferiority margin, analysis plan, and assay sensitivity). When the trial is completed and the final results become available, often an alternative interpretation or conclusion may be of interest. That is, a superiority trial may be "salvaged" to show noninferiority as the lesser objective when it fails to detect a significant difference between the test and active control. Or, a noninferiority trial can be "enhanced" to further demonstrate superiority of the test over the comparator when it satisfies the noninferiority objective. Salvaging a trial from superiority to noninferiority or enhancing a trial from noninferiority to superiority may be feasible when a trial was designed prospectively with switching objectives in mind and well conducted with high quality. However, it is recognized that enhancing is easier while salvaging is more difficult because of the inherent nature of noninferiority trials. Often, the latter should be considered on a case-by-case basis. The issues of switching trial objectives have been well contemplated in CPMP Points to Consider on Switching between Superiority and Noninferiority[11] and Hwang.[12] In fact, the only relevant switching possible is between superiority and noninferiority.

A. SWITCHING FROM NONINFERIORITY TO SUPERIORITY

In an active-controlled noninferiority trial, assuming it is properly designed with adequate power and well conducted with high quality when noninferiority is established (i.e., shows that the lower bound of the CI exceeds or excludes the predefined noninferiority margin, $-\delta$), one can take a stepwise approach to further test whether superiority can be demonstrated (i.e., shows that the lower bound of the CI also exceeds 0). The procedure is straightforward and there is no multiplicity adjustment necessary, because it corresponds to a simple stepwise (in two steps) closed test. If the active control was chosen suitably per HESDE, showing noninferiority will deduce proof of test treatment efficacy. Demonstration of superiority will further enhance or strengthen the fact that the test treatment is not only an effective treatment, but also is more effective than the standard effective control. The size of additional treatment effect needs to be estimated and properly discussed in clinical terms.

In practice, successful switching from noninferiority to superiority first needs the noninferiority to be established via the per protocol (PP) analysis set, and then to have superiority demonstrated via the intention to treat (ITT) analysis set. Because the analyses involve double switching (i.e., switching analysis sets in switching objectives), it is advisable that the PP and ITT analysis sets should be used to ensure robust interpretation, in particular, when patient noncompliance/dropout is severe. For safety analysis no switching of analysis sets should be done and the ITT set should be used throughout.

B. SWITCHING FROM SUPERIORITY TO NONINFERIORITY

When a trial is designed as a superiority trial, it intends to detect a difference between treatments; there is generally no provision to predefine a noninferiority margin. However, it becomes a critical prerequisite as soon as switching objectives emerges as an option. In general, switching from superiority to noninferiority will be more difficult because of the inherent difficulties of noninferiority trials, despite the fact that there remains no multiplicity adjustment because a stepwise closed test is involved. In fact, the switching is only prudent when the analysis fails to yield the superiority objective. A lesser objective to demonstrate noninferiority may be feasible by switching the objectives, provided that a noninferiority margin was predefined and the trial was well conducted with high quality and adequate power. In rare cases where the margin can be chosen and well justified *post hoc*. Nonetheless, a putative placebo approach with preservation of a certain fraction of active control effect remains applicable, provided that the CA of the chosen active control effect holds (or closely holds). It should be noted again that this approach may demonstrate that the test treatment is more effective than placebo (putative), but one cannot conclude that the test treatment is noninferior to the active control by a certain amount because a noninferiority margin was not defined.

Because the switching is from superiority to noninferiority, the analysis set to be used will be that of the ITT set for superiority testing and PP set for noninferiority. Again, to maintain data robustness, both analysis sets should be used for efficacy and the ITT set for safety evaluation. An example in docetaxel (Taxotere) in second-line treatment of patients with locally advanced or metastatic breast cancer is described in Durrleman and Chaikin[43] and From the FDA.[44] In this real-life example not only switching objectives (*post hoc*) was carried out successfully in one of its adequate and well-controlled Phase III trials, but also the approval by the FDA was elevated from accelerated approval to full approval with an expanded indication in the U.S. under the Clinton–Gore oncology initiative.

Comments. Switching objectives between superiority and noninferiority further adds complexity to the inherent difficulties of the noninferiority trials. Nonetheless, switching objectives is a viable option either to enhance or salvage a trial, but the best intention is that it is predefined in the protocol during trial design. Switching from noninferiority to superiority is easier, but not *vice versa*. It should be remembered that switching from superiority to noninferiority *post hoc* will always be problematic and be considered on a trial-by-trial basis. The successful switch in the case of docetaxel was merely an exception.

VIII. ANALYSIS ISSUES

Analyzing data from placebo and active-controlled trials are similar with subtle differences tied in with their respective objectives and formulations of hypotheses.

A. HYPOTHESIS TESTING VS. CONFIDENCE INTERVAL (CI)

As discussed previously the hypothesis testing and its equivalent CI approaches are used in the analysis of data from superiority, noninferiority, and equivalence trials. In superiority trials the emphasis tends to be more on testing and p-values, though point estimates and CIs are routinely reported, in particular, the control is placebo. The key will be the estimated effect size, variability, and p-values. On the other hand, in active-controlled noninferiority trials the CI approach is preferred, i.e., demonstration of noninferiority by showing that the lower limit of the CI excludes the predefined noninferiority margin. Less attention is usually paid to the p-values.

B. ANALYSIS SETS

In a superiority trial the analysis based on ITT analysis set is usually considered as the primary analysis. The analysis derived from the PP analysis set is supplementary or secondary. It has been well recognized that the ITT approach is conservative and is the analysis of choice in superiority trials. However, in a noninferiority trial, the reverse is true, because it is believed that the ITT approach tends to bias results toward no difference. Some authors[3,17] have challenged this assertion. Nonetheless, it is agreed that in a noninferiority trial a robust interpretation can only be reached when analyses based on the PP and ITT analysis sets lead to a similar conclusion. A switch of objectives in analysis would require this difference of emphasis to be recognized.[11]

C. SWITCHING OBJECTIVES

Analysis in switching objectives between superiority and noninferiority will involve the proper choice of analysis sets (as discussed above) and analytic methods for noninferiority assessment. Assessing superiority is straightforward. Demonstration of noninferiority will depend on how the noninferiority objective is defined. A routine CI approach will do if an appropriate fixed noninferiority margin is predefined, otherwise a more difficult *post hoc* justification of the margin or demonstration of preservation of a certain faction of the active control effect via putative placebo[32] based on a meta-analysis on the historical trials will be needed. An equivalent Baysian analysis[41] can also be used, despite the ambiguity about the utility and acceptance of the Baysian approach by the regulatory authorities. It is rather clear that there will be no multiplicity adjustment necessary, regardless of the direction of objectives switching, because it corresponds to a simple stepwise closed test.

It should be noted that prespecification of trial objective switching between superiority and noninferiority in active-controlled trials can be very difficult, in particular when the test treatment effect may be overrated or the active control effect is known to be high. One might be able to use an adaptive group sequential closed testing procedure to study the superiority and noninferiority hypotheses.[45]

D. Interim Analysis and Sample Size Reestimation

Superiority trials are often designed with *interim* analysis for midstream trial conduct modification (e.g., early termination of the trial for overwhelming efficacy, futility, or harm) via group sequential methods,[46,47] in particular, the α spending function approach.[48,49] Sample size reestimation[50,51] has also been utilized in the event that the sample size originally estimated becomes inadequate with amendment of trial assumptions while the trial is in progress. The α spending function and conditional power[52] approaches are useful methods for performing interim analysis and sample size reestimation in superiority trials. Such methods are equally applicable to noninferiority and equivalence trials, in particular the group sequential confidence approach proposed by Jennison and Turnbull.[53,54] (Extensive discussion on interim analysis and sample size reestimation can be found in Chapter 14.)

Midstream sample size adjustment remains a valuable tool for restoring a positive superiority or noninferiority trial when the planned power is on the short side. Friede and Kieser[55] demonstrated blinded sample size reassessment in noninferiority and equivalence trials utilizing an internal pilot design.

In situations where superiority is uncertain and noninferiority is more plausible, an adaptive group sequential closed testing procedure[45] can be used. In this adaptive procedure, the superiority and noninferiority hypotheses can be tested concurrently. The sample size can initially be planned for superiority and readjusted (increased) for demonstrating noninferiority when it is deemed more plausible than showing superiority based on interim data. They showed via simulation studies that this adaptive procedure allowing for concurrent superiority and noninferiority testing has sample size saving over the traditional group sequential test designed solely for testing either superiority or noninferiority.

E. Multiple Endpoints/Treatments

Most analyses on the active control noninferiority and equivalence trials have been involved in two treatments on a univariate endpoint. There is limited research in assessing noninferiority and equivalence in trials on multiple endpoints or multiple treatments.

When an active-controlled trial involved multiple primary endpoints, Quan et al.[56] suggested a closed procedure for equivalence assessment on multiple endpoints with prespecified equivalence margins on the individual endpoints. Their approach extends the intersection-union test discussed in Berger and Hsu.[57] They used an example with three equally important primary endpoints in demonstrating efficacy for a selective COX-2 inhibitor in osteoarthritis. Equivalence of the test treatment (COX-2) to an active control treatment (a nonsteroidal antiinflammatory drug — NSAID) on three endpoints was demonstrated. The step-down procedure can be used to demonstrate whether equivalence is achieved for all of, any two of, or one of the three endpoints. (Note that the last option in demonstrating equivalence in an individual endpoint may be plausible mathematically; it may not be clinically attractive.) For assessing equivalence of all three endpoints simultaneously, $(1 - 2\alpha) \times 100\%$ CIs (or slightly smaller CIs) are used. For assessing at least two of the three endpoints, $(1 - \alpha) \times 100\%$ CIs are used. For selecting an individual endpoint on which equivalence may be demonstrated, $(1 - 2\alpha/3) \times 100\%$ CIs are used. The closed step-down procedure controls the experimentwise error rate as shown in simulation studies. The procedure can be easily generalized to multiple endpoints greater than three and to a noninferiority assessment as well. Note that the step-down procedures proposed by Hochberg[58] and Simes[59] in significance testing are not readily applicable to cases of equivalence assessment in multiple endpoints. Their tests do not necessarily control the experimentwise error rate for all cases pending study power and correlation structure among the endpoints.

For showing noninferiority or equivalence in active-controlled trials involving more than two treatments, similar closed stepwise test or pairwise procedure applies. Giani and Strassburger[60] considered testing multiple test treatments for equivalence to an active control treatment for all or nothing analysis or for subset comparisons. Wiens and Iglewicz[61] considered equivalence in three treatments where three lots of the vaccine product being equivalent would establish the consistency of the manufacturing process. Procedures are extended stepwise to select pairs of treatments that are equivalent to each other when all three treatments are not shown to be equivalent. This equivalence testing may not be applicable in the vaccine consistency study that requires all or nothing equivalence testing, but may be applicable in other situations.

IX. SOME CAVEATS

A. TRIAL QUALITY

In a superiority trial to show difference between treatments, there is always a strong imperative to design and conduct the trial with high quality to enhance the likelihood of demonstrating assay sensitivity. Whereas, in a trial to show noninferiority of the test treatment to an effective active control, there is relatively weaker stimulus to design and conduct a high-quality study because of the expectations of patients and investigators on receiving active treatments.

Many clinical researchers including Temple[62,63] believed that trial sloppiness (poor trial quality) in a noninferiority trial, would bias toward no difference and, in turn, increase the likelihood that an ineffective treatment would be falsely concluded effective.

The above assertion is generally true, but not necessarily always the case. Hauck and Anderson[17] questioned whether any bias introduced is strictly toward no difference. In fact, trial sloppiness introduces noise. Noise implies increased variability with wider CI and in turn it biases toward the null (inferiority). In addition, sloppiness introduces bias. Bias may happen in either direction (i.e., reduced or increased observed difference). Therefore, sloppiness may bias toward either the null (inferiority) or alternative (noninferiority), though the latter is the major concern in conducting a noninferiority trial. Hwang[64] and Hwang and Morikawa[3] compared the hypotheses (null vs. alternative) and test statistics of the superiority vs. noninferiority trials and demonstrated that good trial design and conduct with large observed differences and small standard errors are necessary regardless of whether a trial is designed to show superiority or noninferiority. Moreover, through the test statistics in a noninferiority trial, it was shown that rejecting the null hypothesis to conclude noninferiority depends on the relative magnitude of the ratio of the predefined fixed margin divided by the standard error of the treatment difference, even when the observed difference is biased toward zero. Therefore, good trial quality is necessary for any trial to show positive results regardless of whether it is intended to show superiority or noninferiority.

B. ISSUE OF TRANSITIVITY AND DRIFT

Transitivity is expressed in the following mathematical expression:

$$A > B \quad \text{and} \quad B > C \Rightarrow (\text{implies}) \, A > C.$$

It simply means that if A is greater than B and B is greater than C then it automatically implies that A is greater than C. Transitivity works well in a superiority trial setting. Unfortunately, transitivity assertion does not necessarily hold in the noninferiority or equivalence settings. Hauck and Anderson[17] gave a simple example and it goes like this: given a common margin to be five units, C is noninferior (three units inferior, but less than the margin of five units) to B and B is also noninferior (again three units inferior, but less than the margin of five units) to A. Now C cannot be concluded noninferior (six units inferior, exceeded the margin of five units) to A.

In fact, in the above simple example, C has drifted away from A. The phenomenon of drift or biocreep may happen when a noninferior (slightly inferior — not much worse per predefined margin) test treatment becomes the active control for the next series of noninferiority trials and so on till the new generation active control drifts far away and becomes almost a placebo. The drift or biocreep problem can be avoided if one always chooses the most effective or the most prescribed active control with well demonstrated HESDE.[19]

C. Useful Alternatives

A few useful alternatives[2,3] are available if an appropriate active-controlled noninferiority trial cannot be designed or conducted. These alternatives will be briefly summarized as follows:

- Include a placebo arm in addition to the active control treatment if ethical concerns are not major. Such a three-arm trial provides a straightforward solution to establishing AS. This design directly measures the test treatment effect (test vs. placebo) and establishes AS when a difference between the test treatment and placebo is detected. It also allows for noninferiority comparison of the test treatment to the active control in a setting where AS is established by the active control vs. placebo comparison. In fact, the active control vs. placebo comparison in such a trial provides internal evidence of AS of the trial. It is particularly informative even when the test treatment and placebo are nondistinguishable in the trial. If the active control is superior to placebo, the trial does have AS and will provide evidence that the test treatment is indeed ineffective. On the other hand, if neither the test nor the active control can be distinguished from placebo, the trial is proved as not having AS. That is, this three-arm trial can readily evaluate whether a failure to distinguish the test treatment from placebo is due to ineffectiveness of the test, or simply the trial does not have AS to detect a difference when it exists. An article by Piegot et al.[24] provided an excellent discussion on the subject of assessing noninferiority in a three-arm trial with placebo.
- Show superiority of the test treatment to a standard active control at an effective or low dose, if the test treatment in the phase II trials has shown to be highly effective. Demonstration of superiority in the former is straightforward if the test treatment is indeed highly effective. One can predefine an appropriate noninferiority margin (if feasible) and the possibility of switching objectives from superiority and noninferiority in the protocol if one is not particularly confident about showing superiority. The latter uses a low dose, either of the active control or of the test drug, which may provide a pseudo-placebo. Demonstration of superiority to a pseudo-placebo would establish test treatment effects and trial AS.
- Design a trial to establish a clear dose–response relationship for the test treatment and demonstrate pairwise differences between doses (e.g., the highest vs. the lowest) of the test treatment. A trial may be less useful for dose determination, if the trial failed to show a significant difference between doses, despite that a significant trend in dose–response is established. In this case, a therapeutic dose will be difficult to establish. Again, the inclusion of a placebo (zero dose) will be very useful, in particular, if a significant difference between any

dose and placebo is detected. This will demonstrate AS and establish a test treatment effect.

- In many cases variations of placebo-controlled designs such as an add-on, replacement, early escape, or randomized withdrawal trial has been shown to be very useful. An add-on trial is a placebo-controlled trial in which a test treatment is compared with placebo in patients also receiving effective standard treatment. It is commonly used in cancer, antiepileptic, hypertension, CHF, and lipid-lowering trials for second-line therapy. This design is useful when the first-line standard treatment is not fully effective or additional effect is desirable, and the added test treatment as the second-line therapy will provide evidence of improved effectiveness. A variation of this design is the replacement trial, in which the test treatment or placebo is added by random assignment to conventional therapy and then the conventional therapy is withdrawn, usually by tapering. This design has often been used in trials to study steroid-sparing/replacement and antiepileptic drugs. Another design is an early-escape trial. Early escape refers to prompt withdrawal of trial patients whose clinical status worsens or fails to improve to a predefined level. In such cases, the need to change therapy becomes a trial primary endpoint. Another modification is a randomized withdrawal trial, in which patients receiving a test treatment for a fixed time period are then randomized to continue treatment with the test treatment or placebo. The observed difference between the test treatment and placebo would establish the test treatment effects. All these designs would demonstrate AS when a difference between the test treatment and placebo is detected.

X. DISCUSSION

There is no doubt that the WMA Helsinki Declaration in 2000[8] has rendered a brand new challenge in clinical trials, in particular the active-controlled trial is gaining more attention with marked increase in applications. The Guidance of ICH E9,[36] E10,[2] and CPMP Points to Consider,[11,37] as well as The European regulatory experience[65] have indeed provided better understanding regarding superiority, noninferiority, and equivalence trials. Recognition of the relevancy of demonstrating therapeutic noninferiority than equivalence is emerging. Emphasis on trial AS has also enhanced the likelihood of success in design and conduct of positive trials regardless of the trial objective. AS can be measured directly in a superiority trial, whether the control is placebo or an active control. However, it can only be demonstrated indirectly or rather deduced in an active-controlled noninferiority trial. The deduction will be based on proved HESDE of the chosen active control from similarly designed historical placebo-controlled trials, degree of the CA of the control effect that holds, and quality of the current trial.

As described in ICH E10, a successful active-controlled noninferiority trial requires four critical steps: 1. determining that the HESDE for the chosen active control drug exists, 2. designing the current trial similar to the historical trials, 3. setting an acceptable margin, and 4. conducting the trial with high quality. In determining that HESDE of the active control did exist, one needs to evaluate and estimate the control effect size from the historical placebo-controlled trials if it is not known or readily available in a disease area of interest. Estimating the active control effect size in practice can be problematic, e.g., which trials to include, which estimate to adopt, and what model to use? In the estimation process bias can be introduced and the control effect can be over- or underestimated. Most often the presence of quality historical trials is rare or in certain disease areas such as depression, HESDE is hardly in existence for any active control treatments. Problems may also arise in designing the current trial to be closely similar to the historical trials since patient population, standard care, and medical practice are changing over time. Next, in determining a fixed noninferiority margin or a certain fraction of control effect to be preserved or retained for indirect comparison of the test treatment to a putative placebo, there is not yet a logical and consistent approach available. Because of the uncertainty surrounding some unverifiable assumptions (e.g., constancy of active control effect), defining the appropriate margin or right level of fraction for preservation can be highly subjective and logically, may be on a case-by-case basis. Nonetheless, the margin or fraction preservation chosen ought to be clinically relevant and statistically sound — it remains the key issue in noninferiority trials not yet satisfactorily resolved. The 2004 CPMP Points to Consider draft[37] offers general guidance on designing noninferiority trials and assessing test treatment effectiveness, but it fails to provide adequate and in-depth account on the choice of the margin. Continued research in this area is necessary and it remains to be seen whether the approach of prespecification of a fixed noninferiority margin or preservation of a fraction of active control effect will be the preferred method for noninferiority trials. An approach, suggested by Giani and Strassberg[58] and further explored in Wiens,[18] which sets the margin to be proportional to the variance obtained via the meta-analysis on historical trials seems to have some statistical appeals. Again, the right constant to apply and its justification remained unclear.

When switching objectives between superiority and noninferiority becomes an option, one must pay attention to the features of the superiority and noninferiority trials, particularly the latter. In fact, switching objectives will further add complexity to the inherent difficulties of the noninferiority trials. Nonetheless, switching is a viable alternative either to enhance or salvage a trial, but the intention is best to be predefined in the protocol at the trial design. Be aware that switching from superiority to noninferiority *post hoc* will always be problematic and the choice of analysis sets (i.e., ITT on superiority and PP on noninferiority) can also be confusing. The best approach is to put equal weight on both analyses to reach robust interpretation. In general, switching from noninferiority to superiority is easier, but the reverse is rather difficult and it should be considered on a trial-by-trial basis.

In addition to trial assay sensitivity, HESDE and constancy of the active control, and trial quality, issues of nontransitivity and drift (or biocreep) phenomenon in noninferiority trials also need to be recognized. Designing an acceptable noninferiority trial can be a frustrating experience in some disease areas. Merely showing noninferiority to deduce efficacy of a test treatment may not be enough, in particular in the region of European Union (EU) or Japan, where evidence of relative effectiveness of test to standard treatments is usually required for pricing and reimbursement needs. Useful alternatives to a noninferiority trial (e.g., an add-on design) or an active-controlled superiority trial may be necessary for a novel new treatment.

Finally, like any positive clinical trial the clinician and statistician play important roles. Whether the task is to determine the margin or fraction preservation, the clinician, and statistician need to work closely together. Rigorous efforts should be put in defining the purpose of the trial, investigating relevant historical data, and designing the trial appropriately. The statistician, in particular, should not and must not act merely like a bench technician or a number cruncher. One must utilize his/her well-honed statistical training and background to design, conduct, analyze, and report a positive adequate and well-controlled trial according to good clinical practice (GCP) and good statistical practice (GSP).

REFERENCES

1. FDA CFR Title 21, Part 314.126, Adequate and well-controlled studies, Revised as of April 1, 2000, U.S. Government Printing Office, Washington, DC, 2000.
2. ICH E10 Guidance, Choice of control group and related issues in clinical trials, Guidance for Industry, CDER/CBER, Food and Drug Administration, pp. 1–48, May 2001, http://www.fda.gov/cder/guidance/4155fnl.htm
3. Hwang, I.K. and Morikawa, T., Design issues in noninferiority/equivalence trials, *Drug Inf. J.*, 33, 1205–1218, 1999.
4. Hwang, I.K., Selection of control group, In *Encyclopedia of Biometrics*, 2nd ed., Chow, S.C., ed., Dekker, New York, pp. 921–926, 2003.
5. Rothman, K.J. and Michels, K.B., The continued unethical use of placebo controls, *N. Engl. J. Med.*, 331, 394–398, 1994.
6. Freedman, B., Weijer, C., and Glass, K.C., Placebo orthodoxy in clinical research. I: empirical and methodological myths, *J. Law Med. Ethics*, 24, 243–251, 1996.
7. Freedman, B., Weijer, C., and Glass, K.C., Placebo orthodoxy in clinical research. II: ethical, legal, and regulatory myths, *J. Law Med. Ethics*, 24, 252–259, 1996.
8. WMA Declaration of Helsinki, Ethical principles for medical research involving human subjects, *J. Am. Med. Assoc.*, 284, 3043–3045, 2000.
9. Temple, R. and Ellenberg, S., Placebo-controlled trials and active-controlled trials in the evaluation of new treatments. Part 1: ethical and scientific issues, *Ann. Int. Med.*, 133(6), 455–463, 2000.
10. Ellenberg, S. and Temple, R., Placebo-controlled trials and active-controlled trials in the evaluation of new treatments. Part 2: practical issues and special cases, *Ann. Int. Med.*, 133(6), 464–470, 2000.

11. CPMP Points to Consider on switching between superiority and noninferiority, EMEA July 2000, CPMP/EWP/482/99, pp. 1–10, 2000.
12. Hwang, I.K., U.S. prospective on switching between superiority and noninferiority, Presented at *2002 DIA 38th Annual Meeting*, Chicago, IL, June 2002.
13. Blackwelder, W.C., Proving the null hypothesis, *Control. Clin. Trials*, 3, 345–353, 1982.
14. Ng, T-H., A specification of treatment difference in the design of clinical trials with active controls, *Drug Inf. J.*, 27, 705–719, 1993.
15. Morikawa, T. and Yoshida, M., A useful testing strategy in phase III trials: combined test of superiority and test of equivalence, *J. Biopharm. Stat.*, 5(3), 297–306, 1995.
16. Röhmel, J., Therapeutic equivalence investigation: statistical considerations, *Stat. Med.*, 17, 1703–1704, 1998.
17. Hauck, W.W. and Anderson, S., Some issues in the design and analysis of equivalence trials, *Drug Inf. J.*, 33, 109–118, 1999.
18. Wiens, B.L., Choosing an equivalence limit for noninferiority or equivalence studies, *Control. Clin. Trials*, 23, 2–14, 2002.
19. D'Agostino, R.B., Massaro, J.M., and Sullivan, L.M., Noninferiority trials: design concepts and issues — the encounters of academic consultants in statistics, *Stat. Med.*, 22, 169–186, 2003.
20. Hung, H.M.J., Wang, S.-J., Tsong, Y., Lawrence, J., and O'Neill, R.T., Some fundamental issues with noninferiority testing in active-controlled trials, *Stat. Med.*, 22, 213–225, 2003.
21. Rothmann, M., Li, N., Chen, G., Chi, G.Y.H., Temple, R., and Tsou, H.H., Design and analysis of noninferiority trials in oncology, *Stat. Med.*, 22, 239–264, 2003.
22. Chi, G.Y.H., Chen, G., Rothmann, M., and Li, N., Active control trials, In *Encyclopedia of Biometrics*, 2nd ed., Chow, S.C., ed., Dekker, New York, pp. 9–15, 2003.
23. Laster, L.L. and Johnson, M.F., Noninferiority trials: the "at least as good as" criterion, *Stat. Med.*, 22, 187–200, 2003.
24. Pigeot, I., Schäfer, J., Röhmel, J., and Hauschke, D., Assessing noninferiority of a new treatment in a three-arm clinical trial including a placebo, *Stat. Med.*, 22, 883–899, 2003.
25. Schuirmann, D.J., A comparison of the two one-sided tests procedure and the power approach for assessing the equivalence of average bioavailability, *J. Pharmacokinet. Biopharm.*, 15, 657–680, 1987.
26. Dunnett, C.W. and Gent, M., An alternative to the use of two-sided tests in clinical trials, *Stat. Med.*, 15, 1729–1738, 1996.
27. Chow, S.-C. and Shao, J., A note on statistical methods for assessing therapeutic equivalence, *Control. Clin. Trials*, 23, 515–520, 2002.
28. Blackwelder, W.C., Showing a treatment is good because it is not bad: when does "noninferiority" imply effectiveness? *Control. Clin. Trials*, 23, 52–54, 2002.
29. Lachin, J.M., Introduction to sample size determination and power analysis for clinical trials, *Control. Clin. Trials*, 2, 93–113, 1981.
30. Jones, B., Jarvis, P., Lewis, J.A., and Ebbutt, A.F., Trials to assess equivalence: the importance of rigorous methods, *Br. Med. J.*, 313, 36–39, 1996.
31. Liu, J.P. and Chow, S.C., Sample size determination for the two one-sided tests procedure in bioequivalence, *J. Pharmacokinet. Biopharm.*, 20, 101–104, 1992.

32. Hasselblad, V. and Kong, F., Statistical methods for comparison to placebo in active-control trials, *Drug Inf. J.*, 35, 435–449, 2001.
33. DerSimonian, R. and Laird, N., Meta-analysis in clinical trials, *Control. Clin. Trials*, 7, 177–188, 1986.
34. Wang, S.-J., Hung, H.M.J., and Tsong, Y., Utility and pitfalls of some statistical methods in active-controlled clinical trials, *Control. Clin. Trials*, 23, 15–28, 2002.
35. Parmar, M.K.B., Torri, V., and Stewart, L., Extracting summary statistics to perform meta-analysis of the published literature for survival endpoints, *Stat. Med.*, 17, 2815–2834, 1998.
36. ICH E9 Guidance, Statistical principles for clinical trials, Guidance for Industry, CDER/CBER, Food and Drug Administration, pp. 1–46, September 1998, http://www.fda.gov/cder/guidance/ICH_E9-fnl.PDF
37. CPMP Points to Consider on the choice of noninferiority margin, EMEA February 2004, CPMP/EWP/2158/99 draft, pp. 1–12, 2004.
38. Ng, T.-H., Choice of delta in equivalence testing, *Drug Inf. J.*, 35, 1517–1527, 2001.
39. FDA Points to Consider: clinical development and labeling of antiinfective drug products, FDA Division of AntiInfective Drug Product, Washington, October 26, 1992.
40. Phillips, K., A new test of noninferiority for antiinfective trials, *Stat. Med.*, 22, 201–212, 2003.
41. Simon, R., Bayesian design and analysis of active control trials, *Biometrics*, 55(2), 484–487, 1999.
42. Wang, S.-J. and Hung, H.M.J., TACT method for noninferiority testing in active-controlled trials, *Stat. Med.*, 22, 227–238, 2003.
43. Durrleman, S. and Chaikin, P., The use of putative placebo in active control trials: two applications in a regulatory setting, *Stat. Med.*, 22, 941–952, 2003.
44. From the FDA, Accelerated approval of new drugs in the Division of Oncology Drug Products — Taxotere, *Cancer Ther.*, 1(4), 220–222, 1998.
45. Wang, S.J., Hung, H.M.J., Tsong, Y., Cui, L., and Nuri, W.A., Group sequential test strategies for superiority and noninferiority hypotheses in active control trials, *Stat. Med.*, 20, 1903–1912, 2001.
46. Pocock, S.J., Group sequential methods in the design and analysis of clinical trials, *Biometrika*, 64, 191–199, 1977.
47. O'Brien, P.C. and Fleming, T.R., A multiple testing procedure for clinical trials, *Biometrics*, 35, 549–556, 1979.
48. Lan, K.K.G. and DeMets, D.L., Design and analysis of group sequential tests based on the type I error spending function, *Biometrika*, 74, 149–154, 1983.
49. Hwang, I.K., Shih, W.J., and deCani, J.S., Group sequential design using a family of type I error probability spending functions, *Stat. Med.*, 9, 1439–1445, 1990.
50. Gould, A.L. and Shih, W.J., Sample size reestimation without unblinding for normally distributed outcomes with unknown variance, *Commun. Stat. Theor. Methods*, 21, 2833–2853, 1992.
51. Shih, W.J., Commentary: sample size reestimation — journey for a decade, *Stat. Med.*, 20, 515–518, 2001.
52. Lan, K.K.G., Simon, R., and Halperin, M., Stochastically curtailed tests in long-term clinical trials, *Commun. Stat.*, C1, 207–219, 1982.
53. Jennison, C. and Turnbull, B.W., Repeated confidence intervals for group sequential trials, *Control. Clin. Trials*, 5, 33–45, 1984.

54. Jennison, C. and Turnbull, B.W., Sequential equivalence testing and repeated confidence intervals, with applications to normal and binary responses, *Biometrics*, 49, 31–43, 1993.

55. Friede, T. and Kieser, M., Blinded sample size reassessment in noninferiority and equivalence trials, *Stat. Med.*, 22, 995–1007, 2003.

56. Quan, H., Bolognese, J., and Yuan, W., Assessment of equivalence on multiple endpoints, *Stat. Med.*, 20, 3159–3173, 2001.

57. Berger, R.L. and Hsu, J., Bioequivalence trials, intersection-union tests, and equivalence confidence sets (with discussion), *Stat. Sci.*, 11, 283–319, 1996.

58. Hochberg, Y., A sharper Bonferroni procedure for multiple tests of significance, *Biometrika*, 75, 800–802, 1988.

59. Simes, R.J., An improved Bonferroni procedure for multiple tests of significance, *Biometrika*, 73, 751–754, 1986.

60. Giani, G. and Strassburger, K., Testing and selecting for equivalence with respect to a control, *J. Am. Stat. Assoc.*, 89, 320–329, 1994.

61. Wiens, B.L. and Iglewicz, B., Design and analysis of three treatment equivalence trials, *Control. Clin. Trials*, 21, 127–137, 2000.

62. Temple, R., Government viewpoint of clinical trials, *Drug Inf. J.*, 16, 10–17, 1982.

63. Temple, R., Clinical trials in seriously ill patients — design considerations, *PAACNOTES*, 133–143, 1990.

64. Hwang, I.K., Noninferiority trials: does sloppiness bias toward no difference? *ICSA Bull.*, January, 25–27, 2001.

65. Lewis, J.A., The European regulatory experience, *Stat. Med.*, 21, 2931–2938, 2002.

13 Interim Analysis and Bias in Clinical Trials: The Adaptive Design Perspective

Qing Liu and Gordon Pledger

CONTENTS

I. INTRODUCTION

Some bias is inevitable in controlled clinical trials. The issue relevant to trial modifications based on external or internal data is whether additional bias would be introduced. It is naive to equate blindness with validity, i.e., to accept the premise that the trial organizers are free to make trial modifications without introducing bias if only blinded data are used, while bias is unavoidable but immeasurable when modifications are based on unblinded data. We point out that neither part of this proposition is true. A fruitful approach presented here is to examine how trial modifications would introduce additional bias from various sources. While careful planning and execution are necessary, it is also essential to select appropriate adaptive design and inferential procedures in order to avoid additional bias.

Interim analyses have traditionally been used in classical group sequential designs where the only actions allowed at an interim analysis are to stop or continue the trial according to prespecified stopping criteria. Increasingly in practice, however, these interim analyses also lead to other actions, such as changing the sample size, dropping treatment groups, changing endpoints, or modifying the statistical analysis plan. A less obvious but more common setting is to modify an ongoing trial on the basis of external information or blinded review of the database. What separates these two settings is blinding, i.e., whether modifications are based on comparative unblinded interim results or blinded review of the database. Further discussion on interim analysis can be seen in Chapter 14.

Blinding is undoubtedly important and fundamental to controlled clinical trials. Unfortunately, blinding is also mythicized as being synonymous with validity. It is widely believed that modifications of study designs based on blinded data will not invalidate the study results while bias is unavoidable but immeasurable if modifications, when performed by trial organizers, are based on unblinded data. We point out that the dichotomy of blinding and unblinding does not exist in practice, and stress that the question of fundamental importance is validity. We emphasize that basing changes on blinded data does not ensure validity. On the other hand, changes can be made based on unblinded data without introducing bias if appropriate procedures for adaptive designs are followed.

II. BIAS

Bias is a central concept in the validity of clinical trials. Fleming[2] gave the following broad definition:

> *"Bias can be thought of as anything that systematically impairs the design, conduct, or interpretation of preclinical and clinical studies such that false or unwarranted conclusions result."*

Sackett[1] summarized the sources of bias for clinical trials in six categories:

(1) Reading up on the field
(2) Specifying and selecting the study sample
(3) Executing the experimental maneuver
(4) Measuring exposures and outcomes

(5) Analyzing the data

(6) Interpreting the analysis.

Bias in (1) is frequently called literature bias. For all clinical trials it is a risk that could introduce bias in the design, conduct, analysis, and interpretation of clinical trials, i.e., in sources (2) through (6). Thus, it can be reasonably assumed, solely on this basis, that bias from sources (2) through (6) exists in various degrees in any clinical trial. The question is whether trial modifications will introduce additional bias. To explore the issue, it is important to examine how trial modifications would increase various sources of bias, and how such additional bias can be either avoided, or minimized. The context relevant to this discussion is where unblinded group data are available from interim analysis, and it is assumed that neither patients nor investigators will have access to these data.

For an ongoing trial where patients are enrolled, treated, and evaluated, bias from sources (2) to (4) can arise due to patients' and investigators' involvement, with or without blinding, although the use of double-blinding would minimize the comparative bias between treatment groups. If it could be argued that the release of unblinded group data would introduce additional bias in (2) to (4), then such additional bias should be assumed to exist for the classical group sequential design. This is because continuation of a trial after an interim analysis would indicate to both the patients and investigators that an investigational therapeutic medication has some effect since both would have access to protocol designs. Thus, as compared to the classical group sequential design, concerns for additional bias in (2) to (4) from either the patients or investigators would not arise if modifications, made by either the Data Monitoring Committee (DMC) or trial organizers, do not involve patient enrollment, treatment, or evaluations. Similar issues could exist for sponsor staffs who work closely with the investigators on data collection and safety monitoring, where the above argument applies. The roles of DMC or trial organizers in (2) to (4) are indirect through passing information on unblinded results or decisions on protocol modifications to patients or investigators; when this passage is blocked, additional bias in (2) to (4) is avoidable.

For bias in (6), the main concern is when interpreting the final analysis. Moreover, it is reasonable to assume that additional bias in (6) would not arise if trial modifications would not introduce additional bias in (5). In general, bias in (5) consists of bias in type I error rates and bias in parameter estimates. In our view, the former is of primary interest in assessing the validity of trial results after modification. In clinical trials there is no concrete definition of parameters because of the lack of random sampling of patients from a prespecified population at large. Nonetheless parameter estimation has been perceived by many as meaningful to the "would-be population," which could be better described in the context circumstantial to the trial. Setting aside this philosophical argument, the main discussion in the following sections will be focused on bias in both the type I error rates and parameter estimation.

III. MODIFICATIONS USING "BLINDED" DATA

A. BLINDING

A problematic but largely ignored area is blinded review of the database. It is not unusual that study protocols provide minimal information on statistical methods, with specifics deferred to a statistical analysis plan. But the development of a statistical analysis plan typically coincides with the collection and blinded review of efficacy, safety, and laboratory data, making it impossible to establish that the development of a statistical analysis plan is not data dependent. Often such a statistical analysis plan is accepted by regulatory agencies at face value as long as its finalization occurs prior to releasing the randomization code. The International Conference on Harmonization (ICH E9)[3] states:

> "*One type of monitoring concerns... checking the appropriateness of design assumptions, etc. This type of monitoring does not require access to information on comparative treatment effects, nor unblinding of data, and therefore has no impact on type I error.*"

Even more provocative, a recent draft guidance by the Food and Drug Administration[4] claims:

> "*When a DMC is the only group reviewing unblinded interim data, the trial organizers are free to make changes in the ongoing trial that may be motivated by newly available data outside the trial or by accumulating data from within the trial (e.g., overall event rates).*"

These are overstatements on the credibility of modifications using "blinded" data. In practice, type I error rates can be inflated because blinding may be partial and incomplete.

The fallacy on blindness is the perception that there is a dichotomy of blinding and unblinding. Such a dichotomy exists only mechanistically as the word "blinded" practically means that the randomization code is not released, and "unblinded" means the randomization code is released. Thus, we will assume in the following only the mechanistic interpretation of the terms blinding or blinded data. Between blinding and unblinding, there are partial unblinding and blinding under the null neutral principle. The latter is fundamental to the validity of the trial.

B. PARTIAL UNBLINDING

It is important to recognize that under mechanistic blinding, there are several ways to partially unblind the data, which could result in inflation of type I error rates.

One type of partial unblinding involves construction of a pseudo randomization code that is positively correlated with the true randomization code. There are several ways to achieve this. One scheme, proposed in the literature for sample size adjustment, is to artificially divide patients into different strata and use different randomization ratios for different strata.[5] Trial organizers who have access to stratification information for individual patients can construct unbiased estimates of effects for different treatment groups. However, under the standard operating procedure of any sponsor, the randomization code is not released and the trial would still be called blinded. Another maneuver is to use a secondary variable that is differentially affected by the treatment of the study drug as compared with the control, e.g., the pseudo code based on ranks by the degree of a known side effect from within each randomization block would correlate with the true randomization.

Partial unblinding also results from a fairly standard practice used for sample size adjustment. In order to estimate "nuisance" parameters, the trial organizers send outcome data and the randomization code to an "independent" third party, such as an academic statistician. With all the data needed, the third party calculates the estimates and sends them back to the trial organizers who will then perform sample size adjustment. This procedure is treated as blinded by trial organizers. In many cases regulatory agencies are apparently in agreement. The effect of such sample size adjustment on the type I error rate has been studied and the conclusion has been that such procedures do not materially inflate the type I error rates. But, neither the mathematical formulation nor the stimulation studies in this area have incorporated the fact the trial organizers, in possession of estimates of nuisance parameters, also have access to individual patient outcome data. From elementary statistics courses, it is well known that the calculation of the total sum of squares in an analysis of variance model does not require group information and also the sum of squares due to "error" can be easily calculated from estimates of the variance. Thus, with these two pieces of information, the trial organizers, although formally blinded, have no problem calculating the F-statistic. In a simulation study the type I error rate can be as high as 55% in extreme situations.

Because partial unblinding, either indirect or direct, can inflate the type I error rate, its use should be discouraged by regulatory agencies and prohibited at the policy level via sponsor's standard operation procedures.

C. THE NULL NEUTRAL PRINCIPLE

Despite the potential for inflating the type I error rate, modifications of the design or statistical analysis plan are very common on the basis of other scientific or clinical reasons. Often these reasons are external to the trial. But there are many internal reasons as well. One type of modification that has been studied in the literature is sample size adjustment using only the outcome data (i.e., not requiring the release of randomization code to a third party as described above).

On rare occasions, the primary endpoint is changed from a responder variable at a specified time of followup to a time-to-response variable, if the overall response rate is very high. Often, blinded data are used to fine tune statistical methods for hypothesis testing, e.g., building a regression model to include appropriate covariates, checking or adjusting the distribution of the test statistic to ensure normality, etc.

To assist these types of modifications while being mindful of validity, the use of pseudo randomization code based on *null neutral* variables can be helpful. Specifically, a variable is null neutral if it is uncorrelated with the true randomization under the primary null hypothesis. Certainly, a code obtained by randomly assigning pseudo treatment groups to patients is null neutral, but it is not useful. A more meaningful approach is to use a secondary variable that is null neutral concerning the primary null hypothesis but correlated with the true randomization code under an alternative to the primary null hypothesis. Then a pseudo randomization code can be constructed based on rank values of the null neutral variable within each randomization block. The goal of modifications is to increase the power for rejecting the null hypothesis under the alternative. As under the alternative a pseudo randomization code based on null neutral secondary variables is correlated with the true randomization code, its usefulness is apparent. The *null neutral principle* states that only the null neutral variables should be used in the modifications of the test method. The foundation for the principle is that *the type I error rate under modifications based on null neutral variables can be controlled at a stated significance level.*

To justify the claim, the paradigm for significance tests must be shifted from a sampling based procedure to a randomization based procedure. The advantage is that for randomized experiments, a randomization procedure under which the treatment assignments are random while responses from experimental units are fixed, allows more freedom of choice and therefore increases the power of the test. Specifically, under a sampling procedure, the test method must be specified in advance, while under a randomization procedure, an "optimal" test method can be determined with the accumulating response data. In a randomization procedure, both the primary variable and secondary neutral variables are fixed. In addition, modifications to the test method are also fixed because they are results of reviewing the primary and secondary null neutral variables. By definition, neither the primary nor secondary null neutral variables would correlate with the randomization under the null hypothesis. Thus, the null distribution of the test statistic, selected as a result of modifications, can be easily obtained by rerandomizing treatment groups to patients using the exact randomization procedure used in the actual patient randomization. Since the randomization test, conditional upon the primary and secondary null neutral variables, controls the conditional type I error rate at a stated significance level, the unconditional type I error rate is also controlled. A formal proof can be given using the general adaptation theory of Liu et al.[6]

D. Adaptive Statistical Analysis Planning

The process of reviewing blinded null neutral variables, modifying the test method, and assessing the randomization based p-value of the modified test is called *adaptive statistical analysis planning* (ASAP). A prerequisite for ASAP is the relevancy condition: the rejection of the null hypothesis corresponding to the modified test must imply the rejection of the primary null hypothesis. This requires that the primary null hypothesis be specified in the protocol and that the rejection of the primary null hypothesis is necessary for trial success such that not only is the type I error rate controlled but the result of the test is also interpretable. On the other hand, ASAP recognizes the dilemma facing trial statisticians and provides a valid approach to allow the development of a statistical analysis plan with the accumulation of the data. To balance specificity and flexibility, it is reasonable to follow the advice: *specify what you can and modify what you cannot specify.* Under ASAP, the quoted claims by both the ICH E9[3] and the draft FDA guidance[4] in Section III.A are valid. Apart from its scientific merits, the incorporation of ASAP can also facilitate quality and speed for delivering statistical outputs and clinical reports.

E. Scope and Limitations

Although modification using blinded data is tempting and can be very useful, we warn that the blinded data may not be informative and blinding will hinder the flexibility in the types of modifications to be made. For example, blinded sample size adjustment methods do not provide directional information on the treatment effects, and increasing sample size can be problematic both ethically and economically when the actual effect is negative. The more efficient approach is to base modifications on formal interim analyses built into the trial design.

IV. MODIFICATIONS USING UNBLINDED DATA

A. Bias and Naive Analysis

The terminology "unblinded data" refers to summary statistics for different treatment groups, rather than individual patient outcomes. It is used interchangeably with "unblinded group data." In this section, it is assumed that unblinded interim data will be made available to only the DMC and trial organizers, who will then make decisions regarding trial modifications. Moreover, both the patients and investigators will be blinded to the interim results and decisions concerning trial modifications. This is to confine any potential addition of bias in source (5), i.e., bias in the type I error rates and parameter estimates.

It is generally stated that modifications to an ongoing trial based on unblinded interim data would introduce additional bias. However, it is less well recognized that the additional bias is the result of employing naive methods for testing and estimation. The additional bias is certainly unavoidable but immeasurable if modifications to the trial are kept unknown to trial evaluators, e.g., the FDA reviewers, either intentionally or unintentionally. Even if the modifications were known, the use of incorrect methods would still introduce additional bias. For example, it is not uncommon for the FDA to request a sponsor to specify an alpha-spending rule when the sponsor states that the trial would not stop for efficacy and the purpose of the interim analysis is "administrative." But for various reasons in practice, such "administrative" interim analysis would often trigger modifications of trial designs that are typically documented in protocol amendments. The FDA might be satisfied if the sponsor would spend a rather small alpha, say 0.0001, for the interim analysis. It must be realized that an alpha-spending rule is adequate only for the conventional group sequential design for which the only decision at an interim analysis is to stop or continue. For trials with modifications such a superficial correction does not protect the overall type I error rate.

Thus, to make progress, we assume further that adequate and honest documentation of the modifications to the trial is available to trial evaluators. We then discuss adaptive designs under which any additional potential bias can be quantified and also corrected.

B. THE PHILOSOPHY OF ADAPTIVE DESIGNS

It is well known that in designing a clinical trial numerous assumptions must be made regarding, say, the patient population, treatments, endpoints, effect size, prognostic factors, outcome distributions, etc. In classical nonadaptive designs, the basic premise is that these assumptions, except the effect size of the experimental treatment, are true. In reality, many clinical trials fail not because the experimental treatments are not effective but because the trial designs are based on unrealistic assumptions. To demonstrate treatment effect new trials are designed, which correct the mistaken assumptions used in previous trials.

Adaptive designs recognize that assumptions in a trial design may not be true. Rather than being overly specific with respect to these assumptions, a range of possibilities are permitted in the initial design such that greater specificity can be reached later based on the results of planned interim analysis. In an adaptive design, both "learning" and "confirmation" are allowed, and at the same time, the data for learning and confirmation can be integrated for hypothesis testing and parameter estimation. In multistage adaptive designs, the line between learning and confirmation is blurred as data at a particular stage can serve both purposes. The central issue regarding adaptive designs is how to avoid bias, and specifically, bias in type I error rates and parameter estimates.

C. TWO-STAGE ADAPTIVE DESIGNS

The basic form of adaptive design is a two-stage adaptive design under which a clinical trial is divided into two sequential stages such that data from the first stage can be used to modify certain features of the design or statistical analysis for the second stage. Specific two-stage adaptive designs for sample size adjustment have been studied by various authors.[7-9] A general unified framework for two-stage adaptive designs is given by Liu et al.[6] Under the general framework, modifications of the trial are not limited to sample size adjustment, and can include dropping treatment groups, changing endpoints, and fine tuning the final statistical analysis. Two-stage adaptive designs are important because they are adequate for many practical applications. They also serve as building blocks for multistage adaptive group sequential designs. Below we discuss in greater detail the concept of adaptation and methods for hypothesis testing and estimation.

1. Adaptation

Adaptation is an essential element of a two-stage adaptive design, which can be viewed as a formalization of the process for interim analysis, decision making for modifying the design or statistical analysis, and assessing the final trial outcome as a result of modification. Three critical components are: the interim data, an adaptation rule for modification, and the final trial outcome.

The interim data form the basis for gaining information on those assumptions that are important for the trial's success but cannot be assumed to be true with confidence at the trial's inception. Thus, not only must interim data be relevant to the issue at hand but also informative.

An adaptation rule can be thought of as a transition from the interim data to a decision on the types of modifications for the second stage. In mathematical terms, an adaptation rule is a function of the interim data and its range is the collection of all potential decisions on modifications for the second stage. Technically, the function must be measurable and its range must be enumerable.[6] It is important to realize that for each potential decision on modifications there is a null hypothesis and a corresponding test statistic, and they may or may not be the same depending on the nature of the decisions. Thus, to avoid difficulty in the interpretation and extrapolation of the final results, it must be assumed that modifications are limited such that the rejection of any modified null hypothesis can lead to trial success. A prerequisite is that the success criteria are specified in advance, by which the corresponding primary null hypothesis is also prespecified. This is the relevancy condition. Mathematically, the primary null hypothesis must imply all possible modified null hypotheses and, consequently, rejecting a modified null hypothesis implies logically rejecting the primary null hypothesis. In practice, it is helpful but not necessary to enumerate all possible decisions on modifications in advance to promote understanding, confidence, and smooth execution.

The third essential element of adaptation is assessing the final trial outcome, which is described in the following as hypothesis testing and parameter estimation.

2. Hypothesis Testing

For the first stage, a null hypothesis and the corresponding test statistic must be specified in the protocol. It is required that the null hypothesis be implied by the primary null hypothesis and that the test statistic be a function of the interim data. The null hypothesis can then be rejected at the end of the first stage if the p-value, one-sided in favor of the alternative hypothesis, is less than a prespecified fraction of the overall alpha; the trial will then stop. In many applications, it is also desirable to stop the trial for futility, which occurs when the p-value is greater than a prespecified futility level. Otherwise, the trial will continue and a decision will be made based on interim data regarding the modifications of the first stage null hypothesis and the corresponding test statistic. Among all possible modifications, the default is not to modify the trial. Regardless of the nature of the decision made, a null hypothesis and a test statistic will be formulated for the second stage. Notice that the first stage p-value provides not only the basis for hypothesis testing for the first stage but also a summary of the strength of evidence, which can be incorporated in the hypothesis testing at the end of the second stage. This is achieved via the use of a conditional error function, proposed by Proschan and Hunsberger.[8] A conditional error function essentially defines the conditional type I error rate for the second stage for each realization of the first stage test statistic. In general, a conditional error function is an increasing function of the first stage test statistic; the stronger the evidence in the first stage, the larger the conditional error rate for the second stage and therefore the smaller the size for the second stage. From Liu et al.,[6] the second stage p-value is required to follow a conditional uniform distribution, given the interim data and the choice of null hypothesis and test statistic for the second stage. At the end of the second stage, the second stage null hypothesis is rejected if the second stage conditional p-value is less than or equal to the conditional error rate.

To control the overall type I error rate at the alpha-level, the conditional error function must integrate to alpha. Proschan and Hunsberger[8] proposed conditional error functions for two-stage adaptive designs for sample size adjustment. The procedure is valid for general adaptations as well.[6] In particular, the validity does not depend on the prespecification of an exact adaptive rule except for its possible outcomes, i.e., all possible modified null hypotheses, to ensure that they are all relevant for trial success and that the construction of the second stage conditional p-value is technically achievable for each possible null hypothesis.

One important application of two-stage adaptive designs is for trials with a prespecified "administrative" interim analysis. Although at trial inception a sponsor would insist that the purpose of the interim analysis was to assist designing other trials of the clinical program, it would be irresponsible not to modify the trial if interim data suggest that the protocol assumptions regarding safety and efficacy are overly optimistic or pessimistic. Thus, because the potential exists for modification, neither the naive analysis assuming no modification nor the usual alpha-spending approach mentioned earlier can be proven to control the type I error rate. To resolve the issue, the two-stage adaptive design proposed by Proschan et al.[10] can be used. Such a design protects the type I error rate without the need for specifying in advance whether or not modifications to the trial will be made. If no modification is made, the analysis is asymptotically equivalent to the naive analysis under which no alpha-penalty is necessary.

3. Point Estimation and Confidence Intervals

Pragmatically, parameter estimates are important as treatment effect sizes are routinely reported in drug package inserts and in scientific literature. These estimates are also used for designing future trials as well as by physicians and drug makers to "informally" distinguish one drug from another. Despite the fact that a parameter estimate from a clinical trial would invariably be biased for the patient population at large because of the inclusion and exclusion criteria, it is important to ensure that additional bias will not be introduced through trial modification, which would then make it impossible to compare, again "informally", different drugs even for the "would-be population" from which the patient sample for the trial could be thought of as randomly selected.

Methods for obtaining point estimates and confidence intervals are developed by Liu and Chi[9] for two-stage adaptive designs with sample size adjustment. The theory and methods under general adaptation rules are given by Liu et al.[6]

These methods assume that the parameter in question has the same interpretation in both stages for all possible decisions regarding modifications. That is, the parameter must be invariant to adaptation. Obviously, restricting the adaptation such that the parameter will not change its interpretation can satisfy this assumption. For many applications, however, such a restriction can unnecessarily limit the potential flexibility in hypothesis testing. To balance the need for hypothesis testing and estimation, consider only those "construct" parameters for which their interpretations are not dependent upon the specifics of study design or analytical modeling that are subject to adaptation. In contrast, "nonconstruct" parameters are design-specific, and their estimates can be difficult to interpret beyond the confines of the trial design, and there is less interest in practice to report their estimates. Two notable examples of such nonconstruct parameters are the linear trend parameter for a linear trend test for dose response studies and the common odds ratio for a series of 2×2 tables.

The estimation methods also assume that data for the construct parameters are always available regardless of whether the trial stops early and regardless of decisions concerning modifications. For practical applications, these data are naturally available if patient enrollment continues during the period between the time of last patient enrollment for the interim analysis and the time of delivering the interim results. In fact, it is entirely reasonable to establish a policy on the minimal sample size for the second stage.

Thus, for practical applications, it is advisable that the construct parameters and policies on adaptation and a minimum sample size for the second stage be specified in the protocol to guarantee interpretability of construct parameters and also the availability of data for these parameters.

D. ADAPTIVE GROUP SEQUENTIAL DESIGNS

The two-stage adaptive designs can be easily extended to multistage adaptive group sequential designs. In a two-stage adaptive design, the conditional error rate is the conditional type I error rate for the second stage. In a multistage design, it is the conditional type I error rate for the remaining experiment that may contain one or more stages.[11] At any stage the cumulative interim data will be reviewed and the trial may be designated to stop at the end of the next stage regardless of the outcomes. If the trial is designated to stop, the conditional error rate is spent in the final hypothesis testing, and if the trial is to continue, the conditional error rate is the total type I error rate for designing a new "two-stage" trial with its own conditional significance and futility levels. This process continues until the trial stops either because it stops at the designated stopping time or it hits a stopping boundary for either significance or futility.

This concept of adaptive group sequential designs has its origin in the self-designing procedures of Fisher[12] and Shen and Fisher[13] where a "designated stopping time" is determined on the basis of ongoing data. In contrast, the conventional group sequential designs have a *fixed* designated stopping time, which is 100% of the "information time." While both approaches control the type I error rate, they differ in how the type I error rate is controlled: in an adaptive group sequential trial, the conditional error rates are spent dynamically on the basis of ongoing data, whereas a conventional group sequential design spends the overall alpha-rate according to a prespecified spending function at prespecified information times.

In a general formulation, data from different stages are not required to be independent to permit much wider applications where the Brownian motion process, which underlies the conventional group sequential designs, is not adequate. At each stage, decisions on other types of modifications for the remaining trial are also allowed, in addition to decisions for trial stopping for the next stage. The result is a very general and flexible framework, which is justified by martingale theory and the adaptation theory of Liu et al.[6] Special cases for sample size adjustment under the assumption of "independent" increments are proposed by various authors.[14-16] For statistical inference, methods proposed by Liu and Chi,[9] Liu et al.,[6] and Proschan et al.[10] can be extended for calculation of overall p-value, point estimates, and confidence intervals.

V. DISCUSSION

We have assumed that decisions on trial modifications would not be made known to patients and investigators, in order to avoid additional bias in the event that knowledge of the decisions would lead to further modifications in patient enrollment, treatment, or evaluation. It must be pointed out that this assumption is "sufficient" but not absolutely necessary for the trial to be valid and interpretable. In certain therapeutic areas, such as oncology, not only are the treatments tailored according to patients' prognoses at diagnosis but also they are constantly modified on the basis of observed safety and efficacy responses to treatments. The effect sizes would therefore depend heavily on the exact circumstantial context of the trial. Because the circumstances cannot be replicated, the observed effects cannot be generalized to the patient population at large. This view was also expressed by Leber,[17]

> *"Comparisons of drug performance based upon results obtained in different clinical trials are always of arguable validity and reliability. Because studies are conducted at different times, with different samples of patients, by different investigators, employing different criteria and/or different conditions (dose, dosing regimen, etc.), quantitative estimates of treatment response and the timing of response may be expected to vary considerably from study to study. Accordingly, estimates of treatment effects obtained from a single study or small series of studies have limited value as estimates of the likely effect of a drug in the population as a whole."*

In the oncology setting, restricting trial adaptation for the sake of estimating effect sizes makes little sense. Here the trial organizers should act responsibly in modifying certain aspects of the trial, including enrollment criteria, treatments, and perhaps methods of evaluation, etc. To avoid comparative bias, it is necessary that the trial outcomes be based on objective criteria such as time of death, or that patient evaluators be blinded to other information that might reveal the identity of the underlying treatment. The bias in type I error rates can then be controlled at a prespecified alpha-level using scientifically valid adaptive designs and analysis procedures.

Finally, we point out that adaptation is not new to clinical trials. Under the conventional clinical development paradigm where confirmatory phase 3 trials follow smaller scale phase 2 trials, the transition from phase 2 to phase 3 is an adaptation process. What is new is how to combine data that are used for "learning" with data that are for confirmation. Thus, at the clinical development level, trial organizers now have the flexibility to integrate different phases of the clinical development, e.g., phase 2 and phase 3,[18] into a coherent development program under which clinical trials can be conducted more effectively and efficiently.

REFERENCES

1. Sackett, D.L., Bias in analytic research (with discussion) (Com: pp. 64–68), *J. Chron. Dis.*, 32, 51–63, 1979.
2. Fleming, Z., Efficacy Review. In: *Regulatory Science Course*, FDA/CDER internal training course, 1997.

3. International Conference on Harmonization. Guidance on statistical principles for clinical trials. In: *Federal Register*, Vol. 63, No. 179, 49583–49598, 1998.

4. Food and Drug Administration. Draft guidance for clinical trial sponsors: on the establishment and operation of clinical trial data monitoring committees, 2001, http://www.fda.gov/cber/gdlns/clindatmon.pdf

5. Shih, W.J. and Zhao, P.L., Design for sample size re-estimation with interim data for double-blind clinical trials with binary outcomes, *Stat. Med.*, 16, 1913–1923, 1997.

6. Liu, Q., Proschan, M.A., and Pledger, G.W., A unified theory of two-stage adaptive designs, *J. Am. Stat. Assoc.*, 97, 1034–1041, 2002.

7. Bauer, P. and Köhne, K., Evaluations of experiments with adaptive interim analyses, *Biometrics*, 50, 1029–1041, 1994.

8. Proschan, M.A. and Hunsberger, S.A., Designed extension of studies based on conditional power, *Biometrics*, 51, 1315–1324, 1995.

9. Liu, Q. and Chi, G.Y.H., On sample size and inference for two-stage adaptive designs, *Biometrics*, 57, 172–177, 2001.

10. Proschan, M.A., Liu, Q., and Hunsberger, S.A., Practical midcourse sample size modification in clinical trials, *Control Clin. Trials*, 24, 4–15, 2003.

11. Müller, H. and Schäfer, H., Adaptive group sequential designs for clinical trials: combining the advantages of adaptive and of classical group sequential approaches, *Biometrics*, 57, 886–891, 2001.

12. Fisher, L., Self-designing clinical trials, *Stat. Med.*, 17, 1551–1562, 1998.

13. Shen, Y. and Fisher, L., Statistical inference for self-designing clinical trials with a one-sided hypothesis, *Biometrics*, 55, 190–197, 1999.

14. Cui, L., Hung, J.H.M., and Wang, S.J., Modification of sample size in group sequential clinical trials, *Biometrics*, 55, 853–857, 1999.

15. Lehmacher, W. and Wassmer, G., Adaptive sample size calculations in group sequential trials, *Biometrics*, 55, 1286–1290, 1999.

16. Brannath, W., Posch, M., and Bauer, P., Recursive combination tests, *J. Am. Stat. Assoc.*, 97, 236–244, 2002.

17. Leber, P. and Zomig (zolmitriptan) P., File NDA 20-768, 1997, http://www.fda.gov/cder/foi/nda/97/020768ap_Zomig_admindoc.pdf

18. Liu, Q. and Pledger, G.W., Phase 2 and 3 combination designs to accelerate drug development. *J. Am. Stat. Assoc.*, 100, 493–502, 2005.

14 Interim Analysis and Adaptive Design in Clinical Trials

Irving K. Hwang and K. K. Gordon Lan

CONTENTS

I. INTRODUCTION

Double-blind, randomized clinical trials (RCTs) in the 1960s had emerged as the gold standard for evaluation of new drugs or therapeutic procedures in medical research since Sir Austin Bradford Hill introduced the trial design in 1946. Almost all of these RCTs were based on fixed design. These trials were primarily nonsequential and made no allowance for repeated testing (i.e., interim look/analysis of accumulating data and early decision making on trial design and conduct). Interim examinations of data were performed, formally or informally, but usually lacked documentation. The scientific issues of performing repeated testing and methodology for group sequential designs had drawn special attention in the statistical and clinical trial literature during the 1970s and 1980s. In particular, the work of Pocock,[1] O'Brien and Fleming,[2] Lan and DeMets,[3] and Lan et al.,[4] suggested viable methodological solutions for problems of inflation of error probabilities due to repeated testing and early trial stopping.

Medical research in the United States prior to the 1970s was predominantly conducted by academic institutions via government funding under the auspices of National Institutes of Health (NIH) and Veterans Administration (VA). Performing interim analyses and making early decisions were promoted primarily by scientific and ethical reasons. Over the past three decades the center of gravity of clinical research has slowly shifted to the pharmaceutical industry,[5] which has additional needs. One such need is to shorten the drug development cycle so as to have a new drug approved and marketed sooner to provide a competitive edge commercially. Time and resource management are crucial. Interim analysis and designs of adaptive nature, therefore, are now becoming important tools for the pharmaceutical companies in managing critical trials in drug development process.

Drug development involves both early-phase (Phases I to IIa) exploratory trials and late-phase (Phases IIb to III) confirmatory trials. The major concern is for the latter where the performance of interim analysis, in particular, with midcourse adaptation, may skew/bias the results or their interpretation when conducted improperly. Therefore, we focus our attention in this chapter primarily on issues of interim analysis and adaptive design in large late-phase confirmatory trials, although the principles remain valid for small early-phase exploratory trials.

In this chapter we begin by addressing the distinctive issues between interim analysis and data monitoring in Section II, since these two are not considered synonymous in the pharmaceutical industry. In Section III, we address the Data Monitoring Committee (DMC) including its role and responsibility in interim analysis of clinical trials. In discussion of the methodologies for interim analysis and adaptive design, we concentrate on two most popular and flexible approaches, namely, the error rate spending function[3,6] and Conditioning Power (CP)[4] approaches. The readers will find that these two approaches are theoretically interrelated and can be used independently or complementarily. Sections IV and V discuss the essence of error rate spending function and CP approaches, respectively. In these two sections we review both the fundamental theories as well as practical issues involved in interim analysis. Examples of landmark clinical trials are given for illustration of the use of these effective approaches. Before closing with general discussion, we also briefly review advances in adaptive design in Section VI. Relevant references are provided for readers with further interests. This chapter can be viewed as an expanded summary of many selected papers published by the authors as well as many others on the topic related to interim analysis and adaptive design.

II. INTERIM ANALYSIS VS. DATA MONITORING

Interim analysis and data monitoring in the pharmaceutical industry are generally considered nonsynonymous. The distinction is best described in "Interim Analysis in the Pharmaceutical Industry" by PMA Biostatistics and Medical Ad Hoc Committee on Interim Analysis.[7] In this PMA Position Paper, interim analysis was defined as: "Unmasked (blinded) data analysis of response variable while the trial is in progress and before the response data are available for all patients. The test statistics on the response variable are calculated and significance testing (or confidence intervals) is often performed." Whilst data monitoring is defined as: "An active process involving the completely masked (blinded) review of the clinical data while the trial is in progress. This is performed to monitor the progress and conduct of the trial." The focus of the PMA Position Paper definitions was on whether the analysis is performed on "unblinded" or "blinded" data. A followup paper[8] further defined interim analysis as: "Any analysis, summary or inspection of unblinded trial data prior to the end of data collection phase of the trial. The data collection phase encompasses the entire duration of the trial up to the finalization and locking of the trial's database. This phase includes the treatment phase, as well as the data cleanup period, the period in which data related questions are being addressed." Along the same vein data monitoring was defined as: "Any completely blinded review, analysis, summary or inspection of the trial data prior to the end of the data collection phase of the trial."

ICH E9 Guidance: Statistical Principles for Clinical Trials[9] classifies trial monitoring into two distinct types. One type of monitoring concerns the oversight of the quality of the trial (i.e., data monitoring) and the other type involves breaking the blind in making treatment comparisons (i.e., interim analysis). It further defines interim analysis as: "Any analysis intended to compare treatment arms with respect to efficacy or safety at any time prior to the formal completion of a trial. … Interim analysis requires unblinded (i.e., key breaking) access to treatment group assignment (actual treatment assignment or identification of group assignment) and comparative treatment group summary information. … Any interim analysis that is not planned appropriately … may flaw the results of a trial and possibly weaken confidence in the conclusion drawn. Therefore, such analyses should be avoided."

Current practice in the pharmaceutical industry is that interim analysis would include any analysis performed on unblinded data prior to database finalization. In addition, grouping patients according to randomization or treatment received is considered unblinding, even if the actual treatment identification is not revealed. Using arbitrary labels for treatments (e.g., A, B, C) should also be considered tantamount to unblinding. Interim analysis involves unblinded data. Unblinding data prior to trial completion may introduce both patient selection and evaluation bias and may also introduce trial operational bias before database finalization. What would make things worse is one's inability to determine whether or not bias was actually introduced, let alone to assess quantitatively and/or qualitatively its impact.

We have made a distinction between interim analysis and data monitoring based on whether or not the identity of the treatment is revealed and/or patients are grouped according to randomization or treatment received. In fact, data monitoring is a necessary process in clinical trials without unblinding the data to assure that the quality of trial conduct is maintained and the safety of the participating subjects is ensured (e.g., checking the recruitment status, aggregating the overall mortality rate, and/or reviewing serious AEs and elevated laboratory tests). In particular, ICH E9 defines data monitoring as: "Trial monitoring concerning the oversight of the quality of the trial includes whether the protocol is being followed, the acceptability of data being accrued, the success of planned accrued targets, the checking of the design assumptions, success in keeping patients in the trials, etc. This type of monitoring does not require access to information on comparative treatment effects, not unblinding of data and therefore has no impact on Type I error. … The period of this type of monitoring usually starts with the selection of the trial sites and ends with the collection and cleaning of the last subject's data." In principle, because data monitoring does not involve unblinding data, there should be no concern for bias introduction. In reality, however, this is not always the case. For example, certain aspects of the data, such as a typical AE or laboratory test, may associate with certain treatment but not with the others, would essentially reveal the treatment identity. In certain response variables or endpoints (e.g., dichotomous/binomial or survival), knowledge of the variance virtually reveals the treatment effect since the variance and expectation are stochastically dependent. This problem is of particular concern when sophisticated computerized data monitoring browsing tools are available. Nonetheless, because data monitoring is an essential activity, there are no simple solutions to this problem. Many sponsors address this problem with strict standard operating procedures (SOPs) on data monitoring and interim analysis in close concert with data blinding and unblinding procedures.

It is well known that performing interim analyses on accumulating data may inflate the type I and II error probabilities above the prespecified levels associated with the testing of hypotheses[10,11] regardless whether the trial is double-blind or open-label. For example, if we set $\alpha = 0.05$ and perform repeated tests at the same level, then the true Type I error probability would be inflated drastically with the increased number of tests (e.g., 0.05 for testing once, 0.08 twice, 0.11 three times, 0.14 five times, 0.19 ten times, and 0.25 twenty times — a five fold of the true 0.05 level). To protect the error probabilities, group sequential methods (GSMs) such as the Pocock boundary,[1] the O'Brien–Fleming boundary,[2] and an error rate spending function approach of Lan and DeMets[3] were proposed. The approach of Lan and DeMets generalizes both the boundaries of Pocock and O'Brien–Fleming with much greater flexibility and has now emerged as the mainstream tool in GSMs and applications. A parallel methodology to the GSMs is the CP or stochastic curtailing approach by Lan et al.[4] Another development is the Bayesian approach.[12-14]

In this chapter we focus on the frequentist viewpoint and concentrate our discussions on two most popular and flexible approaches — namely the error rate spending and CP approaches in Sections IV and V, respectively, following the review of DMC in the next section. (Note: Chapter 15 provides a regulatory perspective on data monitoring and interim analysis.)

III. DATA MONITORING COMMITTEE (DMC)

Ongoing trial monitoring is an ethical responsibility of a trial's investigators and sponsor to their trial participants. Such monitoring of trial data is required not only to protect the safety and well-beings of human research subjects, but also to ensure the scientific integrity of trials under investigation. ICH E6 Good Clinical Practice (GCP). Consolidated Guidance[15] recommends: "The sponsor may consider establishing an independent data monitoring committee (IDMC) to assess the progress of a clinical trial, including the safety data and the critical efficacy endpoints at intervals, and to recommend to the sponsor whether to continue, modify, or stop a trial. The IDMC should have written operating procedures and maintain written records of all its meetings." Consequently, a critical clinical trial that has a formal interim analysis plan in the protocol usually establishes an independent DMC. The DMC monitors subject recruitment, evaluates interim results (safety and efficacy), and relevant external information regularly, as well as safeguards the blinding and objectivity so as to ensure the integrity of the trial.

A DMC is a group of experts with pertinent knowledge and experience external to the sponsor that reviews trial accumulating data from an ongoing trial on a regular basis. (In some situations, a DMC may be formed within a sponsor, but independent of the project team that runs a particular trial.) The DMC advises the sponsor regarding the patient safety and ongoing trial conduct per ethics and scientific merit. The name of DMC varies — most often it is called Data and Safety Monitoring Committee/Board (DSMC/DSMB). It has been also named as Ethical Review Committee (ERC) and a few others. DMCs were initially used in the 1960s exclusively in large landmark mortality and/or irreversible morbidity trials sponsored by NIH and VA in the U.S. Few trials sponsored by the pharmaceutical industry involved DMC oversight until late 1970s and 1980s. The very first one of such trials was The Blocadren Myocardial Infarction Study[16] in which an independent ERC was involved. The involvement of external advisors in interim analyses led to the recommendation of early termination of BMIS for overwhelming efficacy. The use of DMCs in industry-sponsored trials has increased ever since and they are currently used in a variety of situations with slightly variant models of operations.

All clinical trials require safety monitoring, but not all trials require monitoring by a formal committee or board external to the trial organizers, sponsors, and investigators. The need for a DMC and its role may vary depending on the size of the trial, the phase, and the potential risk of the intervention under investigation. Most Phase I and Phase IIa studies of low risk interventions do not require an independent DMC, since they tend to be exploratory and stepwise in nature. Usually, the trial investigator can accomplish the sponsor's safety monitoring duty jointly with the sponsor's Clinical Monitor or Safety Officer. For large scale Phases IIb to III confirmatory trials or in trials that patients are at higher risk of unexpected serious adverse events (SAEs), a DMC is often deemed required to provide more vigorous data monitoring and review. In particular, it is generally agreed that a DMC should be established for an adequate and well-controlled trial with mortality and/or irreversible morbidity as a primary or major secondary endpoint. Because the ultimate responsibility for monitoring trial progress and safety belongs to the trial sponsor, a DMC may be appointed to serve this function for the sponsor. In fact, the sponsor may delegate this responsibility to a trial organizer or Contract Research Organization (CRO), in which case the DMC selection, meetings, and other activities may be coordinated by that CRO. Once an independent DMC is established to assume the sponsor's monitoring responsibility, a special relationship is established between the DMC, sponsor, CRO, and other trial governing bodies such as the Steering Committee (SC) or Policy Board (PB), Data Coordination Center (DCC), IRBs of the clinical trial centers/sites, and the investigators, as appropriate.

A. DMC Role and Responsibilities

The responsibilities of the DMC can be broadly grouped into three areas.

1. Performance Monitoring

The DMC regularly reviews the performance of clinical centers/sites and the trial in aggregate with respect to:

  i. Subject recruitment relative to target goals
 ii. Adherence to inclusion/exclusion criteria
iii. Timely submission and completeness of data forms
 iv. Subject followup compliance
  v. Data errors.

These performance criteria should be monitored continuously by the trial manager and investigators, but should be reviewed by the DMC at scheduled intervals.

2. Safety Review

Safety review is an ongoing process. There are usually several potential formats for presentation of this data to the DMC:

  i. Aggregate (pooled) data
 ii. By treatment group (semiblinded, e.g., A, B, C)
iii. By treatment group (unblinded)
 iv. Individual patient/event listings.

The frequency and exact method of data review should be formulated in a monitoring plan. The adverse and/or endpoint events reviewed by the DMC will depend on the investigative therapy and patient population being studied. In addition to scheduled DMC safety review, provision should be made for *ad hoc* reviews, which may be triggered by unexpected adverse events or an increase in a particular event above a specified threshold.

3. Interim Analyses on Efficacy and Safety

In addition to routine safety monitoring, the protocol may also stipulate formal interim analyses for evaluation of safety and/or efficacy periodically. If interim analyses are warranted, the study protocol should include a formal plan, indicating when the analyses will be conducted, the expected consequences of these analyses, a discussion of whether p-values will be adjusted, and methods of controlling the overall Type I error rate. In contrast to ongoing safety reports that represent snapshots of live data, the interim analysis is a formal process that is usually included in the study's statistical analysis plan (SAP) and sample size calculations. This plan should be reviewed carefully and approved by the DMC as it will define the DMCs recommended action based on the findings from this analysis. As noted above, however, the DMC may modify the timing of interim analyses, the types of events, or request additional data included in these analyses based on routine observations or on an *ad hoc* basis.

B. DMC MEMBERSHIP AND RELATIONSHIPS

The DMC finds itself serving as an extension of the sponsor from a regulatory perspective, but required to be independent and free of potential conflict of interests from an ethical and trial conduct viewpoint. Careful selection of the DMC members and a clear understanding in the monitoring plan of how the DMC will relate to the sponsor, investigators, SC, DCC, and regulatory agencies will allow for the DMC to perform its primary function without compromise.

The chairperson of the DMC must have experience with the conduct of clinical trials, strong leadership skills, and the confidence of the sponsor and the SC chairperson. The individual members of the DMC are in general chosen with input from the DMC chairperson, approved by the sponsor and the SC. The DMC members should possess the necessary expertise to allow the DMC as a whole to perform all of its functions, including monitoring trial performance, reviewing safety data with an understanding of its relevance to the condition and treatment being studied, and recognizing when the observed outcomes are alarmingly beyond those expected. In most cases, a DMC may have three to five members to handle reasonably complex issues. Its membership is generally recommended in the following:

- Clinician or other scientist preferably in an area related to the condition under study with experience in clinical trial conduct, DMC function, and GCP guidelines to serve as the chairperson. A person with experience, statue, and integrity is preferred.
- Statistician — not associated with the SC, the sponsor, or the DCC, and preferably with prior DMC experience.
- Two or three experts in the conditions and/or treatments under study.
- In certain situations epidemiologist or trial ethicist may also be included.

C. DMC STATISTICAL CONSIDERATIONS

There are two areas of statistical concerns for the DMC. The DMC statistician should have a thorough and in depth knowledge of these issues but all members should have at least an elementary understanding.

1. Statistical "Penalty" for Repeated Testing

Ongoing data monitoring may result in statistical issues with so-called multiple tests/looks of the data. If repeated tests of the data are planned, however, each test can no longer be considered significant at the nominal $\alpha = 0.05$. Rather, the nominal α level at each interim analysis needs to be adjusted downward (the so-called statistical penalty for multiple testing) to preserve the overall Type I error probability. Statistical methodologies have been well developed in this area. Namely, the GSMs (in particular, the error rate spending approach) and the CP approach, as will be discussed in the following sections. Repeated testing of the data can also affect the power of a study, and the sequential design will need to have a sample size larger than the fixed design, if interim analyses are planned.

Safety review by the DMC is less affected by this concern than formal interim analyses. That is, ongoing safety review without endpoint comparisons in order to assess for potential safety concerns is an obligation of the trial. Once a concern is established, a more formal and thorough analysis via the spending of the Type I and/or Type II error rates (α and/or β) may need to be considered.

2. Early Stopping Guidelines

The major purpose of interim safety analysis or formal interim analysis from the DMC perspectives is to allow the DMC to perform its function of recommending to the trial governance body (i.e., the SC and/or sponsor) whether the trial conduct should continue or modify including early stopping. A "stopping guideline" specifies the significance level for observed differences that would warrant consideration of stopping the trial for overwhelming efficacy, futility, or harm. Stopping guidelines should be specified *a priori* in the protocol and agreed upon during the initial meeting of the DMC. The guidelines for the DMC should not be invoked without consideration of other trial data and external trial information that may affect the assumptions used to derive the guidelines originally. The guidelines also are not intended to reflect all potential scenarios that may arise during the trial. The DMC may need to create additional rules or exercise judgment to terminate a trial prior to its scheduled end based on safety or efficacy considerations beyond reasonable doubt. The Coronary Drug Project Research Group[17] asserted: "... decision making in clinical trials is complicated and often protracted. ... no single statistical decision rule or procedure can take the place of well reasoned consideration of all aspects of the data by a group of concerned, competent, and experienced persons with a wide range of scientific backgrounds and points of view."

Relevant references on DMC issues can be found in Fleming and DeMets,[18] Armstrong and Furberg,[19] DeMets et al.,[20] and Guidance for Clinical Trial Sponsors — On the Establishment and Operation of Clinical Trial Data Monitoring Committee.[21] The EMEA also proposed to develop a CPMP Points to Consider on Data Monitoring Committee to provide the EU a consensual viewpoint in a concept paper.[22]

IV. THE ERROR RATE SPENDING FUNCTION APPROACH

As discussed earlier two key issues in interim analysis are of concern. One is bias and the other is the effect on error probabilities. Bias in clinical trials can be minimized via randomization and blinding. It can be dealt with further through vigorous GCP training and strict SOPs execution. The effect on inflation of error probabilities can generally be controlled via sequential methodology. Significant research and development have been advanced in this field during the past three decades. Excellent methodology review literature can be found in DeMets and Lan,[23–25] Hwang,[26] Davis and Hwang,[27] PMA Biostatistics and Medical Ad Hoc Committee on Interim Analysis,[7] Whitehead,[28] Jennison and Turnbull,[29] and Shih.[30] Pocock[1] and O'Brien and Fleming[2] independently introduced an approach referred as "GSMs," which extended the work of repeated significant testing pioneered by Armitage.[31] Lan and DeMets[3] applied the concept of Brownian motion process termed it as "α (error rate) spending" to the GSMs. The error rate spending approach rendered a break-through extension with great flexibility and controls the overall error level while allowing number and timing of analyses unfixed *a priori*.

The essence of GSMs is to control the error probabilities, in particular, the Type I error rate or significance level, α. The error rate spending function allocates a portion of the fixed Type I error probability to each interim analysis based on the fraction of trial information or statistical information (e.g., patients or events) accrued during the trial according to the prespecified shape of the spending function. This trial information fraction is usually termed as the information time $\tau, 0 \leq \tau \leq 1$, which is defined as the amount of trial information accrued at an interim analysis over the total trial information expected at the end of the trial. The α spending must be equal to 0 at $\tau = 0$ and equal to α at $\tau = 1$. We first review some group sequential methodology fundamentals prior to the discussion on the error rate spending functions as follows.

A. THE FUNDAMENTALS

Assume we have i.i.d. random variables $Y_{ij} \sim N(\mu, \sigma^2)$, $i = 1, ..., M$; $j = 1, ..., n_i$, where i indicates stage (i.e., ith interim analysis), j represents patient (i.e., jth patient), and σ^2 is known. The maximum sample size is $N = \sum_{i=1,M} n_i$ ($= Mn$ when $n_i = n, i = 1, ..., M$). Without loss of generality, we plan to perform an M-stage group sequential test of the null hypothesis H_0: $\mu = 0$ vs. H_1: $\mu > 0$. For simplicity we perform a one-sided test in a one-group case. (Note that the between-group comparison can be easily conformed into a one-group case.) We now review the various interim analysis processes as introduced in Lan and Wittes[32] and Lan and Zucker.[33]

1. Partial Sum Process (S-Process)

Let $X_i = \sum_{j=1,n_i} [Y_{ij}/(\sigma\sqrt{n_i})]$, then X_i is also i.i.d. and $X_i \sim N(\Delta, 1)$, $\Delta = \mu\sqrt{n_i}/\sigma$, $i = 1,...,M$.

Now,

$$S_0 = 0, \ S_1 = X_1,...,$$
$$S_i = X_1 + \cdots + X_i,...,$$
$$S_M = X_1 + \cdots + X_i + \cdots + X_M,$$
$$\text{where } S_i = \sum_{k=1,i} X_k \sim N(i\Delta, i), \ i = 1,...,M$$

and the statistic $[(S_i - i\Delta)/\sqrt{i}] \sim N(0, 1)$ and $E(S_i) = i\Delta$, $V(S_i) = i$, and $\text{COV}(S_i, S_j) = \min(i,j)$. Here $\{S_i\}$ is a Partial Sum Process (S-Process) with a noncentrality parameter Δ. $\{S_i\}$ has the following properties:

i. $\{S_i\}$ has independent increments.

$$S_0 = 0, \ S_1 = X_1,$$

$$S_2 = X_1 + X_2 = S_1 + (S_2 - S_1),$$

$$S_3 = (X_1 + X_2) + X_3 = S_2 + (S_3 - S_2),...,$$

$$S_i = (X_1 + X_2 + \cdots + X_{i-1}) + X_i = S_{i-1} + (S_i - S_{i-1}).$$

That is, S_1 and $(S_2 - S_1),..., S_{i-1}$ and $(S_i - S_{i-1}),...,$ and S_{M-1} and $(S_M - S_{M-1})$ are mutually independent and $\{S_i\}$ has independent increments.

ii. $S_{i-1} \sim N((i-1)\Delta, i-1)$, $S_i \sim N(i\Delta, i)$, and $(S_i - S_{i-1}) \sim N(\Delta, 1)$. That is, the increments in $\{S_i\}$ are equal, simply because $i = 1,...,M$ has equal increments.

2. Standardized S-Process (Z-Process)

Let $Z_i = \sum_{k=1,i} X_k/\sqrt{i} = S_i/\sqrt{i}$, then $Z_i \sim N(\sqrt{i}\Delta, 1)$, $i = 1,...,M$ and

$$E(Z_i) = \sqrt{i}\Delta, \ V(Z_i) = 1, \ \text{and} \ \text{COV}(Z_i, Z_j) = \sqrt{(i/j)} \ \text{for } i < j.$$

Now, $\{Z_i\}$ is a Standardized S-Process (Z-Process).

3. Discretized Standard Brownian Motion Process (B-Process)

Let $B_i = S_i/\sqrt{M} = (S_i/\sqrt{i})\sqrt{(i/M)} = Z_i\sqrt{\tau_i}$, then

$$B_i \sim N(\tau_i\theta, \tau_i), \ \tau_i = i/M, i=1,...,M \quad \text{with} \quad \theta = \sqrt{M}\Delta \quad \text{and}$$
$$E(B_i) = \tau_i\theta, \ V(B_i) = \tau_i, \quad \text{and} \quad \text{COV}(B_i, B_j) = \min(\tau_i, \tau_j).$$

Here $\{B_i\} = \{B(\tau_i)\}$, $0 \le \tau_i \le 1$, $i = 1,...,M$ is called a Discretized Standard Brownian Motion Process (B-Process) with a linear drift parameter θ.

Now, $\{B_i\}$ has the following properties:

i. $\{B_i\}$ has independent increments. For example, $B_i = B_{i-1} + (B_i - B_{i-1})$ or $B(\tau_i) = B(\tau_{i-1}) + [B(\tau_i) - B(\tau_{i-1})]$. That is, B_{i-1} and $(B_i - B_{i-1})$ are independent and $\{B_i\}$ has independent increments.

ii. $B_{i-1} \sim N(\tau_{i-1}\theta, \tau_{i-1})$, $B_i \sim N(\tau_i\theta, \tau_i)$, and $(B_i - B_{i-1}) \sim N((\tau_i - \tau_{i-1})\theta, \tau_i - \tau_{i-1})$.

That is, the variance increments in $\{B_i\}$ depend on the information time intervals of $\tau_i - \tau_{i-1}$, $i = 1, ..., M$, which can be equal or unequal, though the increments in $i = 1, ..., M$ are equal. The B-Process, therefore, provides the very much needed flexibility for unequally-spaced interim analyses, which will be discussed further later.

Recall that

$$S_i = \sum_{k=1,i} X_k \sim N(i\Delta, i) \text{ (Partial Sum or S-Value)},$$

$$Z_i = (S_i/\sqrt{i}) \sim N(\sqrt{i}\Delta, 1) \text{ (Z-Value), and}$$

$$B_i = (S_i/\sqrt{M}) = (S_i/\sqrt{i})\sqrt{(i/M)} = (Z_i\sqrt{\tau_i}) \sim N(\tau_i\theta, \tau_i) \text{ (B-Value)},$$

$$\tau_i = i/M; \ i = 1, ..., M \text{ with } \theta = \sqrt{M}\Delta.$$

Hence, we have defined the following processes involved in interim analysis:

$\{S_i\}$ is an S-Process with a noncentrality parameter Δ,
$\{Z_i\}$ is a Z-Process, and
$\{B_i\}$ is a B-Process with a drift parameter $\theta, i = 1, ..., M$.

The relationships are simply

$$S_i = Z_i\sqrt{i},$$

$$Z_i = S_i/\sqrt{i}, \text{ and the B-Value}$$

$$B_i = (S_i/\sqrt{M}) = (Z_i\sqrt{\tau_i}) \sim N(\tau_i\theta, \tau_i), \ \tau_i = i/M; \ i = 1, ..., M \text{ with } \theta = \sqrt{M}\Delta.$$

Now, we can display the interim analysis process in a straightforward group sequential framework as follows:

Group Sequential Analysis

Interim analysis, i	1	$\cdots$	i	$\cdots$	M
Information time, τ_i	τ_1	$\cdots$	τ_i	$\cdots$	$\tau_M = 1$
Z-Value	Z_1	$\cdots$	Z_i	$\cdots$	Z_M
B-Value	B_1	$\cdots$	B_i	$\cdots$	B_M
or	$B(\tau_1)$	$\cdots$	$B(\tau_i)$	$\cdots$	$B(\tau_M)$
Boundary	c_1	$\cdots$	c_i	$\cdots$	c_M

B. GROUP SEQUENTIAL BOUNDARIES

For a one-sided boundary, to control the overall Type I error rate, it requires that

$$P[Z_1 \geq c_1, \quad \text{or} \quad Z_2 \geq c_2, ..., \quad \text{or} \quad Z_i \geq c_i, ..., \quad \text{or} \quad Z_M \geq c_M | H_0]$$
$$= \sum_{i=1,M} P[Z_i \geq c_i; Z_j < c_j, j \leq i - 1 | H_0]$$
$$= \sum_{i=1,M} P[(B_i/\sqrt{\tau_i}) \geq c_i; (B_j/\sqrt{\tau_j}) < c_j, j \leq i - 1 | H_0] = \alpha.$$

That is, the overall boundary crossing probability equals to the prespecified level α. For a two-sided symmetric boundary one simply replaces α by $\alpha/2$ and applies symmetrically. (Discussion for asymmetric boundaries for controlling both Types I and II error rates (α and β) and other approaches will be covered later.) Now, the group sequential tests can be simply summarized as:

- Compute the test statistic (i.e., the Z_i value) at each interim analysis i $(1, ..., M)$, which corresponds to the information time τ_i $(0 < \tau_1, ..., \tau_M = 1)$ based on the accumulated fraction of trial information (interim data) sequentially.
- Compare the test statistic Z_i to a predefined critical value or boundary value c_i such that the overall error probability (α) is maintained.
- Reject the null hypothesis H_0 and stop the trial early if the boundary is crossed. Otherwise, the interim analysis process continues till the final analysis.
- At the final analysis (at the scheduled trial end) either reject the null hypothesis H_0 if $Z_M \geq c_M$ or do not reject H_0 if $Z_M < c_M$.

An *ad hoc* rule, not based on precise theoretical model, was proposed by Haybittle[34] and later by Peto et al.[35] It suggested the use of a two-sided critical values of $c_i = 3.0$ at interim analyses for $i < M$, but retains $c_M = 1.96$ at the final analysis. This *ad hoc* rule may be simple to use for interim analyses, but it does not precisely maintain the prespecified error probabilities. In the following we will review the "one-sided" versions of the original two classical group sequential boundaries:

1. The Pocock Boundary[1]

The Pocock boundary can be formulated via the Z-process as finding the boundary value of $c_i = c$ — a constant value for $i = 1, ..., M$ such that

$$P[Z_1 \geq c, \quad \text{or} \quad Z_2 \geq c, ..., \quad \text{or} \quad Z_i \geq c, ..., \quad \text{or} \quad Z_M \geq c | H_0]$$
$$= \sum_{i=1,M} P[Z_i \geq c; Z_j < c, j \leq i - 1 | H_0] = \alpha.$$

The value of c can be calculated via iterative numerical integration.[36] For example at $\alpha = 0.025$ (one-sided), the constant boundaries of Pocock are

$\{c\} = \{2.178, 2.178\}$, $M = 2$; $\{c\} = \{2.289, 2.289, 2.289\}$, $M = 3$; $\{c\} = \{2.361,$ $2.361, 2.361, 2.361\}$, $M = 4$; and $\{c\} = \{2.413, 2.413, 2.413, 2.413, 2.413\}$, $M = 5$. Note that the Pocock boundaries are equally spaced.

2. The O'Brien–Fleming Boundary[2]

The O'Brien–Fleming boundary, on the other hand, is best formulated via the B-process as finding the boundary value of $c_i = c$ for $i = 1, ..., M$ such that

$$P[B_1 \geq c, \quad \text{or} \quad B_2 \geq c, ..., \quad \text{or} \quad B_i \geq c, ..., \quad \text{or} \quad B_M \geq c | H_0]$$

$$= \sum_{i=1,M} P[B_i \geq c; B_j < c, j \leq i - 1 | H_0] = \alpha.$$

Recall that $B_i = Z_i \sqrt{\tau_i}$ and for $B_i \geq c$ it will be equivalent to have

$$Z_i \geq (c / \sqrt{\tau_i}) = c_i, \quad i = 1, ..., M.$$

Again, via iterative numerical integration the boundaries of O'Brien–Fleming (one-sided) can be calculated at $\alpha = 0.025$ with $c = 1.978$, $\{c_i\} = \{2.797, 1.987\}$, $M = 2$; $c = 2.004$, $\{c_i\} = \{3.471, 2.454, 2.004\}$, $M = 3$; $c = 2.024$, $\{c_i\} = \{4.049, 2.863, 2.338, 2.024\}$, $M = 4$; $c = 2.040$, $\{c_i\} = \{4.562, 3.226, 2.643, 2.281, 2.040\}$, $M = 5$. It should be noted that the original development of the O'Brien–Fleming boundary was not based on the B-Process, but rather the S-Process and therefore, its boundaries are equally spaced.

The interim analyses for the Pocock boundary are performed at the same critical value throughout. Early stopping is possible; however, it pays large penalty for the final analysis, if it was not stopped early. For the O'Brien–Fleming boundary, on the other hand, interim analyses are performed at decreasing critical values. Early stopping is extremely difficult, but only pays little penalty for the final analysis. It should be noted that both the Pocock and O'Brien–Fleming boundaries are based on fixed and "equally spaced" times, i.e., the number and timing of analyses are predefined and cannot be changed. That is, these boundaries require "equal" variance increments or placed in equally spaced information times. At trial design it may be convenient to plan for fixed M analyses at calendar times or equally spaced information times. However, during the course of a trial, changes often occur for both frequency and timing of interim analyses. Actual analyses seldom take place at fixed numbers with equally spaced information times. So a more flexible and practical procedure is needed. The error rate spending approach proposed by Lan and DeMets[3] meets this important requirement well and it has since emerged as the mainstream procedure in group sequential methodology.

C. Error Rate Spending Functions (Lan and DeMets,[3] Hwang et al.,[6] Chang et al.[37])

The concept of the Lan–DeMets error rate spending function was motivated by the continuous boundary crossing probabilities of the B-process. They suggested employing the discretized version to construct sequential boundaries for interim analyses. The α spending function $\alpha(\tau)$ is defined such that $\alpha(\tau = \tau_0 = 0) = 0$ and $\alpha(\tau = \tau_M = 1) = \alpha$. The group sequential boundaries (or critical values) can be determined according to the spending function $\alpha(\tau)$ at the span of interim analyses. The total α or Type I error rate can be spent over the information time $\tau, 0 < \tau \leq 1$ accordingly. Lan and DeMets[38] gave an intuitive discussion on calendar vs. information time in GSMs. In the B-Process the variance $V(B_i) = \tau_i$, where τ_i(information time) $= i/M$, $\sum_{k=1,i} n_k / \sum_{k=1,M} n_k$ (fraction in patients), or $\sum_{k=1,i} e_k / \sum_{k=1,M} e_k$ (fraction in events), $i = 1, \ldots, M$. Note that when τ_i is defined in terms of $\sum_{k=1,i} n_k / \sum_{k=1,M} n_k$ or $\sum_{k=1,i} e_k / \sum_{k=1,M} e_k$ the increments between analyses are independent, but may not necessarily need to be equal. Now, we will show how the error rate spending function approach works as follows.

Recall that

$$P[Z_1 \geq c_1, \quad \text{or} \quad Z_2 \geq c_2, \ldots, \quad \text{or} \quad Z_i \geq c_i, \ldots, \quad \text{or} \quad Z_M \geq c_M | H_0] = \alpha.$$

We can decompose the total rejection region and α based on the interim analyses at information times into increments as

$$P[Z_1 \geq c_1 | H_0] = \alpha(\tau_1) \text{ and } P[Z_1 \geq c_1, \text{ or } Z_2 \geq c_2 | H_0] = \alpha(\tau_2),$$

the increment $P[Z_1 < c_1, Z_2 \geq c_2 | H_0] = \alpha(\tau_2) - \alpha(\tau_1)$ represents the additional α that is spent when the 2nd interim analysis is performed when the boundary was not crossed at the 1st analysis. At the ith analysis

$$P[Z_1 \geq c_1, \quad \text{or} \quad Z_2 \geq c_2, \ldots, \quad \text{or} \quad Z_i \geq c_i | H_0] = \alpha(\tau_i) \text{ and}$$
$$P[Z_1 < c_1, Z_2 < c_2, \ldots, Z_{i-1} < c_{i-1}, Z_i \geq c_i | H_0] = \alpha(\tau_i) - \alpha(\tau_{i-1}).$$

$\alpha(\tau_i) - \alpha(\tau_{i-1})$ represents the additional α that is spent when the ith analysis is performed. The process may stop early when the boundary is crossed or may continue till the final analysis such that

$$P[Z_1 \geq c_1, \text{ or } Z_2 \geq c_2, \ldots, \text{ or } Z_i \geq c_i, \ldots, \text{ or } Z_M \geq c_M | H_0]$$
$$= \sum_{i=1,M} P[Z_i \geq c; Z_j < c, j \leq i - 1 | H_0]$$
$$= \sum_{i=1,M} [\alpha(\tau_i) - \alpha(\tau_{i-1})] = \alpha(\tau_M) = \alpha(1) = \alpha$$

That is, the boundary crossing probability α equals to the sum of all alpha increments spent at interim analyses. For a fixed design, $P[Z_{M=1} \geq c_{M=1} | H_0] = \alpha(\tau_{M=1} = 1) = \alpha$. That is, the total α is spent once all at one analysis at the end of the trial.

TABLE 14.1
Interim Analyses via Equally-Spaced Pocock and O'Brien–Fleming Boundaries

Analysis	i	1	2	3	4	5
Inf. time	τ_i	0.2	0.4	0.6	0.8	1.0
Pocock	c_i	2.413	2.413	2.413	2.413	2.413
	$\alpha(\tau_i) - \alpha(\tau_{i-1})$	0.0079	0.0059	0.0045	0.0036	0.0031
	$\Sigma[\alpha(\tau_i) - \alpha(\tau_{i-1})]$	0.0079	0.0138	0.0183	0.0219	0.025
O'Brien–Fleming	c_i	4.562	3.226	2.634	2.281	2.040
	$\alpha(\tau_i) - \alpha(\tau_{i-1})$	0.0000	0.0006	0.0039	0.0083	0.0122
	$\Sigma[\alpha(\tau_i) - \alpha(\tau_{i-1})]$	0.0000	0.0006	0.0045	0.0128	0.025

To solve for the boundary values c_is, numerical integration of multivariate normal distribution using the method of numerical quadrature is required. Note that in

$$P[Z_1 < c_1, Z_2 < c_2, ..., Z_{i-1} < c_{i-1}, Z_i \geq c_i | H_0] = \alpha(\tau_i) - \alpha(\tau_{i-1}), \ i = 1, ..., M$$

and evaluation of c_is will only depend on $\alpha(\tau_j), j = 1, ..., i$. That is, for $i = 2, ..., M$ only the joint distribution of $(Z_1, Z_2, ..., Z_i)$ is needed for numerical integration. This demonstrates the flexibility of this α spending function approach for interim analysis because there is no requirement for a given M, the total number of analyses, or equally spaced τ_i. All that is needed is $0 = \alpha(\tau_0) < \alpha(\tau_1) < \cdots < \alpha(\tau_M) = \alpha(1) = \alpha$, a strictly increasing function $\alpha(\tau)$, known as the error rate or α spending function, which needs to be prespecified to guide how the α is to be spent over the information time.

Though the equally spaced Pocock and O'Brien–Fleming boundaries were not originally developed via the α spending concept, we can reconstruct their α spending increments, e.g., $M = 5$, $\alpha = 0.025$ (one-sided) shown in Table 14.1 as follows. (The α spending patterns can be found in Figure 14.1.)

Lan and DeMets[3] provided continuous α spending functions approximately for the O'Brien–Fleming and Pocock boundaries, respectively, as

$$\alpha_1^*(\tau) = \alpha_{O'B-F}(\tau) = 2[1 - \Phi(z_{1-\alpha/2}/\sqrt{\tau})] \text{ (one-sided) and}$$
$$\alpha_2^*(\tau) = \alpha_P(\tau) = \alpha \ln[1 + (e - 1)\tau],$$

where $\Phi(\cdot)$ represents the c.d.f. of the standard normal.

A couple of general families of α spending functions have also been proposed in the literature. One is the "power function" spending family $\alpha(\tau) = \alpha\tau^\rho, \rho > 0$ proposed by Lan and DeMets[3] and Kim and DeMets.[39] The other is the

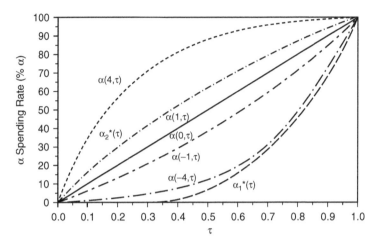

FIGURE 14.1 γ Family of α spending function.

"truncated exponential distribution" or "γ" spending family by Hwang et al.[6]:

$$\alpha(\gamma, \tau) = \begin{cases} \alpha[(1 - e^{-\gamma\tau})/1 - e^{-\gamma})], & \gamma \neq 0 \\ \alpha\tau, & \gamma = 0 \end{cases} \quad \text{for } 0 \leq \tau \leq 1.$$

A few members of the γ family of α spending functions are plotted in Figure 14.1.

Note that many popular boundaries are in fact members of the rich γ family. For example, the continuous Pocock boundary $\alpha_2^*(\tau)$ is virtually identical to $\alpha(1, \tau)$; the continuous O'Brien–Fleming boundary $\alpha_1^*(\tau)$ is also a member of the γ family with approximately $\gamma = -4$ or -5; the power function members $\alpha(\tau) = \alpha\tau^{3/2}$ is closely approximated by $\alpha(-1, \tau)$ and $\alpha(\tau) = \alpha\tau^2$ by $\alpha(-2, \tau)$. Two landmark clinical trials: The "4S"[40,41] and "AFCAPS/TexCAPS"[42] both adopted O'Brien–Fleming-like boundaries based on a member of the γ family, i.e., $\alpha(-4, \tau)$. Both trials were designed as the so-called "total information" trial instead of the traditional "fixed sample size" or "maximum duration" trial. An information-based trial would maintain statistical power regardless of the realized event rate, though in general, study duration may need to be extended, or in some cases the sample size increased.

We will not discuss boundary optimality, because optimality in group sequential designs is usually not well defined. In fact, the choice of boundary is based more on the nature of trial design and clinical judgment than on strict statistical properties. In general, choosing a member (e.g., $1 \leq \gamma \leq 4$) with a concave α spending function will be suitable for trials with immediate response and short patient follow up such as single-dose analgesic studies or for accelerated early stopping in early phase exploratory studies. For large mortality/irreversible morbidity trials where patient recruitment is massive and follow up is long term, the choice of a convex member (e.g., $-5 \leq \gamma \leq -1$) would be appropriate. In situations where greater α is to be preserved for the final analysis, an extremely small γ (e.g., $\gamma = -15$ or even -20) has also been adopted. The power of the group sequential test generally increases with the convexity of the α spending function. A few statistical packages are available commercially for group sequential designs and analysis. (These packages will not be listed or discussed in this manuscript.) Nonetheless, a versatile yet free program is available named LANDEM.[43] This program and its relevant documents are accessible at "www.medsch.wisc.edu/landemets." All these packages have been updated to include the power function and γ families of α spending functions.

A natural extension to the use of flexible Type I error rate spending function approach is to use both Type I (α) and Type II (β) error rate spending functions from Chang et al.[37] in constructing the rejection (upper) and acceptance (lower) boundaries, respectively. A trial can be stopped early for overwhelming efficacy when the upper rejection boundary is crossed. The trial can also be stopped early when the lower acceptance boundary is crossed for futility or harm. The null hypothesis can be either two-sided or one-sided. The boundaries can be symmetric or asymmetric. In practice, the latter makes more clinical sense because there is usually less threshold or tolerance for futility or safety than for efficacy. Emerson and Fleming[44] proposed two-sided symmetric boundaries with equal α and β spending. Pampallona and Tsiatis[45] suggested unequal α and β spending. Chang et al.[37] constructed both symmetric and asymmetric boundaries via the γ family spending functions for unequal α and β spending. For asymmetric boundaries using both α and β spending functions it requires that

$$\sum_{i=1,M} P[Z_i \geq c_i; b_j < Z_j < c_j, j \leq i-1|H_0] = \alpha \text{ and}$$

$$\sum_{i=1,M} P[Z_i \leq b_i; b_j < Z_j < c_j, j \leq i-1|H_a] = \beta,$$

where $c_i > b_i$, $i = 1,...,M-1$; $c_M = b_M$. Symmetric boundaries can easily be constructed by imposing absolute values on Z_i (i.e., $|Z_i|$) and have $|c_i| > |b_i|$, $i = 1,...,M-1$; $|c_M| = |b_M|$.

It should be noted that before employing the α and β spending functions to construct group sequential boundaries, the following conditions must be fully understood:

(i) The upper and lower boundaries depend on both H_0 and H_a specified *a priori* in the protocol. This set of boundaries should *not* be changed after interim analyses. Otherwise, it will cause inconsistency between the use of the sequential boundary and the actual recommendation of the DMC to the sponsor on early termination.

(ii) The lower boundary, if crossed, should *not* be overruled.

For further discussion on overruling of the group sequential boundary, refer to Lan et al.[46]

Futility analyses (i.e., accepting the null hypothesis of no treatment difference) can also be conducted at interim analyses using CP (stochastic curtailment) methodology.[32,47] The CP approach will be discussed in essence later in Section V.

It should be emphasized that in constructing boundaries via the error rate spending function approach there is no requirement to predefine M, the total number of analyses. However, for design purpose some number M and an alpha spending function must be prespecified. Both frequency and timing of analyses can be changed as trial proceeds forward. The analyses can be unequally-spaced in information time and boundaries can be reconstructed based on the prespecified error rate spending function. The error rate spending over the information time cannot be changed during the trial, but frequency and timing can be changed based on recent results and the impact on the overall error level is generally very small. Accurate estimation of the total information is necessary to maintain power. The γ family of error rate spending functions is versatile and it generalizes the well-known boundaries.

D. Applications

The GSMs are well developed. Although the Lan–DeMets error rate spending approach provides the flexibility in group sequential design and analysis, at study design it does require that the number and times of analyses and how the error rate is to be spent (i.e., the error rate spending function) be prespecified. Once the group sequential boundary and the sample size based on the trial design are established and the trial proceeds forward, the frequency and timing of the interim analyses may be changed as practice dictates without significant impact on the overall error rate. In design and analysis applications via the error rate spending approach one can compare means, proportions, survival curves, repeated measures, and multiple endpoints, etc., in performing repeated hypothesis tests. We will provide a general review on some of these applications in this chapter. For specific and/or detailed discussions one can refer to Kim and DeMets,[39] Pocock et al.,[48] Lan and Lachin,[49] Lee and DeMets,[50] Wu and Lan,[51] Lan and Zucker,[33] Lan et al.,[52] DeMets and Lan,[25] Jennison and Turnbull,[29] Reboussin et al.,[43] and Shih,[30] to name just a few.

Classical GSMs[1,2] were developed based on a partial sum process with independent increments on immediate response, either continuous or dichotomous. Tsiatis[53,54] and others showed that the logrank statistic (as well as a general class of linear rank statistics) computed sequentially behave (asymptotically) like a partial sum of independent normal random variables. Lan and DeMets[3] introduced the error rate spending concept via the Brownian motion process. Lan and Wittes[32] and Lan and Zucker[33] further demonstrated that the S-Process (partial sum process) can be mapped into the B-Process (Brownian motion process). Jennison and Turnbull[55] later ratified the theory that explains the independent increments structure in group sequential test statistics. Scharfstein et al.[56] further demonstrated that sequential Wald statistics behave asymptotic multivariate normal. All these advances extend the GSMs to more complicated cases in survival analysis models and correlated observations including repeated measures in longitudinal data analysis.

In general, group sequential design and analysis can proceed as follows.

1. First determine the total number of planned interim analyses M and the times of the analyses in information time. The trial information can be patient, event or other surrogate depending on the nature of the trial and the increments can be either equal or unequal pending preference in practice.

2. Choose a specific error rate spending function and generate the group sequential boundary accordingly for the M interim analyses at the predefined times in information time under the null hypothesis H_0 to maintain a prespecified overall α error level. One-sided, two-sided, symmetric, or asymmetric boundaries can be generated based on the chosen error rate spending function(s), to maintain the overall α level or the overall α and β levels as appropriate.

3. Under the alternative hypothesis H_a and the sequential boundary generated, obtain the value of Δ (the expected value of the test statistic under H_a) to achieve a desired power $1 - \beta$.

4. Determine the values of n (assume $n_i = n$, $i = 1, ..., M$ for equal increments) or n_i, $i = 1, ..., M$ (unequal increments) that determines the total sample size $N = Mn$ or $N = \sum_{1,M} n_i$. Note that the information time is $\tau_i = i/M$ or $i(n/N)$ for equal increments or $\tau_i = \sum_{1,i} n_k/N$ for unequal increments, $i = 1, ..., M$ with $\tau_0 = 0$, $\tau_1 > 0$, and $\tau_M = 1$. It has been shown that the sequential methods developed for the comparison of the means are also applicable to the survival distribution comparisons. However, the concept of trial information needs some modification, because it corresponds to the variance of the linear rank statistics and has different interpretations for different tests. We use the logrank test for illustration. In general, for survival analysis or event-based trial, sample size in number of patients alone is not enough to reflect the trial information, one must further determine the total expected number of events (e.g., deaths). When survival data are compared the corresponding information fraction is $\tau_i = \sum_{k=1,i} e_k / \sum_{k=1,M} e_k$, $i = 1, ..., M$. The number in the numerator is the expected number of events at τ_i, while the number in the denominator is the total expected number of events for the whole trial. Because the expected number of events at τ_i is not observable, we usually use the observed number of events as the substitute in practice. In general, there is no simple interpretation of trial information for the Wilcoxon test. Nonetheless, when event rate is low the information fraction for the logrank test provides a good approximation. Further discussions can be found in Lan et al.[57]

5. Perform the scheduled interim analysis at τ_i, $i = 1, ..., M$. At time τ_i compare the computed test statistic to the group sequential boundary value.

Reject the null hypothesis H_0 and recommend early trial stopping if the boundary is crossed. Otherwise, the interim analysis process continues till the final analysis. At the final analysis either reject or do not reject the null hypothesis H_0 pending whether the final test statistic exceeds the final boundary value.

1. An Example

We give herein a brief description of the use of the γ-family of α spending functions in planning interim analysis and early stopping guidelines with a landmark trial — the 4S.[40] Some preliminary discussion on interim analysis and group sequential boundary was also given by Hwang et al.[6] The final study results were published in the Lancet.[41]

Briefly, the 4S was a multicenter, randomized, triple-blind, placebo-controlled trial, conducted in Scandinavia, to confirm the efficacy of simvastatin (a statin-HMG CoA Reductase inhibitor) in secondary prevention of total mortality of all causes in patients with ischemic heart disease and hypercholesterolemia. The total sample size planned was approximately 4000 patients to provide a 95% power at $\alpha = 0.05$ (two-sided). The estimated total trial information was 380 deaths. Three analyses ($M = 3$; two interims and one final) were planned at unequal information times ($\tau_1 = 0.50$, 190 deaths; $\tau_2 = 0.80$, 300 deaths; $\tau_3 = 1.00$, 380 deaths). The corresponding group sequential boundary was $\{2.753, 2.343, 2.020\}$, an O'Brien–Fleming-like boundary constructed by using the α spending function $\alpha\,(-4, \tau)$ of the γ family. 4444 patients were randomized at 94 centers in Scandinavia between May 1988 and August 1989. At the very first DMC (was actually named DSMC for the 4S) meeting prior to the first scheduled interim analysis, the DMC requested that an additional interim analysis be conducted at 100 deaths to ascertain that smivastatin treatment would not render harm in early stages of the trial. Accordingly, 4444 patients were actually randomized and the trial information was reestimated to be approximately 440 deaths and the total number of analyses was revised to four ($M = 4$; three interims and one final). The 4S was then planned as a minimum of one-year recruitment period and a three-year follow up period on the last randomized patient or the total trial information of 440 deaths were reached, whichever came last. The revised plan for analyses were again at unequal information times ($\tau_1 = 0.23$, 100 deaths; $\tau_2 = 0.46$, 200 deaths; $\tau_3 = 0.80$, 350 deaths; and $\tau_4 = 1.00$, 440 deaths). The group sequential boundary was revised to $\{3.200, 2.885, 2.341, 2.022\}$ based on the predefined $\alpha(-4, \tau)$ spending function.

Having examined the 3rd interim analysis results thoroughly, the DMC (May 27, 1994) advised that the 4S should be stopped as soon as possible because of overwhelming efficacy in primary endpoint as evidenced in boundary crossing. After careful consultation with the SC chairman, August 1, 1994 was chosen as the cutoff date at which it was anticipated approximately that the protocol-specified total trial information target of 440 deaths would be reached. Highly significant results were observed for both the primary endpoint — total mortality (hazard ratio — simvastatin to placebo: HR = 0.70, $p = .0003$) and secondary endpoints (e.g., major coronary events: HR = 0.66, $p = .00001$; any coronary events: HR = 0.74, $p = .00001$).

The error rate spending function approach indeed provided the flexibility in revising the interim plan and early stopping guidelines as needed for the 4S while the trial was ongoing. Most importantly, the DMC of the 4S was able to perform its chartered duty and maintained not only the high ethics, but also the total integrity of the landmark trial.

There are also other developments in GSMs such as repeated confidence intervals and sequential estimation following stopping that are worth noting as follows.

Jennison and Turnbull[58] developed a repeated confidence interval (RCI) approach in the group sequential setting. Simply, the RCIs can be constructed by inverting the group sequential tests into a sequence of confidence intervals $[\mu_{Li}, \mu_{Ui}]$, $i = 1,...,M$ such that the overall coverage probability for the unknown μ is $1 - \alpha$. In inverting the RCIs the same boundary or critical values c_is for repeated hypothesis tests are used. The uses of the RCI and hypothesis testing approaches will yield the same conclusion regarding the null hypothesis H_0: $\mu = 0$. However, the RCIs provide more information. The error rate spending approach application to the RCI approach has the same advantages as in group sequential testing in that either the timing or the number of interim analyses via the RCIs can be flexible. Similarly, the total expected information must be determined for the design and used to calculate the information fraction for a prespecified error rate spending function. The RCIs are especially useful for group sequential equivalence trials that are designed to test whether two treatments have an effect within a specified equivalence margin and thus can be considered interchangeable.

Once a trial is stopped or completed, one would like to estimate the treatment effect. Hughes and Pocock[59] pointed out that clinical trials that stopped early are prone to overestimate the true treatment effect. In fact, the naïve estimates are biased after a sequential trial has been stopped and appropriate adjustments are needed. Different proposals[60–63] have been made to construct confidence intervals with correct coverage probability following a group sequential design. These proposals suggest different ways to order the sample space for sequential trials and none is considered universally superior. Hughes and Pocock[58] proposed a Bayesian "shrinkage" approach, which would require the choice of an appropriate prior distribution. (The Bayesian approach is beyond the scope of this discussion.)

One particular issue of interest is what to do when the group sequential boundary is crossed, but the independent DMC decides for some compelling reasons (e.g., to gain extended patient experience on safety and/or efficacy) that the trial should continue. One simple and straightforward approach[64] is to recapture the already spent α and redistribute it over the remainders of the trial.

Overall, the error rate spending function approach generalizes the classic GSMs, which provides not only the control of error probabilities, but also the flexibility in performing interim analyses in practice. The traditional GSMs have been primarily focused on early termination of a trial, for ethical and/or economic reasons. Recently, considerable interest has also been placed in possibly extending a trial beyond its originally planned sample size and/or duration, based on findings of interim data. It also includes converting a fixed design into a sequential trial. These important topics will be reviewed in the following sections, in particular, in the discussions of CP and adaptive design.

V. THE CONDITIONAL POWER (CP) APPROACH

Next, we will discuss the CP approach, which also has made major impact on design and conduct of clinical trials for the past two decades.

A. CURTAILMENT VS. STOCHASTIC CURTAILMENT

The method of curtailment was used often in sampling plans.[65] In a simple sampling plan, a fixed number N items of a batch are inspected, and if n ($< N$) or more items are found defective, the batch will be rejected. This process can be curtailed if n items are found defective before all N items have been examined. However, it is important to note that this curtailment can be made only for the purpose of rejection or acceptance. To estimate the probability of an item being defective, curtailment may cause bias and reduction of information.

A similar idea can be applied to hypothesis testing. For example, to test whether a coin is bias, we may conduct an experiment of tossing the coin 400 times. The test statistic is

$$Z = (H - 200)/\sqrt{(400 \times 0.5 \times 0.5)},$$

where H = the total number of heads. If we choose a two-sided α-level of 0.05, we may reject the null hypothesis that the coin is unbiased, if $|Z| \geq 1.96$, or $|H\text{-}200| \geq 20$. Now, suppose after flipping the coin 350 times and having observed 220 heads, we can predict for sure that $H \geq 220$. For the purpose of hypothesis testing, the experiment can then be curtailed. In clinical trials, curtailment rarely occurs. By the time the final decision can be predicted with certainty, it is close to the end of the trial, and people involved in the trial usually choose to finish it. Instead, a modification of curtailment, called stochastic curtailment or the use of CP, is the subject of interest.

As discussed in previous sections that before the GSMs were introduced in the 1970s, data were monitored periodically in many NIH-sponsored clinical trials, even if the study was a fixed design. In many of those long-term clinical trials, the concept of CP was found to be a helpful statistical tool to answer questions raised by the clinicians. CP is the probability, conditional on the accrued data that the final Z-value will fall into the rejection or acceptance region. If the final outcome of a trial can be predicted with a high probability (i.e., if the CP is very high or very low), perhaps the trial should be terminated early.

Even in preclinical studies, the concept of CP was often discussed during the course of an experiment. For example, when a NIH intramural scientist requests for 100 rats to evaluate a new compound, the Animal Use Committee may grant only 50. Another 50 will be granted, if the results from the first 50 rats are "promising." Here, "promising" can be translated loosely as "if the trend of the data continues, the probability of obtaining a positive result is high."

Conceptually, simulations can be used to evaluate CP even under fairly complicated settings. However, in many practical situations, CP can be computed easily if the underlying statistic follows the Brownian motion process. To simplify our discussion, again, we follow the B-value approach of Lan and Wittes[32] and start with the simplest one-sample case for one-sided hypothesis testing. This statistical framework can be generalized to many more complex settings for two-sample comparisons in clinical trials, as discussed in the previous section.

Now, let us first assume that we have extensive experience with a standard treatment, and the distribution of the patients' responses, after standardization, are known to be normal with zero mean and unit variance. A new test treatment is being tested for benefit. Denote the response of a new test treatment group patient by $X \sim N(\mu, 1)$. Assume that a larger response is a better outcome, so the hypothesis being considered is

$$H_0 : \mu = 0 \text{ vs. } H_a : \mu = \mu_0 > 0;$$

and the test statistic is

$$Z = (X_1 + X_2 + \cdots + X_N)/\sqrt{N}.$$

If $\alpha = 0.025$, the rejection region is $Z \geq 1.96$. Suppose the anticipated treatment effect is $\mu = \mu_0 > 0$, then under this simple alternative,

$$E(Z) = \theta = N\mu_0/\sqrt{N} = \sqrt{N}\mu_0.$$

To reach a power of, say, 85% for this given treatment effect, the sample size required is obtained by solving the equation

$$E(Z) = \sqrt{N}\mu_0 = z_\alpha + z_\beta = 1.96 + 1.04 = 3.0.$$

Note that for this choice of sample size N, the power is 85% only if the treatment effect is indeed $\mu = \mu_0$ as stated in the protocol. The "real power" depends on the real treatment effect μ, which is unfortunately "unknown."

After n observations ($n < N$) are made, the interim Z-value, $Z_n = \sum_{1,n} X_i/\sqrt{n}$, provides us some information for projecting the behavior of Z_N. Unconditionally, the expected value of Z_n is $\mu_0\sqrt{n}$, which increases with n along a square root trend. If Z_n is greater (less) than $\mu_0\sqrt{n}$, then the "observed treatment effect ($\bar{X}$)" will be greater (less) than μ_0. Obviously, a linear trend is a lot easier to deal with, and a square root trend can be converted to a linear trend by multiplying another square root of the time parameter. This will be the motivation for introducing the B-value again as follows.

Following the decomposition suggested by Lan and Wittes,[32] we rewrite

$$Z_N = \sqrt{(n/N)} \cdot \left(\sum_{1,n} X_i/\sqrt{n} \right) + \left(\sum_{n+1,N} X_i/\sqrt{N} \right) = \sqrt{\tau} Z_n + \left(\sum_{n+1,N} X_i/\sqrt{N} \right).$$

If we define information time $\tau = n/N$ ($0 \le \tau \le 1$), and rewrite Z_n as Z_τ and $B_\tau = Z_\tau \sqrt{\tau}$ (note that to simplify the presentation, the symbols and expressions used for the B-values herein are slightly different from those shown in the previous section), then $Z_N = Z_1 = B_1$ at $\tau = 1$ and the above expression becomes

$$Z_1 = B_1 = B_\tau + (B_1 - B_\tau).$$

Once again, three important properties of this decomposition are listed below:

(i) B_τ and $B_1 - B_\tau$ are normal and independent.
(ii) $E(B_\tau) = \tau\theta$ and $E(B_1 - B_\tau) = (1 - \tau)\theta$.
(iii) $V(B_\tau) = \tau$ and $V(B_1 - B_\tau) = 1 - \tau$.

These are the basic properties of a Brownian motion process with a linear drift θ. (For the serious readers, refer to the excellent textbook by Siegmund[66] for details.) Note that during the interim analysis, because $X_1, X_2, ..., X_n$ are fixed, Z_τ and B_τ are also fixed. Only the future observations $X_{n+1}, ..., X_N$ are random. Therefore, part of the $(100 \times \tau\%)$ variation of Z_1 is fixed, and the unconditional variance $V(Z_1) = 1$ is reduced to a conditional variance of $V_C(Z_1) = 1 - \tau$ according to (iii) above. Similarly, because B_τ is fixed, (ii) implies that the conditional mean $E_C(Z_1) = B_\tau + E(B_1 - B_\tau) = B_\tau + \theta(1 - \tau)$. Note that the value of $E_C(Z_1)$ depends on $\theta = \mu\sqrt{N}$, which contains the unknown treatment effect μ as a factor. A graphic explanation of this approach to an interim analysis is given in the example below.

Example 1. (The reader should refer to Figure 14.2 while reading the example.)
Consider a study with $\mu_0 = 0.2$. If the desired power is 85%, then solve for N from $0.2 \times \sqrt{N} = 3 \Rightarrow N = 225$. Assume interim data were analyzed at $n = 90$ with a Z-value of 2.864, then the information time $\tau = 90/225 = 0.4$ and $Z_{0.4} = 2.864$, a very encouraging result. The corresponding B-value is $B_{0.4} = 2.864 \times \sqrt{0.4} = 1.8$.
This trial starts at $(\tau = 0, B_{\tau=0}) = (0, 0)$, and the interim position is $(\tau, B_\tau) = (0.4, 1.8)$ at $\tau = 0.4$. From this point on, the trend of the data depends on the unknown parameter θ. Let us consider three relevant trends:

(i) The hypothetical trend $\theta = 3$. This one assumes that the treatment effect $\mu = \mu_0 = 0.2$ as assumed and stated in the protocol. During the design stage, we expect the B-value goes up along the straight line with slope $= 3$, and reaches $B_1 = Z_1 = 3$ at the end of the study ($\tau = 1$).

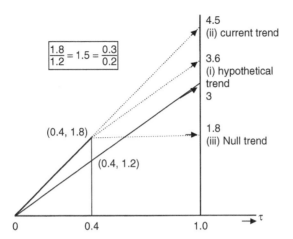

FIGURE 14.2 Example of trends.

The expected value of B_τ at $\tau = 0.4$ is $3 \times 0.4 = 1.2$. Currently, we take an interim look and observed $B_\tau = B_{0.4} = 1.8$, which is 50% greater than 1.2. This indicates that the observed treatment effect $\bar{x}$ is 50% greater than the hypothetical treatment effect μ_0 stated in the protocol (i.e., 0.3 vs. 0.2). Note that our current position at $(0.4, 1.8)$ is fixed. From this point on, the trend of the data depends on the true value of $\theta = \sqrt{N}\mu$. Under $\mu = \mu_0$, $\theta = 3$ and the future B-values will move along a line with slope $= 3$, or, parallel to the line starting at $(0, 0)$ heading toward $(1, 3)$. At the end of the trial $(\tau = 1)$, we expect the final Z-value to be $E_C(Z_1) = 1.8 + 0.6 \times 3 = 3.6$, i.e., at an expected position $(1, 3.6)$.

(ii) Similarly, under the current trend of $\theta = 4.5$, $E_C(Z_1) = 1.8 + 0.6 \times 4.5 = 4.5$.

(iii) Under the null trend $\theta = 0$, $E_C(Z_1) = 1.8 + 0 = 1.8$.

Once the conditional mean and variance are determined, the evaluation of CP is straightforward.

(i) $P[Z_1 = B_1 \geq 1.96 | B_{.4} = 1.8,\ \theta = 3]$

$$= P\left[\frac{B_1 - 3.6}{\sqrt{.6}} \geq \frac{1.96 - 3.6}{\sqrt{.6}} \Big| B_{.4} = 1.8,\ \theta = 3\right]$$

$$= P[N(0, 1) \geq -2.12] = 0.9830$$

(ii) $P[Z_1 = B_1 \geq 1.96 | B_{.4} = 1.8,\ \theta = 4.5]$

$$= P\left[\frac{B_1 - 4.5}{\sqrt{.6}} \geq \frac{1.96 - 4.5}{\sqrt{.6}} \Big| B_{.4} = 1.8,\ \theta = 4.5\right]$$

$$= P[N(0, 1) \geq -3.28] = 0.9995$$

(iii) $P[Z_1 = B_1 \geq 1.96 | B_{.4} = 1.8, \theta = 0] = P\left[N(0,1) \geq \dfrac{1.96 - 1.8}{\sqrt{.6}}\right]$

$= P[N(0,1) \geq 0.21] = 0.4168$

For given B_τ at the interim information time τ and the linear drift (trend) parameter θ, the above computations for the CP that $Z_1 = B_1 \geq c$ can be summarized by the following equation:

$$CP = P[B_1 \geq c | B_\tau; \theta] = P\left[\frac{B_1 - B_\tau - (1 - \tau)\theta}{\sqrt{1 - \tau}} \geq \frac{c - B_\tau - (1 - \tau)\theta}{\sqrt{1 - \tau}} | B_\tau; \theta\right]$$

$$= \Phi\left[\frac{B_\tau + (1 - \tau)\theta - c}{\sqrt{1 - \tau}}\right]. \tag{14.1}$$

B. EFFECT ON TYPE I ERROR RATE

Even though the use of CP as a statistical tool in interim analysis is very natural, it may affect the α-level and the power of the trial. We only present this effect on the α-level. (The effect on the power will be similar.) Note that α is evaluated under the null hypothesis, and therefore, to evaluate the effect of stochastic curtailment on α, we need to evaluate CP at $\theta = 0$. Consider the simple case with only one interim analysis at $\tau = 0.5$ taken, and the DMC decides to stop early and claim beneficial effect of the new treatment if:

$P[Z_1 \geq 1.96 | Z_{\tau=0.5}, \theta = 0] \geq \gamma = 0.8$ or applying Eq. (14.1) above, $Z_{0.5} \geq 3.61$.

Note that the rejection region for the fixed design is $\{Z_1 \geq 1.96\}$. With the stopping potential during interim analysis at information time $\tau = 0.5$, the rejection region becomes $\{Z_{0.5} \geq 3.61$ or $Z_1 \geq 1.96\}$. It is obvious that the α-level will be inflated to a value greater than 0.025. For this specific example, the α-level is 0.02502 — the inflation is almost negligible.

More generally, we may take interim analysis more than once, and it helps to explore its impact on the inflation of α. Let us consider the case where M interim analyses were performed at $\tau = 1/M, ..., M/M = 1$, and conclude that the treatment is better, if at any interim analysis,

$P[Z_1 \geq 1.96 | Z_\tau, \theta = 0] \geq \gamma$ for some prespecified γ (say 0.8) $> \alpha = 0.025$.

The effect of stochastic curtailment on the probability of Type I error for $\gamma = 0.8$ is shown in Table 14.2.

The final row gives the upper bound of the α inflation. The proof of this upper bound can be found in Lan et al.[4]

In practice, a few interim analyses on accumulating data via stochastic curtailment the inflation on α is relatively small. However, most people

TABLE 14.2
Stochastic Curtailment on Type I Error Rate

M	Type I Error Rate (α)
1	0.0250
5	0.0255
8	0.0259
12	0.0263
...	...
$\rightarrow \infty$	$\rightarrow \alpha/\gamma = 0.0250/0.8 = 0.03125$

feel uncomfortable with any α inflation, and stochastic curtailment is rather conservative for early termination and therefore, is rarely used to stop a trial early for benefit. (It may sometimes be used in corroboration with the group sequential boundary described earlier.) Let us consider this α inflation from another point of view, and try to find a remedy in practice to maintain the α-level. Try to imagine 0.025 is the amount of Type I error probability allowed to be spent for the entire trial. For a fixed design, we plan to spend all the $\alpha = 0.025$ at the end of the study ($\tau = 1$). To allow for early termination for benefit, we increase the chance of committing a Type I error, or, spend additional α during interim analyses. Therefore, to allow for early termination and maintain the same $\alpha = 0.025$, it is natural to plan on spending the total amount of 0.025 during the course of the study. This idea has already been elaborated in the previous section on the GSMs and α spending function approach. It should be noted that CP is used mostly for early termination of a trial for futility, though recently it has been often applied in sample size reestimation (SSR).

C. Two-Sample Comparisons

The idea of B-value introduced for the one-sample case can be extended to various two-sample comparisons. Let us consider some cases where the method applies.

1. Comparisons of Two Means

Let us assume that the response from a test treatment group patient $X \sim N(\mu_X, \sigma^2)$ and the response from a control treatment group patient $Y \sim N(\mu_Y, \sigma^2)$. We are interested in testing

$$H_0 : \mu_X = \mu_Y \text{ vs. } H_a : \mu_X > \mu_Y.$$

Assume the target sample size is N and there will be $(N/2)$ patients equally randomized to each of the new treatment and standard treatment groups, and σ is known. In practice, σ is replaced by the sample standard deviation. The test statistic in this case is simply

$$Z = \frac{\bar{X} - \bar{Y}}{\sigma\sqrt{1/M + 1/M}} = \frac{\bar{X} - \bar{Y}}{\sigma\sqrt{N/4}} \text{ and}$$

$$EZ = \frac{\mu_X - \mu_Y}{\sigma}\sqrt{N}\sqrt{\frac{1}{2} \times \frac{1}{2}} = \Delta\sqrt{N}\sqrt{\frac{1}{2} \times \frac{1}{2}}.$$

The first factor Δ is sometimes called "Cohen's delta" — a standardized treatment effect. In fact, it is simply the anticipated treatment difference expressed in units of standard deviations. Inside the square roots, the first factor N is the total sample size, and the second factor $(1/2) \times (1/2)$ is the two-sample factor indicating that the patients are equally allocated to the new test and standard treatment groups. For a "1:2" allocation of patients, the two-sample factor will become $(1/3) \times (2/3) = 2/9$.

To evaluate the sample size for given α, β and Δ, solve for N from the equation

$$E(Z) = \Delta\sqrt{N}\sqrt{(1/2 \cdot 1/2)} = \Delta\sqrt{(N/4)} = z_\alpha + z_\beta.$$

During interim with n combined observations, $\tau \approx n/N$. This approximation formula is very accurate in practice, assuming the randomization allocates about the same number of patients into each group. A rigorous definition of τ can be found in Lan and Zucker[33] and Lan et al.[52]

2. Comparison of Two Survival Distributions

Denote the hazard functions as λ_T and λ_C, respectively, for the new test and the standard control treatment groups. Under the proportion hazards assumption, $\lambda_c/\lambda_t = HR$ is a constant over follow up time. Under this framework,

$$E(Z_{\text{logrank}}) = \ln(\lambda_c/\lambda_t)\sqrt{(D/4)} = \Delta\sqrt{(D/4)},$$

where D is the expected number of events (e.g., deaths) in the trial. To evaluate the sample size N for given α, β, and Δ, we first solve for D from the equation

$$E(Z) = \ln(\lambda_c/\lambda_t)\sqrt{(D/4)} = z_\alpha + z_\beta.$$

Randomize N patients into the study and follow them until D events are observed. Note the equation above is similar to that for the comparison of two means. The treatment effect Δ is replaced by $\ln(\lambda_c/\lambda_t)$ and N is replaced by D, the expected number of events in the study.

Example 2. The Beta-Blocker Heart Attack Trial (BHAT)[67,68] was a randomized trial sponsored by the National Heart, Lung, and Blood Institute (NHLBI). The trial compared propranolol (a β-blocker) with placebo in 3,837 patients and the primary endpoint was total mortality of all causes. On October 2, 1981,

BHAT was terminated 9 months earlier than scheduled because of an observed benefit of propranonol. Right before the final DMC meeting, the observed number of events was $d = 318$, and the final number of events was estimated to be $D = 398$. The information time for the DMC meeting was $\tau = 318/398 = 0.8$, with $Z_{0.8}(\text{logrank}) = 2.82$ and a B-value $B_{0.8} = 2.82 \times \sqrt{0.8} = 2.52$. If the proportional hazards assumption was valid, then:

(a) Under the current trend, $E_C(Z_1) = 3.15$ and CP $= 99.61\%$.
(b) Under the null trend, $E_C(Z_1) = 2.52$ and CP $= 89.44\%$.

3. Comparison of Two Proportions

Same as in the case of two means, except that the Xs are Bernoulli (p_X) and the Ys are Bernoulli (p_Y). The role of σ is replaced by $p(1 - p)$. Again, during interim analysis with n combined observations, $\tau \approx n/N$.

a. Bayesian Intuition

Note that during interim analysis, the CP depends on the unknown value of the treatment effect, θ, which determines the distribution of future observations.

During the DMC meetings, the DCC may present CP(θ) for a spectrum of values of θ. The DMC members then use this information to determine whether the trial should be terminated early. A Bayesian approach would use the predictive probability[69] — a weighted average of CP(θ) by the posterior distribution of θ — for consideration of early termination. In practice, we have found that this Bayesian approach has been applied frequently in some informal way.[70] First, the DMC members have different scientific backgrounds, and each member uses his/her own prior distribution, which may not be the same for all the members. Second, these members may have different exposure to the new test treatment. Note that the clinicians on the board are experts in the therapeutic areas being studied; they may have access to external information about the new treatment, which they may not be allowed to share with other members of the DMC. Finally, when a DMC member gathers all the information available, the member probably may not formally derive a predictive power, but may derive some intuitive value, and therefore, the somewhat Bayesian decision may well be reflected in the vote on early termination.

To control the α-level, CP should be evaluated at $\theta = 0$. If CP(0) is high, then the use of CP to stop early for benefit will only inflate the α-level slightly. This special aspect is only a small part of the CP consideration during the discussion in the DMC meetings. The informal Bayesian modification as described above and other medical considerations frequently carry much more weight than the control of the α-level in the early stopping decision process.

D. SAMPLE SIZE REESTIMATION (SSR)

The CP approach can be easily extended to modify the sample size in midcourse of a trial when the treatment effect size Δ is estimated from the interim data. If the CP is used to stop a trial early to claim futility, the α-level will be reduced. This reduction can be used to compensate for the inflation of the α-level caused by the modification of the sample size during the trial.

Now, consider a design with an interim analysis where the data are analyzed at the information time τ, use the sample estimates for μ_x, μ_y, and σ (in a simple case of comparison of two means) to evaluate the CP under the current trend and apply the following rules:

1. If CP $\leq \gamma_L$ (lower limit), stop the trial and accept H_0.
2. If CP $\geq \gamma_U$ (upper limit), continue to the scheduled end of the trial and reject H_0 if the final $Z \geq z_\alpha$.
3. If $\gamma_L < $ CP $< \gamma_U$, then reestimated the sample size to mN ($m > 1$) and extend the trial so that CP_{mN} (the CP under the current trend after trial extension to mN patients) $= \gamma_U$. Reject H_0 if the final $Z \geq z_\alpha$.

A simulation study by Lan and Trost[71] demonstrated that under very general conditions, the Type I error rate can be preserved.

VI. ADAPTIVE DESIGN

What is "adaptive design"? Simply, adaptive design is used loosely to capture the entire process of taking an interim look/analysis at the accumulating data of an ongoing clinical trial, then modify aspects of the trial design, conduct, and/or analysis in midstream of the trial based on feedback or learning from the interim results. This allows one to improve expected trial outcomes during the experiment, while still being able to carry out GCP and reach good statistical decisions in a timely fashion. Therefore, adaptive design sometimes can offer significant ethical and cost advantages over standard fixed design. Historically, there has not been enough statistical research to support the need for an adaptive design in clinical trials. The major concern lies in that potential bias may be introduced by a midcourse change in clinical practice resulting from the interim analysis. Nonetheless, the bias can be minimized and the integrity of the trial can be preserved when dissemination of the unblinded interim results is restricted and is on a "need to know" basis. That is, the interim results should not be made available to those directly involved in the operations of the trial (e.g., investigators, monitors, and some key clinical project members).

Undoubtedly, adaptive design and interim analysis are closely related. Via interim analysis the adaptive design injects appropriate midstream trial design and conduct modifications (see Whitehead et al.,[72] Hwang,[73] Wittes,[74]). These may involve the following, for example:

- Fine tune patient entry (inclusion/exclusion) criteria.
- Switch trial objectives and/or change trial endpoints.
- Extend a trial in upward sample size adjustment (SSR) or trial duration.
- Drop treatment groups/arms and reallocate patients.
- Stop trial early for overwhelming efficacy, futility, or harm.
- Select doses.
- Modify analytic methods.

Any adaptive design features should be defined in the protocol *a priori* closely in junction with the interim analysis plan. Adaptive design can be grossly classified into two categories: Interim adaptation and stagewise adaptation. We will briefly review these designs without technical details as follows.

A. INTERIM ADAPTATION

This class of adaptive designs involves the use of an internal pilot[74–77] or an interim analysis to evaluate accumulating data in midstream using GSMs, CP, or combination. (Because both the GSMs via error rate spending and CP approaches were discussed extensively in Sections IV and V, no further discussion will be given herein.) The data of the internal pilot or interim analysis are considered as an integral part of the accumulating data of the trial. At conclusion of the trial all data are pooled for analysis as a whole. Internal adaptation is applicable to both early phase exploratory as well as late phase confirmatory trials with more use in the latter. In particular, extensive work has been engaged by many authors in sample size reestimation and/or trial extension (Gould,[78] Gould and Shih,[79] Herson and Wittes,[80] Proschan and Hunsberger,[81] Shih and Gould,[82] Lan and Trost,[71] Cui et al.,[83] Gould,[84] Denne,[85] Li et al.,[86] Proschan et al.,[87] Jennison and Turnbull,[88] to name just a few). Few others have also researched in interim change of objectives and/or endpoints.[89] Estimation of parameters can be carried out via interim analysis based on either blinded or unblinded data. The effects on both the Type I error rate (α) and power ($1 - \beta$) are in general small in magnitude. When using the GSMs for sample size reestimation the need for modification in α spending and information time should be incorporated. While the CP approach via the B-values is simple to use, one must choose an appropriate trend (currently observed, null, or hypothetical one) to follow. It is unclear as to how many adaptations are feasible and acceptable, though in general, the consensus is once in the early or midstage, but not in the very late stage of the trial. Many authors prefer sample size reestimation be performed on blinded data to minimize possible bias and maintain trial credibility. Nonetheless, without knowing the observed treatment effect at interim, sample size reestimation might be "shooting darts in total darkness." In particular, if the observed treatment effect is in fact substantially smaller than expected, it is doubtful whether one should increase the sample size at all, regardless of the observed variance.

B. STAGEWISE ADAPTATION

Stagewise (external) adaptation involves a stepwise testing scheme. In a simple and straightforward two-stage design it begins with a small pilot study and follows up with an extended large main study. Then, global results are obtained and decision making is reached by combining p-values, not pooling data of the pilot and main studies. The small pilot study is "external" to the main study and the pilot and main are considered independent studies. Stagewise adaptation can be two- or multi-stage, but it seldom goes beyond three stages in practice. In early phase of new drug development the following situations *a priori* may be relevant for use of the stagewise adaptation design:

- The objectives of the trial are not well defined.
- The clinically relevant endpoints are not well known.
- The treatment effect size or clinically meaningful difference is unsure.
- The variance is uncertain.
- The therapeutic or effective doses are not readily determined.

The stagewise adaptation design, in contrast to group sequential designs, allows for an estimation of the final sample size using the results of the pilot study. The approach is based on the combination of the independent one-sided p-values of the sequence of pilot and main studies by Fisher's combination test. This procedure is well described by Bauer and Köhne[90] and it can be briefly summarized for a two-stage design as follows:

- Plan and conduct two independent randomized studies in sequence: namely, a small external pilot study and an extended large main study.
- Utilize information from the pilot study to adapt the main study for refined design and conduct (e.g., relevant objectives, endpoints, patient entry criteria, sample size, effect size, variance, and dose). Also, obtain the p-value, p_1, of the pilot study.
- Let $\alpha_L, c_\alpha \leq \alpha_L \leq \alpha$ be the lower critical limit so that $p_1 \leq \alpha_L$ rejects the null and stops at the end of the pilot study (claim effect early), where c_α is the critical value for the combination test at the end of trial. Let $\alpha_U, \alpha \leq \alpha_U \leq 1$ be the upper critical limit so that $p_1 \geq \alpha_U$ accepts the null and stops (claim no effect at all). Otherwise, adapt the main study for the second stage.
- At the end of the main study combine the p-values of both the pilot (p_1) and main (p_2) studies to a global test by Fisher's product criterion so that reject the null, when $p_1 p_2 \leq c_\alpha$. A practical choice for early phase exploratory trials could be $\alpha_U = 0.5$, $\alpha_L = 0.0233$, and $c_\alpha = 0.0087$ at $\alpha = 0.05$. For an experiment wise Type I error rate ($\alpha = 0.10, 0.05,$

0.025, 0.01) possible values for α_L, α_U, and the corresponding c_α can be found in Table 1 of Bauer and Köhne.[90]

Stagewise adaptation design represents a flexible alternative to fixed design in the case of uncertainty to make a definitive decision. In particular, it adapts to the experimental paradigm of clinical pharmacology — stepwise and flexibility. A price to pay is statistical power loss due to combining p-values instead of data pooling as well as potential time increase due to stagewise design. For additional work in stagewise design, refer to Bauer and Röhmel,[91] Hothorn and Martin,[92] Posch and Bauer,[93] Liu and Chi,[94] and Posch et al.[95] Also, Chapter 13 provides the adaptive design perspective on interim analysis and bias in clinical trials.

VII. DISCUSSION

Performing planned interim analyses on accumulating data in clinical trials is a frequent and often necessary practice. Recent development of sequential methodology has had a major impact on the design and analysis of controlled clinical trials. This is evident in large clinical trials with long term patient follow up, in particular, the confirmatory trials that are government or industry sponsored. For ethical, economic, and/or administrative reasons (not strongly recommended), interim analyses are often planned and conducted in clinical trials for evidence of safety and efficacy. Undoubtedly, interim analysis, planned or unplanned, in particular the latter, may introduce bias and inflate the error probabilities. ICH E9 Guidance[9] has raised serious concerns about improper planning and conduct of interim analysis. Specifically, it calls for "all interim analyses should be carefully planned in advance and described in the protocol. Special circumstances may dictate the need for an interim analysis that was not defined at the start of a trial. In these cases, a protocol amendment describing the interim analysis must be completed prior to unblinded access to treatment comparison data. ... The execution of an interim analysis must be a completely confidential process because unblinded data and results are potentially involved. The staff involved in the conduct of the trial should remain blind to the results of such analyses, because of the possibility that their attitudes to the trial will be modified and cause changes in the characteristics of patients to be recruited or biases in treatment comparisons. ... Any interim analysis that is not planned appropriately ... may flaw the results of a trial and possibly weaken confidence in the conclusions drawn. Therefore, such analyses should be avoided. If unplanned interim analysis is conducted, the study report should explain why it was necessary, the degree to which blindness had to be broken, provide an assessment of the potential magnitude of bias introduced, and the impact on the interpretation of the results."

Recent developments in sequential methods have been fruitful. In particular, the error rate spending function and CP approaches (either used independently or in combination) have rendered useful and flexible tools. Along with the global regulatory guidance and education in clinical trial conduct have brought better understanding and thus provided logical avenues of planning and conducting interim analysis in clinical trials. Involving independent DMC that charters data and safety monitoring and trial decision-making recommendations (e.g., early trial stopping) for the sponsor further has strengthened the credibility and integrity of the trial.

No one could foresee all aspects of a trial in advance, particularly, in cases where the trial involves brand new therapeutic/disease areas and therefore, adaptive design in many situations is a necessity. It is possible to rescue or salvage a costly critical trial in midcourse via adaptive design and interim analysis. Most often, it involves sample size reestimation or trial extension. Occasionally, it may involve switching trial objectives or curtailing ineffective or toxic treatments/ doses. Again, the error rate spending function and CP approaches are proven useful.

It is possible to salvage a trial in midcourse (e.g., for lack of power), but the adaptability to do this always has a price (e.g., bias, error probability inflation, more patients, longer duration, more costly, and trial credibility compromise). Therefore, it is advisable to think through all aspects of the trial including the power requirement fully in advance before finalizing and launching a trial. It should be borne in mind that adaptive design is by no means a cure all - it mends mild deficiency at midcourse of a trial, but it would not cure a poorly designed and executed trial. Regardless of the design or sequential methods chosen, it should be planned *a priori* at trial design and executed according to GCP and good statistical practice (GSP); the ultimate goal should always be to minimize bias and control error probabilities to maintain the scientific and ethical integrity of the trial.

REFERENCES

1. Pocock, S.J., Group sequential methods in the design and analysis of clinical trials, *Biometrika*, 64, 191–199, 1977.
2. O'Brien, P.C. and Fleming, T.R., A multiple testing procedure for clinical trials, *Biometrics*, 35, 549–556, 1979.
3. Lan, K.K.G. and DeMets, D.L., Discrete sequential boundaries for clinical trials, *Biometrika*, 70, 659–663, 1983.
4. Lan, K.K.G., Simon, R., and Halperin, M., Stochastically curtailed tests in long term clinical trials, *Commun. Stat. Seq. Anal.*, 1, 207–219, 1982.
5. Williams, G.W., Davis, R.L., Getson, A.J., Gould, A.L., Hwang, I.K., Matthews, H., Shih, W.J., Snapinn, S.M., and Walton-Bowen, K.L., Monitoring of clinical trials and interim analyses from a drug sponsor's point of view, *Stat. Med.*, 12, 481–492, 1993.
6. Hwang, I.K., Shih, W.J., and deCani, J.S., Group sequential designs using a family of type I error probability spending functions, *Stat. Med.*, 9, 1439–1445, 1990.

7. PMA Biostatistics and Medical Ad Hoc Committee on Interim Analysis, Interim analysis in the pharmaceutical industry, *Controlled Clin. Trials*, 14, 160–173, 1993.

8. Anbar, D., Enas, G.G., Given, S.V., Hwang, I.K., Johnson, J.D., Tandon, P.K., Trost, D.C., and Zerbe, R.L., Interim analysis: further considerations in the conduct of controlled clinical trials in drug development, *Stat. Med.*, A98-040, 22 1997, Unpublished manuscript 1997.

9. ICH E9 Guidance. Statistical Principles for Clinical Trials. Guidance for Industry, CDER/CBER, Food and Drug Administration, September 1998, pp. 1–46. http://www.fda.gov/cder/guidance/ICH_E9-fnl.PDF

10. Armitage, P., McPherson, C.K., and Rowe, B.C., Repeated significance tests on accumulating data, *J. R. Stat. Soc., Ser. A*, 132, 235–244, 1969.

11. McPherson, C.K. and Armitage, P., Repeated significance tests on accumulating data when the null hypothesis is not true, *J. R. Stat. Soc., Ser. A*, 134, 15–25, 1971.

12. Berry, D.A., Interim analysis in clinical trials: classical vs. Bayesian approaches, *Stat. Med.*, 4, 521–526, 1985.

13. Freedman, L.S. and Spiegelhalter, D.J., Comparison of Bayesian with group sequential methods for monitoring clinical trials, *Controlled Clin. Trials*, 10, 357–367, 1989.

14. Freedman, L.S. and Spiegelhalter, D.J., Application of Bayesian statistics to decision making during a clinical trial, *Stat. Med.*, 11, 23–35, 1992.

15. ICH E6 Guidance. Good Clinical Practice. Consolidated Guidance. CDER/CBER, Food and Drug Administration, March 1998, pp. 1–63. http://www.fda.gov/cder/guidance/ICH_E6-fnl.PDF

16. The Norwegian Multicenter Study Group, Timolol-induced reduction in mortality and reinfarction in patients surviving acute myocardial infarction, *N. Engl. J. Med.*, 304, 801–807, 1981.

17. The Coronary Drug Project Research Group, Practical aspects of decision-making in clinical trials: the Coronary Drug Project as a case study, *Controlled Clin. Trials*, 1, 363–376, 1981.

18. Fleming, T.R. and DeMets, D.L., Monitoring of clinical trials: issues and recommendations, *Controlled Clin. Trials*, 14, 183–197, 1993.

19. Armstrong, P.W. and Furburg, C.D., Clinical trial data and safety monitoring boards: the search for a constitution, *Circulation*, 1 1994, Session 6.

20. DeMets, D.L., Ellenberg, S.S., Fleming, T.R., Childress, J.F., Mayer, K.H., Pollard, R.B., Rahal, J.J., Walters, L., O'Fallon, J., Whitley-Williams, P., Staus, S., Sande, M., and Whitley, R.J., The data and safety monitoring board and acquired immune deficiency syndrome (AIDS) clinical trials, *Controlled Clin. Trials*, 16, 408–421, 1995.

21. Guidance for Clinical Trial Sponsors — On the Establishment and Operation of Clinical Trial Data Monitoring Committee. Draft Guidance. CDER/CBER, Food and Drug Administration, 2003, pp. 1–27 (Posted 07/10/03). http://www.fda.gov/cher/gdlns/clindatmon.pdf

22. Concept Paper on the Development of a Committee for CPMP Point to Consider on Data Monitoring Committees. CPMP/EWP/2459/02 London, February 2004.

23. DeMets, D.L. and Lan, K.K.G., An overview of sequential methods and their application in clinical trials, *Commun. Stat. Theory Methods*, 13, 2315–2338, 1984.

24. DeMets, D.L. and Lan, K.K.G., Interim analysis: the alpha spending function approach, *Stat. Med.*, 13, 1341–1352, 1994.
25. DeMets, D.L. and Lan, K.K.G., The alpha spending function approach to interim data analysis, In *Recent Advances in Clinical Trial Design and Analysis*, Thall, P.F., ed., Kluwer, Boston, pp. 1–27, 1995.
26. Hwang, I.K., Overview of the development of sequential procedures, In *Biopharmaceutical Sequential Statistical Applications*, Peace, K., ed., Marcel Dekker, New York, pp. 3–17, 1992.
27. Davis, R.L. and Hwang, I.K., Interim analysis in clinical trials — part A. methodology, In *Statistics in the Pharmaceutical Industry*, 2nd ed., Buncher, R. and Tsay, J.Y., eds., Marcel Dekker, New York, pp. 267–283, 1993.
28. Whitehead, J., *The Design and Analysis of Sequential Clinical Trials*, 2nd ed., Wiley, Chichester, 1997.
29. Jennison, C. and Turnbull, B.W., *Group Sequential Methods with Applications to Clinical Trials*, Chapman & Hall, Boca Raton, 2000.
30. Shih, W.J., Group sequential methods, In *Encyclopedia of Biopharmaceutical Statistics*, Chow, S.C., ed., Marcel Dekker, New York, pp. 249–258, 2003.
31. Armitage, P., *Sequential Medical Trials*, 2nd ed., Blackwell, Oxford, 1975.
32. Lan, K.K.G. and Wittes, J., The B-value: a tool for monitoring data, *Biometrics*, 44, 579–585, 1988.
33. Lan, K.K.G. and Zucker, D.M., Sequential monitoring of clinical trials: the role of information and Brownian motion, *Stat. Med.*, 12, 753–765, 1993.
34. Haybittle, J.L., Repeated assessment of results in clinical trials of cancer treatment, *Br. J. Radiol.*, 44, 793–797, 1971.
35. Peto, R., Pike, M.C., Armitage, P., Breslow, N.E., Cox, D.R., Howard, S.V., Mantel, N., McPherson, C.K., Peto, J., and Smith, P.G., Design and analysis of randomized clinical trials requiring prolonged observation of each patient, *Br. J. Cancer*, 35, 585–611, 1976.
36. Milton, R.C., Computer evaluation of the multivariate normal integral, *Technometrics*, 14881–14889, 1972.
37. Chang, M.N., Hwang, I.K., and Shih, W.J., Group sequential designs using a family of type I and type II error probability spending functions, *Commun. Stat. Theory Methods*, 27(6), 1323–1339, 1998.
38. Lan, K.K.G. and DeMets, D.L., Group sequential procedures: calendar versus information time, *Stat. Med.*, 8, 1191–1198, 1989.
39. Kim, K. and DeMets, D.L., Design and analysis of group sequential tests based on the type I error spending rate function, *Biometrika*, 74, 149–154, 1987.
40. The Scandinavian Simvastatin Survival Study Group, Design and baseline results of the Scandinavian Simvastatin Survival Study of patients with stable angina and/or previous myocardial infarction, *Am. J. Cardiol.*, 71, 393–400, 1993.
41. The Scandinavian Simvastatin Survival Study Group, Randomized trial of cholesterol lowering in 4444 patients with coronary heart disease: the Scandinavian Simvastatin Survival Study (4S), *Lancet*, 344, 1383–1389, 1994.
42. Downs, J.R., Beere, P.A., Whitney, E., Clearfield, M., Weis, S., Rochen, J., Stein, E.A., Shapiro, D.R., Langendorfer, A., and Gotto, A.M., Design & rationale of the Air Force Texas coronary atherosclerosis prevention study (AFCAPS/TexCAPS), *Am. J. Cardiol.*, 80, 287–293, 1997.

43. Reboussin, D.M., DeMets, D.L., Kim, K.M., and Lan, K.K.G., Computations for group sequential boundaries using the Lan–DeMets spending function method, *Controlled Clin. Trials*, 21, 190–207, 2000.

44. Emerson, S.S. and Fleming, T.R., Symmetric group sequential test designs, *Biometrics*, 45, 905–923, 1989.

45. Pampallona, S. and Tsiatis, A.A., Group sequential designs for one-sided and two-sided hypothesis testing with provision for early stopping in favor of the null hypothesis, *J. Stat. Plann. Inf.*, 42, 19–35, 1994.

46. Lan, K.K.G., Lachin, J.M., and Bautista, O.M., Overruling of a group sequential boundary — a stopping rule versus a guideline, *Stat. Med.*, 22, 3347–3355, 2003.

47. Freidlin, B. and Korn, E.L., A comment on futility monitoring, *Controlled Clin. Trials*, 23, 355–366, 2002.

48. Pocock, S.J., Geller, N.L., and Tsiatis, A.A., The analysis of multiple endpoints in clinical trials, *Biometrics*, 43, 487–498, 1987.

49. Lan, K.K.G. and Lachin, J.M., Implementation of group sequential logrank tests in a maximum duration trial, *Biometrics*, 46, 191–199, 1990.

50. Lee, J.W. and DeMets, D.L., Sequential comparison of change with repeated measurement data, *J. Am. Stat. Assoc.*, 86, 757–762, 1991.

51. Wu, M.C. and Lan, K.K.G., Sequential monitoring for comparison of changes in a response variable in clinical studies, *Biometrics*, 48, 765–779, 1992.

52. Lan, K.K.G., Reboussin, D.M., and DeMets, D.L., Information and information fractions for design and sequential monitoring of clinical trials, *Commun. Stat. Theory Methods*, 23, 403–420, 1994.

53. Tsiatis, A.A., The asymptotic joint distribution of the efficient scores test for the proportional hazards model calculated over time, *Biometrika*, 68, 311–315, 1981.

54. Tsiatis, A.A., Repeated significance testing for a general class of statistics used in censored survival analysis, *J. Am. Stat. Assoc.*, 77, 855–861, 1982.

55. Jennison, C. and Turnbull, B.W., Group-sequential analysis incorporating covariate information, *J. Am. Stat. Assoc.*, 92, 1330–1341, 1997.

56. Scharfstein, D.O., Tsiatis, A.A., and Robins, J.M., Semiparametric efficiency and its implication on the design and analysis of group-sequential studies, *J. Am. Stat. Assoc.*, 92, 1342–1350, 1997.

57. Lan, K.K.G., Rosenberger, W.F., and Lachin, J.M., Use of spending functions for occasional or continuous monitoring of data in a clinical trial, *Stat. Med.*, 12, 2214–2231, 1993.

58. Jennison, C. and Turnbull, B.W., Repeated confidence intervals for group sequential trials, *Controlled Clin. Trials*, 5, 33–45, 1984.

59. Hughes, M.D. and Pocock, S.J., Stopping rules and estimation problems in clinical trials, *Stat. Med.*, 7, 1231–1241, 1988.

60. Siegmund, D., Estimation following sequential tests, *Biometrika*, 65, 341–349, 1978.

61. Tsiatis, A.A., Rosner, G.L., and Mehta, C.R., Exact confidence intervals following a group sequential test, *Biometrics*, 40, 797–803, 1984.

62. Kim, K. and DeMets, D.L., Confidence intervals following group sequential tests in clinical trials, *Biometrics*, 43, 857–864, 1987.

63. Emerson, S.S. and Fleming, T.R., Parameter estimation following group sequential hypothesis testing, *Biometrika*, 77, 875–892, 1990.

64. Lan, K.K.G. and Wittes, J., Data monitoring in complex clinical trials: which treatment is better? *J. Stat. Plann. Inf.*, 42, 241–255, 1994.

65. Wetherill, G.B., *Sequential Methods in Statistics*, 2nd ed., Chapman & Hall, Boca Raton, 1975.
66. Siegmund, D., *Sequential Analysis: Test and Confidence Intervals*, Springer, New York, 1985.
67. Beta-Blocker Heart Attack Trial Research Group, A randomized trial of propranolol in patients with acute myocardial infarction. I. Mortality results, *JAMA*, 246, 1707–1714, 1982.
68. DeMets, D.L., Hardy, R., Friedman, L.M., and Lan, K.K.G., Statistical aspects of early termination in the Beta-Blocker Heart Attack Trial, *Controlled Clin. Trials*, 5, 362–372, 1984.
69. Spiegelhalter, D.J., Freedman, L.S., and Blackburn, P.R., Monitoring clinical trials: conditional or predictive power? *Controlled Clin. Trials*, 7, 8–17, 1986.
70. Lan, K.K.G., Conditional power: a Bayesian approach, *Int. Chin. Stat. Assoc. Bull.*, 43 2000, July.
71. Lan, K.K.G. and Trost, D.C., Estimation of parameters and sample size reestimation, *Proc. Biopharm. Sect.*, 48–51, 1997.
72. Whitehead, J., Whitehead, A., Todd, S., Bolland, K., and Sooriyarachchi, M.R., Mid-trial design reviews for sequential clinical trials, *Stat. Med.*, 20, 165–176, 2001.
73. Hwang, I.K., Adaptive Designs in Clinical Trials: a Discussant's Perspective. Presented at 2001 DIA 37th Annual Meeting, July 8, 2001, Denver, CO.
74. Wittes, J., On changing a long-term clinical trial midstream, *Stat. Med.*, 27, 2789–2795, 2002.
75. Wittes, J. and Brittain, E., The role of internal pilot studies in increasing the efficiency of clinical trials, *Stat. Med.*, 9, 65–72, 1990.
76. Birkett, M.A. and Day, S.J., Internal pilot studies for estimating sample size, *Stat. Med.*, 13, 2455–2463, 1994.
77. Denne, J.S. and Jennison, C., Estimating the sample size for a *t*-test using an internal pilot, *Stat. Med.*, 18, 1575–1585, 1999.
78. Gould, A.L., Interim analysis for monitoring clinical trials that do not materially affect the Type I error rate, *Stat. Med.*, 11, 55–66, 1992.
79. Gould, A.L. and Shih, W.J., Sample size reestimation without unblinding for normally distributed outcomes with known variance, *Commun. Stat. Theory Methods*, 21, 2833–2853, 1992.
80. Herson, J. and Wittes, J., The use of interim analysis for sample size adjustment, *Drug Inf. J.*, 27, 753–760, 1993.
81. Proschan, M.A. and Hunsberger, S.A., Designed extension of studies based on conditional power, *Biometrics*, 51, 1315–1324, 1995.
82. Shih, W.J. and Gould, A.L., Re-evaluating design specifications of longitudinal clinical trials without unblinding when the key response is rate of change, *Stat. Med.*, 14, 2239–2248, 1995.
83. Cui, L., Hung, H.M.J., and Wang, S.-J., Modification of sample size in group sequential clinical trials, *Biometrics*, 55, 853–857, 1999.
84. Gould, A.L., Sample size re-estimation: recent developments and practical considerations, *Stat. Med.*, 20, 2625–2643, 2001.
85. Denne, J.S., Sample size recalculation using conditional power, *Stat. Med.*, 20, 2645–2660, 2001.
86. Li, G., Shih, W.J., Xie, T., and Lu, J., A sample size adjustment procedure for clinical trials based on conditional power, *Biostatistics*, 3, 277–287, 2002.

87. Proschan, M.A., Liu, Q., and Hunsberger, S.A., Practical midcourse sample size modification in clinical trials, *Controlled Clin. Trials*, 24, 4–15, 2003.

88. Jennison, C. and Turnbull, B.W., Mid-course sample size modification in clinical trials based on the observed treatment effect, *Stat. Med.*, 22, 971–993, 2003.

89. Wang, S.-J., Hung, H.M.J., Tsong, Y., and Cui, L., Group sequential test strategies for superiority and non-inferiority hypotheses in active controlled clinical trials, *Stat. Med.*, 20, 1903–1912, 2001.

90. Bauer, P. and Köhne, K., Evaluation of experiments with adaptive interim analyses, *Biometrics*, 50, 1029–1041, 1994, (correction: *Biometrics* 52, 380, 1996).

91. Bauer, P. and Röhmel, J., An adaptive method for establishing a dose–response relationship, *Stat. Med.*, 14, 1595–1607, 1995.

92. Hothorn, L.A. and Martin, U.M., Application of adaptive interim analysis in pharmacology, *Drug Inf. J.*, 31, 615–619, 1997.

93. Posch, M. and Bauer, P., Adaptive two stage designs and the conditional error function, *Biometrical J.*, 41, 689–696, 1999.

94. Liu, Q. and Chi, G.Y.H., On sample size and inference for two-stage adaptive designs, *Biometrics*, 57, 172–177, 2001.

95. Posch, M., Bauer, P., and Brannath, W., Issues in designing flexible trials, *Stat. Med.*, 22, 953–969, 2003.

15 A Regulatory Perspective on Data Monitoring and Interim Analysis

Robert T. O'Neill

CONTENTS

I. INTRODUCTION

The Food and Drug Administration (FDA) is responsible for evaluating the data, statistical analyses, reliability, and validity of conclusions of clinical studies performed by sponsors including the pharmaceutical industry and submitted to FDA in support of the efficacy and safety of new drugs. Also, the FDA reviews and comments on important protocols submitted by the pharmaceutical industry or other sponsors prior to the conduct of these trials, and evaluates the data and conclusions from completed studies submitted in a New Drug Application (NDA). In many situations the appropriateness of an analysis with data monitoring strategies and interim analysis is a critical issue in the evaluation of the evidence.

There has been a tremendous change in the environment for data monitoring and interim analysis of clinical trials over the last decade. While the initial experience with data monitoring occurred in large government-sponsored trials, the recent experience has shown an increase in such trials conducted for the pharmaceutical industry. Much of the early experience gained from

285

government-sponsored trials involved data monitoring carried out by a committee assigned for that function. The data monitoring is a critical function put in place to protect patients in clinical trials and to maintain the integrity of the trial under unmasked access to trial data. The statistical analysis of comparative interim study results is an important strategy that helps in making critical decisions regarding the continued conduct of a clinical trial to meet its intended objective and the termination of trials when the risk to patients is determined to be unwarranted. Several factors have made the early access to and analysis of accruing data a reality. One such factor is the advances in computerization, which ensures timely entry of clinical trial data from case report form into a computer data base, and its timely auditing and cleaning through call backs and visits to the site. Improved electronic data collection strategies are emerging all the time. Another is that virtually all trials for life-threatening diseases are carried out with some type of monitoring and interim analysis, and it is almost standard practice today that such methods are planned in the protocol. Just as important to the increased consideration of interim analysis strategies is the current availability of a variety of statistical methodologies, computer programs to implement them, and the continuing development and refinement of statistical methodologies to guide decision making for trial planning, monitoring, and early termination, including PEST Reading University,[1] EAST 2000 from Cytel Software,[2] and SeqTrial from MathSoft.[3]

Another example of data monitoring strategies receiving attention is the recent research in adaptive designs to deal with midcourse changes of study and sample-size reestimation, but currently there are few examples of actual implementation. For that reason, this chapter will not consider this issue further. Finally, an important stimulus to data-monitoring practices is the monitoring of multiple trials within a drug-development program. Pharmaceutical sponsors are increasingly subject to intensive time pressure in drug-development strategies and there are examples of blending/compressing earlier phase studies, perhaps dose ranging/response studies with later phase efficacy confirmatory trials. In a drug-development environment focused on earliest time to market, especially for new therapies, multiple confirmatory trials may be ongoing simultaneously under vague monitoring strategies. The monitoring function for these broader situations may or may not be carried out by a formally established data-monitoring committee (DMC), but when it is, the methodologies used and the role of the DMC, for both independently externally monitored trials and internal pharmaceutical sponsor monitoring, need written operating standards.

II. A BRIEF REGULATORY HISTORY

The following is a brief regulatory history of the attention given to data monitoring and interim analysis. Federal regulations recognize the role for monitored clinical trials that incorporate interim analysis. Section 314.126(7) of the Code of Federal Regulations[4] concerns the criteria for an adequate and well-controlled study and it states that there should be an analysis of the results of a study adequate to assess the effects of the drug. The regulations state that the effects of any interim analysis performed should be assessed.

In 1985, an amendment to these regulations (CFR 314.50(d)(6)) introduced the requirement for the type and format of documentation of evidence of efficacy and safety that is generally required to be submitted in a NDA by a sponsor. This amendment introduced the requirement for a separate Statistical Section as one of the technical sections to be submitted by a sponsor in a NDA. To implement this change, in July 1988, FDA updated its guidelines for how sponsors prepare these clinical and statistical sections of a NDA. In the *Guideline for the Format and Content of the Clinical and Statistical Sections of a New Drug Application,*[5] the FDA expressed the need for full documentation of all interim analyses, formal or informal, performed for any clinical study. This requirement for documentation of all interim analyses was intended to address those studies that were planned, designed, and analyzed in some formal manner, though FDA was aware that studies were being monitored and analyzed without any formal prospective plan. This guidance has been updated and much of its content incorporated in an international guidance called *ICH E3 Structure and Content of Clinical Study Reports.*[6]

In the early 1990s, most of the discussions in the statistical and clinical trial literature concerned models and methods for monitoring large publicly funded mortality endpoint trials. Because there was little in the literature that concerned the process of data monitoring and interim analysis as carried out by the pharmaceutical industry, it was decided that these evolving issues needed broader input. FDA held a public workshop[7] in conjunction with the Pharmaceutical Manufacturers Association (PMA) on the topic of clinical trial monitoring and interim analysis in pharmaceutical industry-supported trials. It was the first time FDA publicly addressed how the pharmaceutical industry was utilizing data-monitoring strategies including the statistical methods in monitoring clinical trials, and how these processes and procedures for monitoring trials were implemented. A position paper from the industry, under the Writing Committee chairmanship of Ronald Kershner, reflected the issues and concerns at that time, and a meeting in 1993 at the National Institutes of Health (NIH) on data monitoring covered some of the industry[8,9] and regulatory concerns.[10]

A summary of the themes covered at the February 1993 workshop included:

1. Clarifying the purposes and procedures of monitoring industry-sponsored trials for unexpected toxicity and efficacy.
2. Operational aspects of implementing trial monitoring, including the responsibilities, organizational structures, and standard operating procedures (SOPs) for monitoring a study.

3. The statistical aspects of planning interim analyses of an interim analyzed trial with stopping rules (strategies, boundaries) for reaching planned completion of a trial with multiple endpoints and subgroups.
4. Reporting and documentation of how the trial was actually carried out including relevance of the analysis to what was planned as well as to what was actually carried out.
5. What types of communications, interactions, and information flow among the sponsors, DMCs, and FDA are appropriate including types of confidentiality of sharing of the results.
6. What types of trials should have external DMCs.
7. Which types of trial monitoring and situations allow for no penalty statistical looks.

The most visible and perhaps impactful contribution to the regulatory perspective on interim analysis and data monitoring came about during the last part of the 1990s. The International Conference on Harmonization (ICH) of Technical Standards[11–13] is an effort of three regions, viz., the United States, Japan, and the European Union, with the pharmaceutical industry and regulators in those regions to standardize criteria for clinical trials as well as other topics. The ICH E9 Statistical Principles in Clinical Trials[14] is a guidance, finalized and made available in 1998, which addresses mainly statistical concepts including the role of data monitoring primarily from the statistical perspective. There are four sections of the ICH E9 guidance, which address aspects of data monitoring and interim analysis.

The first is Section 3.4, which describes the use of Group Sequential Designs for the purpose of conducting interim analysis. While it is recognized that these designs are not the only designs for this purpose, the practicality of assessing outcomes by treatment group at periodic intervals during the trial is appreciated. In this section there is a description of the need for statistical methods to be fully specified in advance of the availability of the treatment outcomes and subject treatment assignment. This section also contains a discussion of an *independent data-monitoring committee* (IDMC) defined in ICH E6[15] to review or to conduct the interim analysis, and it recognizes that the design used most widely and successfully in large, long-term trials of mortality and major nonfatal endpoints is also used in other trials. In particular, it is recognized that safety must be monitored in all trials and thus the need for formal procedures to cover early stopping for safety reasons is encouraged.

The second is Section 4.1, dealing with trial monitoring and interim analysis. Here there is a distinction made between two types of monitoring. One type concerns the oversight of the quality of the trial, while the other involves the breaking of the blind (unmasking) to make treatment comparisons (i.e., interim analysis). Each type of trial monitoring entails different staff responsibilities and involves access to different types of trial data and information. It is noted that different principles apply for the control of potential statistical and operational bias in each of these situations. Emphasis is made that the protocol or appropriate amendments prior to a first analysis should contain the statistical plans for the interim analysis to prevent bias.

The third is Section 4.5, on interim analysis and early stopping, containing a definition of what is considered an interim analysis, and the various goals of an interim analysis. The concepts of stopping boundaries and flexible alpha spending functions are described. There is a reinforcement of the principle that the execution of an interim analysis should be a confidential process and that all staff (other than the IDMC) involved in the conduct of the trial should be blind to the results of such analyses. This is because of the possibility that their attitudes to the trial will be modified and cause changes in the characteristics of patients to be recruited, thus causing biases in treatment comparisons. Most clinical trials designed to support the efficacy and safety of an investigational product should proceed to full completion of planned sample-size accrual. It is also recognized that only a subset of trials will involve the study of serious life-threatening outcomes or mortality, which may need sequential monitoring of comparative treatment effects. The guidance recognizes the need for external IDMCs for some trials of major public health importance. It also recognizes that when a sponsor assumes the role of monitoring safety and efficacy comparisons with unblinded access to data from a clinical trial that the sponsor financed, special care should be taken to protect the integrity of the trial and limit appropriate sharing of information. A strong recommendation against unplanned interim analysis is given.

The fourth is Section 4.6, which discusses the role of the IDMC. Here there is a call for written operating procedures and the maintenance of records of all its meetings, including interim results that would be available for review at trial completion. The independence of the IDMC is emphasized to control the sharing of important comparative information and to protect the integrity of the trial from adverse impact resulting from access to trial information. Also included is a general statement about composition of the committee containing clinical trial scientists knowledgeable in the appropriate disciplines, including statistics. Finally, there is the clear advice that if pharmaceutical sponsor representatives are on the IDMC, operating procedures of the committee should be defined to control dissemination of interim trial results within the sponsor organization.

In recognition of the increasing attention to the data-monitoring function and the concept of an independent DMC, FDA in 2001 issued for public comment a draft guidance for clinical trial sponsors titled *On the Establishment and Operation of Clinical Trial Data Monitoring Committees*.[16] One of the issues addressed in this draft guidance is the concept of the independence of the committee and especially of the statistician who has access to unmasked or unblinded grouped efficacy and safety comparisons. Here are some of the concerns regarding the potential bias that might be introduced during the interim analysis and data-monitoring process when independence among trial conduct, trial analysis, and monitoring is an issue.

III. INTRODUCING BIAS INTO THE MONITORING PROCESS: SOME CONCERNS

From a statistical perspective there are two sources of bias which may be of more or less concern depending upon the independence of the group charged with monitoring a clinical trial. The first source relates to the process of monitoring a trial that may unblind the trial in subtle or partial ways to participants, investigators, or possibly to management of the trial's sponsor. This may have potential for influencing biased allocation schemes for future patients entered into a trial, changing the outcome or assessment criteria during the trial in a manner to inappropriately optimize observed effects for a treatment, dropping centers or sites that may be experiencing less favorable relative treatment benefits, or changing the protocol in some way that is not taken into account in the ultimate analysis. All these issues impact on the relative treatment comparisons in ways that may produce estimates or inferences not reflecting the true effect of a test drug in the appropriate patient population, especially when not discussed, analyzed, or documented in a trial report.

The second source of bias relates to the appropriate statistical quantification of uncertainty, usually captured in calculation of p-values and more specifically in estimates of treatment effects, confidence intervals for the treatment effects, and other measures of statistical uncertainty. Most clinical trial questions are posed in terms of a hypothesis and the statistical research on repeated significance testing of accumulating data in clinical studies has articulated well the implications on Type I error of excessive statistical tests of hypotheses, the probability of concluding that a drug produces an effect when in fact it does not.[17,18]

Thus, the changes and new guidances that have evolved over the last decade or so can be viewed as the FDA's intent to minimize naive or unknowledgeable clinical trial practices that can potentially adversely impact on the credibility of a trial submitted for regulatory purposes.

The population of controlled clinical trials submitted to the FDA generally fall into three classes:

1. Trials with IDMCs (external to the sponsor), most of which are in life-threatening diseases or use mortality endpoints. These trials should have and almost always do have protocols that use planned interim analysis strategies employing some form of group sequential methods with stopping rules specified in various levels of detail. There are several models followed in these trials, the most frequent of which is along the lines of the large government-sponsored trials by the NIH.

2. Trials in nonlife-threatening diseases, which do not have independent (e.g., internal to the sponsor) DMCs to monitor and may have unplanned analysis or unusual proposals for termination (usually with no published methodology), or questions regarding termination not

planned in the protocol. This is the population of trials that can be problematic and these trials are discouraged.

3. Controlled trials for which the trial sponsor has no expressed intention of terminating earlier than planned completion (assuming this is well stated in a protocol) but which are being monitored for safety but not formally for efficacy outcomes.

The FDA's advice to sponsors for these trials is consistent with the principles in the ICH E9 guidance discussed above. We describe in the next sections the spirit of this advice.

A. PROTOCOL

The monitoring of interim results should be planned in advance, preferably with a limited number of interim analyses focused on key endpoints. A protocol should describe:

Sample size planning assumptions, duration or follow up, and degree of certainty in these planning estimates (e.g., target event rates and minimal difference between treatment and control worth detecting), and also the degree of skepticism regarding the expected treatment effects, etc.

Strategies or contingency plans for stopping the trial earlier than planned in the case of efficacy monitoring and toxicity monitoring (each may require separate decision criteria and boundaries that can be asymmetric) should be described. If group sequential methods are used, there should be some discussion of the timing and number of looks, at least the class or shape of the Type I spending function that is planned to be used and not changed as a result of data-driven analyses.

There are a number of routine situations of interest which must be dealt with. These situations include terminating a trial for better than expected efficacy, terminating a trial for lack of expected efficacy, terminating a trial for unexpected toxicity, modifying a trial design on the basis of comparative results observed during the monitoring of the trial, dropping one arm of a trial in a multi-arm trial, and adjusting the sample size of a trial upwards to maintain planned statistical power because of lower event rates or higher variability than hypothesized.

Statistical methodology is now available to appropriately deal with each of these situations, or at least provide a sensible strategy to follow. However, practitioners may not either be aware of the need for it or ignore it. This is why the training of DMC members in the theory and methods of interim analyses is needed for modern trials that will be subjected to interim analysis. Trial planners should be well trained in these methods and with case studies of other monitored trials as the success and integrity of a clinical trial depends upon how well these concepts are planned and articulated in the protocol and handled in committee decisions.

B. ADMINISTRATIVE LOOKS

The pharmaceutical industry in the late 1980s and early 1990s proposed the concept of administrative looks, which are intended, among other things, to allow for access not only to summaries of patient entry characteristics, accrual patterns, and other administrative data of interest, but also to relative treatment differences on primary and secondary outcomes during the trial but with no expectation to change, modify, or terminate the trial.

The concept of an "administrative" look cannot be separated from the data-monitoring responsibility. Particularly important is the issue of access to unblinded summarized group results of efficacy and safety outcomes and the potential, regardless of intention, of possible early stopping, possible upsizing or downsizing of the trial, changing endpoints in a manner that favors one treatment group, or other variations. As a result of such an administrative look, it is natural to ask questions regarding the practices, procedures, reporting, and documentation requirements regarding unblinding of trial results: who has access to the data in the decision-making chain, what safeguards there are for maintaining the integrity of the trial, which trials deserve internal versus external monitoring groups, or when is it advisable to use external monitoring committees versus internal monitoring committees, etc. Any "administrative look" at accruing study results which is not intended to stop a trial early but which allows for unblinded relative treatment efficacy comparisons should be done cautiously in a manner that does not allow early termination of a trial for rejection of the null hypothesis. This can operationally be accomplished by use of a very conservative spending function during the entire duration of the trial, which essentially leaves one with the same statistical criteria at the completion of a trial as a fixed trial concept would have achieved.

These issues speak to the need for planned SOPs to be in place prior to a trial so as to ensure that unanticipated decisions are made in the context of some planned structure and that all responsible parties are aware of the issues beforehand.

In a broader context, the FDA is concerned about its proper role in the interaction with sponsors, and with IDMCs external to the sponsor and the mechanisms for flow of information, particularly in life-threatening disease areas where special regulations focus on expediting therapies to patients. An evolving consensus is that the FDA does not need to be in any decision-making role for a study or an IDMC. Therefore, the FDA has considered it unwise for staff to be made aware of or have access to unmasked interim treatment effects by group and to be brought into the decision-making process for whether a trial should continue or be terminated. This is a sponsor responsibility in conjunction with the recommendation of its data safety monitoring committee.

REFERENCES

1. PEST, Planning and Evaluation of Sequential Trials, Medical and Pharmaceutical Research Unit, University of Reading. Available at www.reading.ac.uk

2. EaSt-2000, Cytel Software Corporation.

3. S+ SeqTrial, *S-Plus User's Manual*, MathSoft, Inc., Seattle, Washington, 2000, February.

4. Code of Federal Regulations, U.S. Government Printing Office, Washington, 2000.

5. Guideline for the Format and Content of the Clinical and Statistical Sections of New Drug Applications. U.S. Department of Health and Human Services, Public Health Service, FDA, July 1988.

6. *ICH E3 Structure and Content of Clinical Study Reports*, July 1996; An electronic version of this guidance is available via internet using the www.fda.gov/cder/guidance/index.htm

7. PMA/FDA Workshop, Clinical Trial Monitoring and Interim Analysis in the Pharmaceutical Industry, Sheraton Washington hotel, Washington, D.C., February 1992, pp. 24–25.

8. Rockhold, F.W. and Enas, G.G., Data monitoring and interim analyses in the pharmaceutical industry: ethical and logistical considerations, *Stat. Med.*, 12, 471–479, 1993.

9. Interim Analysis in the Pharmaceutical Industry, PMA Biostatistics and Medical Ad hoc Committee on Interim Analysis, *Controlled Clin. Trials*, 14, 160–173, 1993.

10. O'Neill, R.T., Some FDA perspectives on data monitoring in clinical trials in drug development, *Stat. Med.*, 12, 601–608, 1993.

11. D'Arcy, P.F. and Harron, D.W.G., eds., *Proceedings of the Second International Conference on Harmonization, Orlando 1993*, Published at the Queens University of Belfast.

12. D'Arcy, P.F. and Harron, D.W.G., eds., *Proceedings of the Third International Conference on Harmonization, Orlando 1995*, Published at the Queens University of Belfast.

13. D'Arcy, P.F. and Harron, D.W.G., eds., *Proceedings of the Fourth International Conference on Harmonization, Orlando 1997*, Published at the Queens University of Belfast.

14. Guidance for Industry, E9 Statistical Principles for Clinical Trials, U.S. Department of Health and Human Services, April 1998. Available at www.FDA.GOV/CDER/Guidance/Index.htm

15. Guidance for Industry, E6 Good Clinical Practice: Consolidated Guidance, U.S. Department of Health and Human Services, April 1996. Available at www.FDA.GOV/CDER/Guidance/Index.htm

16. On the Establishment and Operation of Clinical Trial Data Monitoring Committees, DRAFT GUIDANCE: Copies available from Office of Training and Communications, Division of Communications Management Drug Information Branch, HFD-210 Center for Drug Evaluation and Research Food and Drug Administration 5600 Fishers Lane, Rockville, MD 20857 (Phone: 301-827-4573) or Internet: http://www.fda.gov/cder/guidance/index.htm

17. McPherson, K. and Armitage, P., Repeated significance tests on accumulating data when the null hypothesis is not true, *J. R. Stat. Soc. A*, 134, 15–25, 1971.

18. O'Neill, R.T., Regulatory perspective on data monitoring, *Stat. Med.*, 21, 2831–2842, 2002.

16 Complex Adaptive Systems, Human Health, and Drug Response: Statistical Challenges in Pharmacogenomics

Kim E. Zerba and C. Frank Shen

CONTENTS

I. THE PROBLEM: INTERINDIVIDUAL HUMAN BIOLOGICAL VARIATION AND DRUG RESPONSE

Traditional drug development from a statistical perspective is focused on the marginal fit of the drug to the average of the population. The entire process of development of compounds during the preclinical phase is based on a mechanistic reductionist approach to human biology which must ignore interindividual human biological variation because of the nature of the process. Towards an attempt to identify compounds that are most likely to succeed in the clinic, during this phase there are numerous, extensive, carefully designed studies on the absorption, distribution, metabolism, excretion and toxicity of compounds.

Despite these extensive efforts there is an industry-wide high failure rate of compounds that reach the clinical phase of development. Compound toxicity and unanticipated biological complexities are two primary reasons often causing failure. Such failure also reflects the pervasive nature of human interindividual variation in the population that is not sampled extensively for safety and rigorous clinical design reasons, during the clinical phases of compound development. It has been recognized that having additional knowledge about relevant features of biology, reflected as biomarkers of drug response, may facilitate higher success rates for compounds which reach the clinic.

Technological advances have resulted in unprecedented capabilities for measuring human biology at the genetic, gene expression, protein and metabolite levels. Such capabilities present innumerable possibilities for these measures on each subject in a study, across different levels in the biological hierarchy from genes to metabolites with the expectation that knowledge and analysis of these vast numbers of measures will facilitate the development of safer, more effective compounds. This expectation comes with the realization that, by studying interindividual variation in such measures in relation to the same in drug response, the possibility that subgroups of subjects in the population that would be more appropriate to receive the drug than others, may be identified. There is a fundamental tension developing between the traditional treatment for the average of the population and the desire to treat the individual. This chapter will focus on key statistical challenges faced by pharmacogenomics studies of human disease and drug response, especially the genetics studies.

II. COMPLEX ADAPTIVE SYSTEMS, HUMAN HEALTH, AND DRUG RESPONSE

The following often ignored features of complex adaptive systems are relevant to the statistical analyses and study design as statisticians are presented with such vast numbers of measures of human biology in studies, conducted to understand the role of interindividual variation in any one or combination of these measures in the risk and progression of disease and drug response. Each individual in the population is a complex adaptive system and the fundamental unit of organization.[1] This means that the functional phenome type of the individual is dynamic with time. At any point of time, the functional phenome type is the product of the interaction between the unique genome type of the individual and suite of internal and external environmental experiences specific to the individual over its lifetime to that point.[2,3] This individual-specific genome type-environment interaction is ignored because the individual is considered as the experimental unit in designed clinical trials, with a necessity to focus on a small number of highly specific features of biological complexity as measures of response or covariates in relation to drug response. Traditionally, the other unmeasured aspects of biological complexity may be simultaneously coupled to the response and other covariates of drug treatment, as part of this genome type-environment interaction for the individual. Such complexities are captured as part of the random error term in the statistical model. To assume the random error term as independent and identically distributed among experimental units, has critical implications when considered in the context of these complex biological interactions and attempts to reveal the aspects relevant to prediction of drug response or risk of disease. The advances in technological capacity to measure human biology now presents a paradox to the statistician in collaborating with physicians, geneticists and biologists, as decisions must be made as to where and how to include many such measures that should not be considered part of the random error term.

Some measures of health or disease or drug response may be emergent features based on interactions among many agents, including genes, proteins, metabolites and environments that include drugs.[1] Emergent features, by definition, are not predictable from the considerations of separate contributions of agents in models. Manifestation of such emergent features is the result of complex, nonlinear, dynamic interactions among agents. One of the most difficult challenges for statisticians is to discover the salient aspects of such emergent features which are detectable in statistical interactions. This is at least partly true because of the vast potential for the considerations of prospective interactions in statistical models where so many agents can now be measured for each subject. These interactions will often be considered in simple, linear, additive models with relatively small sample sizes. Such linear, additive modeling approaches may often fail to detect important interactions and will only serve as first approximations attempting to identify some relevant features of the biology. Of course trade-offs are needed to simplify the complexity in modeling efforts. Solely using such simple approaches might lead to missing much relevant biology, and it is clear that more sophisticated interaction models are needed.[3-6]

The many agents in human complex adaptive systems participate in a dynamic network and most may not be direct causes of disease, health or drug response.[1] Despite the tremendous successes in identifying single genes responsible for human inborn errors of metabolism and mutations, such diseases represent only a small fraction of the noninfectious human disease load. The bulk of the noninfectious human disease load is due to complex, multifactorial disorders.[7] For these diseases, there is likely to be a more extensive, but largely unexplored, role of interindividual genetic variation in the dynamics of network of agents that would facilitate an enhanced understanding of interindividual variation in human disease and drug response.[8,9] The majority of human studies outside the pharmaceutical industry are based on single cross-sectional samples from the population of inference. The longitudinal nature of clinical trial, coupled with its tremendous capacity to measure human biology, presents unprecedented opportunities to model the dynamics of measured aspects of biological networks, relevant to better understanding of interindividual variation in drug response and human disease.

Networks of agents are organized hierarchically and heterarchically[10] into fields that are domains of relational order among agents[11] such that there are stronger relationships among agents within the fields and weaker relationships among fields.[12] The traditional characterizations of molecular pathways reflect this organization to a degree, but as a static view. From the perspective of complex adaptive systems, this organized substructure of networks reflects a dynamic view that is relevant to statisticians, but is largely unexplored, in the development and applications of statistical analyses. Relative to the traditional focus of statistical analyses on first moments, it expands the emphasis of the role of genetic variation in influencing higher moments that include the variance of agents[13,14] and covariance relationships among agents,[1,9] which can be dynamic with time and environmental context, in complex human disease and drug response. It also emphasizes the need to be cognizant that the models used only reflect associations and not causation.

The unique genome type of each individual provides the initial conditions and the capacity for change in response to environmental variation at any point of time. The capacity for change at any point of time has been traditionally referred to as the norm of reaction between genotype and response to environmental change by the geneticists. It is this norm of reaction in the defined time period of a clinical trial, which is the focus of genetic studies of drug response. For enhancing our understanding about the role of genetic variation in risk of disease and drug response, the difficult challenge to statisticians and biologists is to identify the relevant predictive combinations of shared genome type and environment features. There is difficulty at the genome level to identify such shared features, because there are more than 10 million single nucleotide polymorphisms (SNPs) known, the most common type of genetic polymorphism in the human genome, and likely there are more than 30,000 genes from which to sample such features. The complex nature of the problem, with a vast number of possible combinations to consider, makes the traditional linear additive modeling process difficult in comparison to the challenge. It is also clear that new approaches need to include the possibility that many models with different sets of combinations of interacting agents as predictors may have similar predictive capabilities.[15] The statistician has to consider development of many new tools to deal with this problem.

III. FRAMEWORK FOR QUESTIONS

Consideration of these key features of complex adaptive systems that are relevant to understanding the role of genetic variation in complex human diseases and drug response, suggests the simplified framework for defining questions to drive the development of statistical analyses and study design presented in Figure 16.1. This framework represents the complex biological hierarchy in three levels with genetic variation, which contains the DNA polymorphisms including SNPs at the bottom; the intermediate traits represented by gene expression (mRNA), proteins and metabolites and other physiological and biochemistry measures in the middle; and the disease and drug response endpoints at the top of the figure.

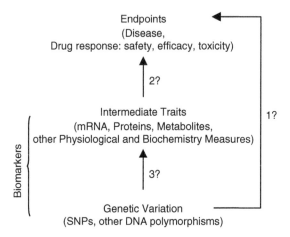

FIGURE 16.1 Framework for questions.

A key question is whether genetic variation at the DNA level can directly predict disease risk and drug response endpoints (Question 1 in Figure 16.1). This is because genotypes representing one or more polymorphisms within and among genes are generally considered fixed over an individual's life history, whereas the intermediate traits are usually in constant flux as part of the homeodynamics of adaptive responses to internal and external environmental changes. The fixed nature of genotypes is an advantage for developing potential diagnostics for disease risk or drug response if predictive genotypes can be identified. Because mRNA expression potentially varies with time, pharmaco-genomics, which includes DNA and mRNA in studies of interindividual variation in disease risk or drug response, is split between the two levels as shown in Figure 16.1. The combination of the DNA and intermediate trait levels represents the collective set of potential agents those are biomarkers of disease risk and drug response. There is also much interest in whether intermediate traits such as gene expression, proteins or metabolites may also be predictive of disease or drug response (Question 2 in Figure 16.1) or whether genotype influences on disease or drug response may be manifested indirectly through influences on the intermediate traits (Question 3 in Figure 16.1). This figure anticipates the upcoming development of systems biology which will attempt to put the "omics" together with an integrated approach to better understand interindividual variation in the complexities of biology that includes drug response.

IV. ADDITIONAL CHALLENGES

There are numerous additional challenges faced by the statistician that are specific to genetic studies, including those related to the fact that particular alleles of genetic polymorphisms are passed together on chromosomes from generation to generation, during the course of evolutionary time.[16–23] This shared evolution among polymorphisms has many implications for the development of statistical methods and design of clinical trial studies. There are many new specific methodologies that have been developed over the last 30 years, and especially in the last 10 years, which attempt to take into account some of the special dependencies among polymorphisms within and among individuals and the consequences for considerations in samples of individuals from the population.

Additional genetic challenges relate to the fact that a clinical trial is composed of individuals from different racial or ethnic populations that may also differ in the frequencies of relevant genetic polymorphisms. The mixture of samples from such populations means that it may be necessary to account for such genetic stratification in the analyses to help avoid spurious associations.[24–26] The traditional self-reported race or ethnicity labels may not be an accurate reflection of the underlying genetic structure and can impact the inferences from genetic association studies that do not consider the potential effects of mixtures of subjects from different population gene pools in the study sample.[27] Familiarity with many advances in statistical genetic methodologies would help the statistician, new to this area, to develop new methodologies required.

The many statistical tests and models which need to be applied in the context of relatively small sample sizes present additional difficulties from the perspective of the tradition of multiplicity adjustment. This challenge is not specific to genetic studies. Although there have also been significant developments in this area (for example, Refs. 28–31), false positive results are likely to be a common feature[32] of such massive studies compared to the relatively small sample sizes which will be typical of most studies for the foreseeable future. Compared with many years ago, there is a strong emphasis now placed on replicating associations of interest in one or more additional independent studies before those are deemed relevant for additional follow-up.

V. CONCLUSION

This is an exciting time for the statisticians in the pharmaceutical industries. The massive amount of data that will be produced at all levels in the biological hierarchy in the near future may be a dream-come-true for many. The challenges described in this paper are daunting but the progress and success in moving away from the fit of the drug for the average of population towards the individual will be measured, in part, by the extent of creativity and innovativeness of the statisticians, in collaboration with physicians, geneticists and biologists towards development of new analytical methodologies for understanding interindividual variation of human disease and drug response by recognizing relevant features and contexts of human complex adaptive systems.

REFERENCES

1. Zerba, K.E., Ferrell, R.E., and Sing, C.F., Complex adaptive systems and human health: the influence of common genotypes of the apolipoprotein E (ApoE) gene polymorphism and age on the relational order within a field of lipid metabolism traits, *Hum. Genet.*, 107(5), 466–475, 2000.
2. Zerba, K.E. and Sing, C.F., The role of genome type-environment interaction and time in understanding the impact of genetic polymorphisms on lipid metabolism, *Curr. Opin. Lipid.*, 4, 152–162, 1993.
3. Sing, C.F., Stengard, J.H., and Kardia, S.L., Genes, environment, and cardiovascular disease, *Arterioscler. Thromb. Vasc. Biol.*, 23(7), 1190–1196, 2003.
4. Cheverud, J.M. and Routman, E.J., Epistasis and its contribution to genetic variance components, *Genetics*, 139, 1455–1461, 1995.
5. Templeton, A.R., Epistasis and complex traits, In *Epistasis and the Evolutionary Process*, Wolf, J., Brodie, I.B., and Wade, M., eds., Oxford University Press, Oxford, pp. 41–57, 2000.
6. Stengard, J.H., Clark, A.G., Weiss, K.M., Kardia, S.L., Nickerson, D.A., Salomaa, V., Ehnholm, C., Boerwinkle, E., and Sing, C.F., Contributions of 18 additional DNA sequence variations in the gene encoding apolipoprotein E to explaining variation in quantitative measures of lipid metabolism, *Am. J. Hum. Genet.*, 71(3), 501–517, 2002.
7. Strohman, R.C., Ancient genomes, wise bodies, unhealthy people: limits of a genetic paradigm in biology and medicine, *Persp. Biol. Med.*, 37(1), 112–145, 1993.
8. Goodwin, B., *How the leopard changed its spots: the evolution of complexity*, Charles Scribner's Sons, New York, 1994.
9. Reilly, S.L., Ferrell, R.E., and Sing, C.F., The gender-specific apolipoprotein E genotype influence on the distribution of plasma lipids and apolipoproteins in the population of Rochester, MN. III. Correlations and covariances, *Am. J. Hum. Genet.*, 55, 1001–1018, 1994.
10. Yates, F.E., Self-organizing systems, In *The Logic of Life: The Challenge of Integrative Physiology*, Boyd, C.A.R. and Noble, D., eds., Oxford University Press, New York, pp. 189–226, 1993.
11. Goodwin, B.C., Toward a science of qualities, In *New metaphysical foundations of modern science*, Harman, W. and Clark, J., eds., Institute of Noetic Sciences, Sausalito, pp. 215–250, 1994.
12. Sing, C.F., Haviland, M.B., and Reilly, S.L., Genetic architecture of common multifactorial diseases. Variation in the Human Genome, *Ciba Found. Symp.*, 197, 211–232, 1996.
13. Reilly, S.L., Ferrell, R.E., Kottke, B.A., Kamboh, M.I., and Sing, C.F., The gender-specific apolipoprotein E genotype influence on the distribution of lipids and apolipoproteins in the population of Rochester, MN. I. Pleiotropic effects on means and variances, *Am. J. Hum. Genet.*, 49, 1155–1166, 1991.
14. Zerba, K.E., Ferrell, R.E., and Sing, C.F., Genotype-environment interaction: apolipoprotein E (*Apo E*) gene effects and age as an index of time and spatial context, *Genetics*, 143, 463–478, 1996.
15. Nelson, M.R., Kardia, S.L., Ferrell, R.E., and Sing, C.F., A combinatorial partitioning method to identify multilocus genotypic partitions that predict quantitative trait variation, *Genome. Res.*, 11(3), 458–470, 2001.

16. Templeton, A.R., Boerwinkle, E., and Sing, C.F., A cladistic analysis of phenotypic associations with haplotypes inferred from restriction endonuclease mapping. I. Basic theory and an analysis of alcohol dehydrogenase activity in *Drosophila, Genetics*, 117, 343–351, 1987.

17. Templeton, A.R., Sing, C.F., Kessling, A., and Humphries, S., A cladistic analysis of phenotype associations with haplotypes inferred from restriction endonuclease mapping. II. The analysis of natural populations, *Genetics*, 120, 1145–1154, 1988.

18. Templeton, A.R., Crandall, K.A., and Sing, C.F., A cladistic analysis of phenotypic associations with haplotypes inferred from restriction endonuclease mapping and DNA sequence data. III. Cladogram estimation, *Genetics*, 132(2), 619–633, 1992.

19. Templeton, A.R. and Sing, C.F., A cladistic analysis of phenotypic associations with haplotypes inferred from restriction endonuclease mapping and DNA sequence data. IV. Nested analyses under cladogram uncertainty and recombination, *Genetics*, 134, 659–669, 1993.

20. Templeton, A., A cladistic analysis of phenotypic associations with haplotypes inferred from restriction endonuclease mapping or DNA sequencing. V. Analysis of case/control sampling designs: Alzheimer's disease and the apoprotein E locus, *Genetics*, 140(1), 403–409, 1995.

21. Templeton, A.R., Cladistic approaches to identifying determinants of variability in multifactorial phenotypes and the evolutionary significance of variation in the human genome, In *Variation in the Human Genome. Ciba Foundation Symposium 197*, Chadwick, D. and Cardew, G., eds., Wiley, Chichester, pp. 259–283, 1996.

22. Weir, B.S., *Genetic Data Analysis II: Methods for Discrete Population Genetic Data*, Sinauer Association, Sunderland, 1996.

23. Seltman, H., Roeder, K., and Devlin, B., Evolutionary-based association analysis using haplotype data, *Genet. Epidemiol.*, 25(1), 48–58, 2003.

24. Devlin, B. and Roeder, K., Genomic control for association studies, *Biometrics*, 55, 997–1004, 1999.

25. Pritchard, J.K. and Rosenberg, N.A., Use of unlinked genetic markers to detect population stratification in association studies, *Am. J. Hum. Genet.*, 65(1), 220–228, 1999.

26. Pritchard, J.K., Stephens, M., and Donnelly, P., Inference of population structure using multilocus genotype data, *Genetics*, 155(2), 945–959, 2000.

27. Freedman, M.L., Reich, D., Penney, K.L. et al., Assessing the impact of population stratification on genetic association studies, *Nat. Genet.*, 36(4), 388–393, 2004.

28. Zaykin, D.V., Zhivotovsky, L.A., Westfall, P.H., and Weir, B.S., Truncated product method for combining P-values, *Genet. Epidemiol.*, 22(2), 170–185, 2002.

29. Devlin, B., Roeder, K., and Wasserman, L., Analysis of multilocus models of association, *Genet. Epidemiol.*, 25(1), 36–47, 2003.

30. Storey, J.D. and Tibshirani, R., Statistical significance for genomewide studies, *Proc. Natl. Acad. Sci. USA*, 100(16), 9440–9445, 2003.

31. Efron, B., Large-scale simultaneous hypothesis testing: the choice of a null hypothesis, *JASA*, 99(465), 96–104, 2004.

32. Hirschhorn, J.N., Lohmueller, K., Byrne, E., and Hirschhorn, K., A comprehensive review of genetic association studies, *Genet. Med.*, 4(2), 45–61, 2002.

17 Phase IV Postmarketing Studies

C. Ralph Buncher and Jia-Yeong Tsay

CONTENTS

I. INTRODUCTION

Experience has taught us that any drug has additional actions besides the efficacy activity for which the medication was approved. If a second activity is also therapeutic, then the sponsor may win approval for an additional indication. More often there is a set of routine side effects that are associated with the drug. A typical set might include dizziness, headaches, dry mouth, and so forth. Occasionally, some years after a drug has been approved, the scientific community discovers that there is a serious side effect such as an increased rate of heart valve problems or an increased rate of strokes or an increased rate of suicide. Depending on the characteristics of each situation, the drug may have new restrictions placed on its use or may be removed from the marketplace.

The statistician recognizes the primary role of sample size in these determinations. A series of a few thousand patients is often sufficient to prove efficacy. Routine side effects are also quite common, effecting in the range of 5% or more of patients, and thus are usually characterized during the efficacy studies. The less common side effects by their very nature involve fewer than 1% of patients, often in the neighborhood of 1 in 1000. Thus, in the voluminous records that are prepared for a New Drug Application (NDA), there may be three cases of a serious problem. Unfortunately, those three cases are surrounded by a dozen other situations in which there are three cases of a serious problem but the other cases are the random occurrences expected when all of the serious problems experienced by a diverse group of sick patients are recorded. The rate of 1 in 1000 will place the situation more in the anecdotal category than in the category in which statistical analysis is conclusive. If the rate is 1 in 10,000, then perhaps no instance of adverse reaction has yet been seen by the time the drug is approved.

Then after approval, the drug is placed in the marketplace and thousands or tens of thousands of patients start using it. With larger numbers, the true statistical facts may start to sort themselves out. Random events will not be higher than background risks but true rare side effects can be found. An exceptionally difficult task is how to find these rare side effects (less than 1 in 1000) with some reasonable expenditure of funds. Randomized controlled clinical trials are in general too expensive and too restricted to provide these answers. The more likely solution is to depend on observational studies in the realm of epidemiology. The field of Pharmacoepidemiology has emerged to resolve these problems. One example of the difficulties involved in these evaluations was given by Psaty et al.[1]

A number of situations can lead to an adverse drug reaction (ADR). The material may accumulate in an individual so the dose to that individual is large. The person may be taking one or more other drugs and the interaction between two or more medications causes the problem. The person may be consuming a particular food and the problem is caused by interaction between the food and the drug. The person may be exposed to an environmental factor and the interaction between that factor and the drug causes the problem.[2] Because the list of possible interacting materials is extensive, it is impossible in a routine system to record enough information to isolate the problem. If there is a specific hypothesis, then a designed study can be created to reveal whether the putative factors cause the reaction or not. No system has ever been universally found to be acceptable.[3] The Food and Drug Administration (FDA) has an Adverse Event Reporting System (AERS) to collect spontaneous adverse event (AE) reports worldwide for FDA approved drugs. The AERS was intended in part to pick up rare AEs, but it may fail when a rare AE is confounded with common population risks.[4]

Postmarketing studies, often called Phase IV studies, are important methods used to obtain more specific information about adverse reactions. For some products, the sponsor arranges to gather information on possible side effects after the drug enters the marketplace. These observational studies are in the realm of epidemiology. Usually there is a particular concern and the studies can be oriented towards answering a particular question. Perhaps a suspicious result appeared in the Phase III studies or other drugs in the same class are known to have characteristic side effects or the follow up period needs to be extended. Then these epidemiological studies, frequently involving thousands of patients, are used to provide answers. Another use is pharmacoeconomic evaluations.[5]

One other method to provide information on side effects is to have an ongoing registry of ADRs. After the thalidomide tragedy,[6] several such systems were established. More recent developments in computers and websites have enabled more modern systems to be functional. The United States FDA established a system called MedWatch in order to monitor "serious adverse reactions."[7] The FDA MedWatch Form can be seen in the last page of the Physicians' Desk Reference.[8] Serious events are any events that are fatal, life-threatening, permanently or significantly disabling, require or prolong hospitalization, cause a congenital anomaly, or need interventions to prevent permanent impairment or damage.

On the nongovernmental side are systems like the Boston Collaborative Drug Surveillance Program which was established in 1966. Cooperation between this unit and the Group Health Cooperative of Puget Sound located in Seattle, Washington and with the General Practice Research Database of the United Kingdom has resulted in more than 200 publications to help "quantify the potential adverse effects of prescription drugs." Also, a web-based database (www.clinicalstudyresults.org) sponsored by Pharmaceutical Research and Manufacturers of America (PhRMA), makes "clinical trial results for U.S.-marketed pharmaceuticals more transparent," including negative studies. Relevant AE information can be found at this site.

Another example is the Canadian database CADRIS (Canada's Adverse Drug Reaction Information System). Experience shows that all of these systems will involve underreporting of the true rate of any reaction. Therefore CADRIS cautions "it is impossible to project true incidence rates of adverse reactions based on the information captured by CADRIS." The Australian Adverse Drug Reactions Advisory Committee of the Therapeutic Goods Administration produces the Australian Adverse Drug Reactions Bulletin six times a year to update readers. All of these systems depend on physicians and patients to report putative adverse reactions so that a careful statistical analysis then has the opportunity, after adjusting for, or accounting for, the many potential biases in the system, to ascertain real problems from the apparent problems.

In the second edition of this book, Kathy Karpenter Wille described "Postmarketing Studies and Adverse Drug Experiences: The Role of Epidemiology."[9] Updated excerpts from that chapter follow to enable the reader to understand more about the advantages and limitations of postmarketing studies.

II. DEFINITION

Epidemiology is the study of the ways in which factors influence the patterns of disease occurrence in human populations.[10] Its application in the pharmaceutical industry can be from two views. First, when applied in the classical sense, descriptive epidemiology can be used during the drug development phase to clearly define the natural history of the disease to be treated. Second, drugs are factors that influence the patterns of disease occurrence in human populations; epidemiologic methods can be used to evaluate the benefits and risks of drugs in the treatment of diseases.

There are three main types of descriptive studies: correlational studies, case reports and case series, and cross-sectional surveys. These, types of studies are valuable in raising hypotheses; however, they are of limited value in testing hypotheses. To test hypotheses, either an observational or an interventional study is required. In observational studies, the investigator cannot allocate patients to exposure or any factors affecting disease status. Differences between groups can only be observed, not created experimentally. In an interventional study, the investigator randomizes the patient to the exposure.[11] In the pharmaceutical industry, observational studies are known as epidemiologic studies, and interventional studies are known as clinical trials. Clinical trials are the gold standard in establishing the efficacy of drugs. However, epidemiology is a tool that is useful in overcoming some limitations of clinical trials. Thus, observational trials complement interventional trials.

A. LIMITATIONS OF CLINICAL TRIALS

The randomized controlled clinical trial is the scientist's most powerful tool in establishing efficacy; however, the clinical trial is an imperfect tool. We can only obtain information in a limited number of patients within a limited spectrum of the disease state.

As information is accumulated prior to approval (Phases I, II, and III), the number of patients studied is only a small fraction of the number of patients that will be treated subsequent to approval. During Phase I trials, perhaps 20 to 40 normal, healthy volunteers will be studied. Phase II studies may involve 100 to 200 patients with the diseases of interest. In Phase III studies, the total number of patients studied rarely exceeds 3000, and this number may be much smaller. Relative to those who will be using the drug after approval, this is typically a small number of patients.

Clinical trials are conducted under strictly defined conditions on a carefully demarcated group of patients who are chosen to be as homogeneous as possible. The drug will be used under much broader conditions in a variety of patients in general use.[12] Because of the limited number of patients studied, it is unlikely that AEs occurring with a low frequency will be detected.

In order to have a 95% probability of observing at least one AE that has a true occurrence rate of 1 in 10,000, you would have to observe nearly 30,000 people. This follows from the Poisson probability law with parameter np, where n is the number of people observed and p is the incidence rate. Table 17.1 gives the study sizes for several combinations of rates and probability of observing at least one event. Note that when the probability of observing at least one event

TABLE 17.1
Number of Persons Required to Observe at Least One Occurrence of an Adverse Event (AE)

Frequency of AE	Probability of Observing at Least One AE			
	95%	90%	85%	80%
1/ 100	300	231	190	161
1/ 500	1498	1151	949	805
1/ 1000	2996	2303	1898	1610
1/ 5000	14,979	11,513	9486	8047
1/ 10,000	29,958	23,026	18,972	16,095
1/ 20,000	59,915	46,052	37,943	32,189
1/ 30,000	89,872	69,078	56,914	48,284
1/ 50,000	149,787	115,130	94,856	80,472
1/100,000	299,574	230,259	189,712	160,944
1/500,000	1,497,867	1,151,293	948,560	804,719

is 95%, the resulting sample size is generally three times the inverse of the rate. This is sometimes known as the "rule of three."[13] The magnitude of these numbers indicates that it would be a logistic nightmare to plan a clinical trial to detect or compare rare AEs.

B. STRENGTHS OF CLINICAL TRIALS

Randomization is the key to the strength of clinical trials. A primary role is to prevent bias in the allocation of treatments. This is the predominant way of controlling for potential confounding variables, particularly confounding by indication.[12] In practice, a physician treats a patient based on the symptoms presented. Most believe that the baseline characteristics of a patient affect the prognosis of that patient. If all patients presenting with similar baseline symptoms are treated with the same drug, and those patients presenting with different symptoms are treated with a different drug, then the association of drug and outcome is confounded by the baseline symptoms. Randomization ensures that patients have an equal probability of receiving the treatments under evaluation.

Compared to observational epidemiologic trials, intervention in the disease process by allocating patients to a treatment makes it easier to evaluate the effect. Prior to approval, the efficacy of the drug must be established; therefore, the clinical trial is the standard. The value of the epidemiologic trial is realized after the drug has been approved. The epidemiologic trial is used to further study the safety of a drug by examining the occurrence of rare AEs. In addition, the epidemiologic trial can also be used to study the economic benefits, health status, and quality of life related to drug treatment.

III. POSTMARKETING STUDIES

A. INTRODUCTION

Phase IV clinical trials are those that conducted after a drug has been approved and marketed. Some Phase IV studies are requested by the FDA as a condition for approval. Others are initiated voluntarily by the manufacturer to further investigate the drug. The typical Phase IV study uses a more heterogeneous population and is designed to more closely recreate the conditions found in general usage. The randomized controlled trial may be used to establish efficacy relative to a competitor or to broaden labeling claims.

As the drug becomes more widely distributed through marketing, previously unreported AEs are likely to be described. Epidemiologic studies provide a methodology for evaluating the risks of AEs that were not detected prior to marketing. Not only should the natural history of the disease be understood, but also the pharmacologic action of a drug needs consideration in the interpretation of the data from such studies.[14] The application of epidemiologic methods to the study of drug effects has emerged as a specialized field of epidemiology, known as pharmacoepidemiology.[12]

Pharmacoepidemiology joins together epidemiology and pharmacology, the study of the properties and reactions of drugs with respect to their therapeutic values. Most research referred to as pharmacoepidemiology occurs once a drug has been approved for marketing.[15] The discipline of pharmacoepidemiology is growing rapidly; there are meetings and journals dedicated to this topic. The application of pharmacoepidemiology will continue to grow as requests by the FDA for postmarketing studies increase and as the FDA comes to a decision about the interpretation of what constitutes the "adequate and well controlled investigations" required for drug approval.[16]

B. OBSERVATIONAL COHORT STUDIES

In observational cohort studies, whether prospective or retrospective, the patients or subjects are classified based on the presence or absence of exposure (to the drug). In a prospective study, patients are followed to a specified endpoint, or until the occurrence of the outcome of interest (an AE or disease). In a retrospective study, patients or subjects are still classified according to exposure; however, enough time has elapsed so the event of interest will have had the opportunity to occur. The controlled cohort study most closely resembles the controlled clinical trial, and it shares many of the same limitations of the clinical trial.[17] To detect differences in the rates of rare AEs, the sample size may be so large as to make this study design impractical. Further, because they are nonrandomized, cohort studies are subject to confounding by indication.[18]

C. CASE-CONTROL STUDIES

A case–control study is an observational study in which cases (those with the disease or outcome of interest) and controls (those without the disease or outcome of interest) are selected. Patients are interviewed or medical records may be reviewed to determine the presence or absence of exposure prior to the development of disease or some other outcome. The exposure in the cases is then compared to the exposure among the controls, and inferences are drawn.[11] Since the participants for case–control studies are selected on the basis of disease status, the design allows for selection of adequate numbers of diseased (and nondiseased) individuals to detect a significant difference. This design is particularly valuable when the disease or side effect being studied is rare.

Case–control studies provided the first clear evidence that oral contraceptives do increase the risk of thromboembolic and thrombotic disease.[19] Based on the results of the case–control studies, which were further substantiated with the results from cohort studies, the product labeling for several oral contraceptives warns of the increased risk of thromboembolic and thrombotic disease users of oral contraceptives.[8]

Major problems encountered with the case–control study are selection bias, resulting from differential selection of cases and controls based on exposure status, and differential recording or reporting of exposure information based on disease status.[11] Ideally, the cases would be all those occurring in a specific population (for example, a case registry, hospital records, or a Health Maintenance Organization) over a well-defined period of time, and the controls should be a sample of the population from which the cases developed.[20]

When studying the role of drugs in relation to disease status, it is important to remember that drug exposure is usually related to some underlying illness. In the more traditional case–control study the exposure (diet, occupation, chemical exposure, smoking history) tends to predate any medical problem. Thus, when evaluating the data from a case–control study in which a drug is hypothesized to be related to a disease, it is important to consider whether the underlying medical condition is related to the illness currently under investigation.[21]

D. EVALUATION OF EPIDEMIOLOGIC STUDIES

The interpretation of results and the conduct of epidemiological studies, particularly case–control studies, are often subjected to criticism and debate.[22–25] The following points should be considered in the evaluation of epidemiologic studies:

(1) The research hypothesis should be stated prior to collecting the data. If a relationship was not a part of the research hypothesis, then associations found subsequent to collection of data should be viewed as hypothesis generating. "Data dredging" brings up all the statistical issues associated with multiple comparisons. Some results

from case–control trials found through data dredging have been contradicted, or the results cannot be confirmed with a cohort study.

(2) In clinical trials, a great deal of effort is expended to ascertain the eligibility of patients; similar effort should take place in epidemiologic trials. For example, the researcher needs to ensure that the disease or AE does not precede exposure. Exposure and disease status should be clearly defined and verified.

(3) The data need to be obtained as objectively as possible. Relying on the memory of individuals to obtain exposure information can be misleading because of "recall bias". Cases may spend more effort searching their distant memory than controls. Studies should involve efforts to verify the patients' reports. For example, if a patient says a medication was taken, can this be verified through prescription records?

(4) To avoid selection bias, diagnosis of disease must be sought with equal rigor in the exposed group and the unexposed group. Preferably, the interviewer will be blinded to the exposure status.

E. AUTOMATED DATABASES

Data sources that link drug histories with medical care records can be used by pharmacoepidemiologists to investigate drugs and their relationship to ADRs in a specific population. If there are regulatory decisions to be made, particularly if there is some question about the safety of a drug, the study should be performed quickly. Automated databases provide a rapid means to identify large numbers of individuals who were exposed to a drug or who developed a disease.

The database should provide information on drug utilization, diagnosis, and demographics. There are many sources available for such data, and it is important to understand the circumstances under which the data were collected if the results are to be interpreted correctly. For example, if outpatient diagnostic codes are related to health insurance reimbursement, the incidence of this code selection may not reflect that of the general population.

The primary advantage of a large linked database is that of speed of access and flexibility.[26] The recorded exposures will include a vast array of drugs, and there will be different types of outcomes. Thus, the study possibilities are virtually limitless. Unfortunately, the large automated database cannot be used to study drugs that are not yet being prescribed, and even these databases cannot be used to detect very rare events (less than 1 in a 1000) with accuracy. However, the automated database is one of the most useful resources for epidemiologic investigations available to the pharmaceutical industry. If there is some indication of a safety issue, say the sponsor is getting reports of a previously unreported AE, the large linked database provides a means for testing a hypothesis in a comparatively short period of time.

IV. SURVEILLANCE/EPIDEMIOLOGIC INTELLIGENCE

A. INTRODUCTION

As discussed earlier, during Phase I through Phase III of drug development, the drug is studied within a limited population, the conditions under which a drug is studied are closely circumscribed and the duration of administration is limited. Thus, adverse reactions that are unlikely to be detected prior to marketing are (i) those that occur with a rare incidence (less than 1 in 10,000); (ii) those resulting from a specific interaction with concomitant drug therapies or a concurrent disease; or (iii) those requiring a long latency. One tool for detecting previously unreported adverse reactions is spontaneous reporting.

B. SPONTANEOUS REPORTING SYSTEM

Faich[27] has defined surveillance as the "systematic detection of drug-induced reactions by practical, uniform methods." One important aspect of this surveillance is the maintenance of a system for the reporting of ADRs. The FDA has a program to monitor ADRs of marketed drugs. The FDA monitoring program is based on reports that arise from the usual practice of medicine. This is experienced during the marketing phase, in contrast to AEs that arise from clinical trials prior to approval of the NDA. Reports can be made directly to the FDA, but more frequently, reports by health professionals and consumers are forwarded directly to the drug manufacturer. The manufacturer is required by law to submit all reports to the FDA. If the reaction is serious and not already listed in the product labeling, it must be submitted to the FDA within 15 working days of initial receipt of the information. All other spontaneous reports are submitted to the FDA periodically. When the FDA receives these reports, they are entered into a computer database. These data are reviewed and analyzed by the Office of Epidemiology and Biostatistics at the FDA, and they are available upon request through Freedom of Information.

C. INTERPRETING AND SUMMARIZING SPONTANEOUS DATA

Spontaneous reporting can provide a timely signal of risk. This early warning system was instrumental in establishing the association between flank pain syndrome (flank pain and transient liver failure) and suprofen, a nonsteroidal antiinflammatory drug.[28] Marketing of suprofen began in the United States in January of 1986, and by mid-March, five or six cases had been reported. In late April a "Dear Doctor letter" was sent out to more than 170,000 physicians. By the end of June, the FDA had received 117 reports of flank pain syndrome. Eventually, 366 cases were reported. In 291 of the 366 cases, the date of onset of flank pain syndrome was available, and it was possible to demonstrate a correlation between the number of cases of flank pain syndrome and suprofen usage.

The early warning system worked well in this context, because the event was unusual in the population not treated with suprofen, and the onset of flank pain syndrome occurred very shortly after taking one or two doses of suprofen. In addition, the individuals taking suprofen were healthy, so there were relatively few underlying diseases or concomitant exposures to confound the results.

The spontaneous reporting system is best used for signaling. One must remember that 'calculated rates' are 'reporting rates,' not 'true incidence rates.' These usually have to be expressed in terms of sales or prescriptions written. Under-reporting is a common problem with this system. Physicians may not be aware of this system, or they may be concerned about possible litigation.[27] The surveillance system was designed to detect possible safety problems with drugs, because they cannot all be known at the time of marketing, so physicians are encouraged to report all suspected adverse reactions. For any given report, there is no certainty that the suspected drug caused the reaction. Comparisons of drugs should not be made from this system; drugs are approved at different times, and they are monitored under different circumstances. The length of time a drug has been marketed, the drug class, recent publicity, or any number of other factors influence reporting.

Manufacturers are required to report an increase in serious, labeled ADRs. An increase in reports could signal a change in awareness or in patterns of use of the medication. An increase could indicate increasing rates of ADRs associated with longer administration of the drug, or an increase in reporting rates could reflect an increase in the occurrence of that disease in the population that is independent of drug administration. An increase in reports might also be a reaction to a media report. The reasons for an increase in the reports of serious, labeled ADRs are many, and probably cannot be discerned from the surveillance system. The surveillance system is a signaling system; an analytic study is frequently required to test the hypotheses it generates.

The reports for labeled ADRs should be reviewed at least as frequently as the cycle for submitting periodic reports. When a significant increase in frequency is found, a narrative summary must be submitted within 15 working days of its detection. Two approaches for detecting increased frequencies have been suggested, an arithmetic approach and a statistically based approach. Briefly, the arithmetic approach calls for reporting a doubling of reports from the comparative reporting period to the current reporting period after an appropriate adjustment for changes in drug usage has been made. Using the statistically based approach, the manufacturer would be required to report an increase in excess of the upper 95% confidence limit for the comparative reporting period after adjustment for drug usage.

The statistical approach uses a large sample approximation that is valid when the number of ADR reports is large. Norwood and Sampson[29] have developed an exact procedure based on a Poisson distribution to monitor ADRs that occur with a low frequency.

V. SUMMARY

One important role of epidemiology in the pharmaceutical industry is to evaluate the safety of a drug. More specifically, epidemiology is used to evaluate the relationship of a drug to AEs. Ideally, a signal would be detected through the spontaneous reporting system. Then, an epidemiologic study might be conducted to test the hypothesis; the data for the study could be drawn from an automated database. An inference would be drawn from the study results based on a scientific rationale. If the conclusion is that there is indeed a risk related to drug treatment, evaluation of the risk then requires an assessment of the benefits of the treatment. Benefit can be measured in terms of quality of life and economic reflections.

Unfortunately, the safety of a drug can easily become an emotional and sensational issue. There are situations in which the data are inadequate for drawing a scientifically supported conclusion, but they are of sufficient interest to attract comments by the press and the public. Once the media have mobilized the public against a drug, the damage is frequently irrevocable, even if the data are shown to be inadequate or subsequent studies exonerate the drug.[30] When there is a safety issue, the pharmaceutical company must act promptly to evaluate the relationship of the adverse drug reports and the drug.

REFERENCES

1. Psaty, B.M., Furgerg, C.D., Ray, W.A., and Weiss, N.S., Potential for conflict of interest in the evaluation of suspected adverse drug reactions. Use of Cerivastatin and risk of rhabdomyolysis, *JAMA*, 292, 2622–2631, 2004.
2. Mills, E., Montori, V.M., Wu, P., Gallicano, K., Clarke, M., and Guyatt, G., Interaction of St John's work with conventional drugs: systematic review of clinical trials, *Br. Med. J.*, 329, 27–30, 2004.
3. Gottlieb, S., Journal calls for new system to monitor post-marketing drug safety, *Br. Med. J.*, 329, 128 2004.
4. The Pink Sheet, pp. 7–8, October 4, 2004.
5. Liang, B.C., The drug development process III: Phase IV clinical trials, *Hosp. Physician*, 38, 42–44, 2002.
6. Lesso, J., The Thalidomide Tragedy: another example of animal research misleading science, Spring 1996 Issue of the CAFMR Newsletter, the Campaign Against Fraudulent Medical Research, Lawson, Australia, 1996.
7. Kessler, D.A., Introducing MedWatch: a new approach to reporting medication and device adverse effects and product problems, *JAMA*, 269, 2765–2768, 1993.
8. Physicians' Desk Reference, 59th ed., Thomson PDA at Montvale, New Jersey, pp. 782, 910, 2528, 3309, 2005.
9. Wille, K.K., Postmarketing studies and adverse drug experiences: the role of epidemiology, In *Statistics in the Pharmaceutical Industry*, 2nd ed., Buncher, C.R. and Tsay, J.-Y., eds., Marcel Dekker, New York, pp. 291–305, Chapter 15, Revised and Expanded, 1994.

10. Lilienfeld, A.M. and Lilienfeld, D.E., *Foundations of Epidemiology*, 2nd ed., Oxford University Press, New York, p. 3, 1980.

11. Hennekens, C.H. and Buring, J.E., *Epidemiology in Medicine*, Mayrent, S.L., ed., Little, Brown and Company, Boston, pp. 16–27, See also pp. 132–149, 1987.

12. Porta, M.S. and Hartzema, A.G., The contribution of epidemiology to the study of drugs, In *Pharmacoepidemiology, An Introduction*, Hartzema, A.G., Porta, M.S., and Tilson, H.H., eds., Harvey Whitney Books Company, Cincinnati, pp. 1–6, 1988.

13. Sackett, D.L., Haynes, R.B., Gent, M., and Taylor, D.W., Compliance, In *Monitoring for Drug Safety*, 2nd ed., Inman, W.H.W., ed., MTP Press, Lancaster, UK, pp. 471–483, 1986.

14. Lawson, D.H., Pharmacoepidemiology: a new discipline, *Br. Med. J.*, 289, 940–941, 1984.

15. Spitzer, W.O., Drugs as determinants of health and disease in the population: an orientation to the bridge science of pharmacoepidemiology, *J. Clin. Epidemiol.*, 44(8), 823–830, 1991.

16. Faich, G.A., Pharmacoepidemiology and clinical research, *J. Clin. Epidemiol.*, 44(8), 821–822, 1991.

17. Edlavitch, S.A., Postmarketing surveillance methodologies, In *Pharmacoepidemiology, An Introduction*, Hartzema, A.G., Porta, M.S., and Tilson, H.H., eds., Harvey Whitney Books Company, Cincinnati, pp. 27–36, 1988.

18. Johnston, S.C., Identifying confounding by indication through blinded prospective review, *Am. J. Epi.*, 154, 276–284, 2001.

19. Stadel, B.V., Oral contraceptives and cardiovascular disease, *N. Engl. J. Med.*, 305, 612–618, 1981.

20. Sartwell, P.E., Retrospective studies. A review for the clinician, *Ann. Intern. Med.*, 81, 381–386, 1974.

21. Jick, H. and Vessey, M.P., Case-control studies in the evaluation of drug-induced illness, *Am. J. Epidemiol.*, 107(1), 1–7, 1978.

22. Feinstein, A.R., Scientific standards in epidemiologic studies of the menace of daily life, *Science*, 242, 1257–1263, 1988.

23. Savitz, D.A., Greenland, S., Stolley, P.D., and Kelsey, J.L., Scientific Standards of Criticism: A Reaction to Scientific Standards in Epidemiologic Studies of the Menace of Daily Life, by A.R. Feinstein, *Epidemiology*, 1(1), 78–83, 1990.

24. Weiss, N.S., Scientific standards in epidemiologic studies, *Epidemiology*, 1(1), 85–86, 1990.

25. Feinstein, A.R., Scientific news and epidemiologic editorials: a reply to the critics, *Epidemiology*, 1(2), 170–180, 1990.

26. Walker, A.M., Large linked data resources, *J Clin. Res. Drug Dev.*, 1–5, 1989.

27. Faich, G.A., Special report: adverse-drug-reaction monitoring, *N. Engl. J. Med.*, 314, 1589–1592, 1986.

28. Rossi, A.C., Bosco, L., Faich, G.A., Tanner, A., and Temple, R., The importance of adverse reaction reporting by physicians: suprofen and the flank pain syndrome, *JAMA*, 259(8), 1203–1204, 1988.

29. Norwood, P.K. and Sampson, A.R., A statistical methodology for postmarketing surveillance of adverse drug reaction reports, *Stat. Med.*, 7, 1023–1030, 1988.

30. Melmon, K.L., Second thoughts: adverse effects of drug banning, *J. Clin. Epidemiol.*, 42(9), 921–923, 1989.

18 The Role of Contract Research Organizations in Clinical Research in the Pharmaceutical Industry

Roger E. Flora and John Constant

CONTENTS

I. INTRODUCTION

Contract Research Organizations (CROs) have played an increasingly important role in pharmaceutical research over the past decade. The role of these organizations within the pharmaceutical industry and their interactions with pharmaceutical companies in development of new drugs have been discussed in this chapter. CROs are defined in accordance with the services they provide and in terms of the organizational structure. The importance of CROs is then assessed by the amount of work they do in support of the clinical research activities by pharmaceutical companies. The underlying reasons for engaging CROs by the pharmaceutical companies and the role of statisticians in CROs keeping the statistical applications requirements in pharmaceutical industry in view are discussed from two different perspectives, viz., the role of statisticians in the pharmaceutical industry in interfacing with a CRO, and the role of CRO statisticians in performing necessary work within their own organizations as well as in interfacing with the client companies.

II. WHAT IS A CRO?

A CRO is defined in the Code *of Federal Regulations* (21 CFR Ch. 1, Sect. 312.3) as follows:

> CRO means a person that assumes, as an independent contractor with the sponsor, one or more of the obligations of the sponsor, e.g., design of a protocol, selection or monitoring of investigations, evaluation of reports, and preparation of materials to be submitted to the Food and Drug Administration.

This definition encompasses a broad range of activities or services but the primary services provided by CROs are those associated with planning and managing of clinical trials, data management, analysis, and reporting of the resultant outcome. More specifically, these services are:

Project planning and management
Design of clinical trial, including protocol and development of case report
 form
Management of clinical trials and in-site monitoring of investigations
Clinical data management
Statistical analysis, reporting, and consultation
Preparation of final clinical study reports and regulatory submissions
Support services at regulatory meetings
Regulatory affairs services

Project planning and management, involves formulating a detailed clinical development plan for a compound, device, or biologic, implementation and managing the execution thereafter. Remaining activities are key elements in the execution of the clinical development plan. The pharmaceutical company that is developing the compound may perform all of these activities, or any subset may be contracted to one or more CROs.

A full-service CRO is one that can provide the *full range* of activities associated with clinical development of a compound, device, or biologic. However only a small proportion of CROs can claim to have these capabilities. The majority of CROs offer some subset out of the complete list of services, or are particularly capable only in certain areas of the clinical development process. Therefore CROs range from very large organizations with clinical research capabilities as good as that of a major pharmaceutical company to a single individual or small organization operating in a narrow niche and offering specific services to the sponsoring company. Based on size of the organization and spectrum of offerings, the structure of a CRO depends on the number of employees and the range of services provided. In general, contrary to pharmaceutical companies even a full-service CRO will have fewer levels of decision-making authorities.

III. IMPORTANCE OF CROs IN PHARMACEUTICAL CLINICAL RESEARCH

CROs have become critical participants in pharmaceutical clinical research. The contract research market continues to grow at 13 to 15% per year.[1] As of December 2003, CROs controlled approximately 70% of the pharmaceutical outsourcing market.[2] Out of an estimated 1000 CROs currently in operation, only a handful have truly global capabilities,[3] but having experienced a six-fold market increase in the past decade, CROs account for some 10% of spending by R&D sponsors and are involved in about two-thirds of clinical projects.[4,5] The recent emergence of trade associations and specialists conferences dealing with CRO issues is another indication of the development and maturation of the CRO industry. In 2002, the Association for Clinical Research Organizations (ACRO) was formed to represent the trade group for large CROs, while another competing organization, yet unnamed, was formed in May 2004 for smaller CROs at "The Partnerships with CROs (and Other Outsourcing Providers)" conference in Orlando, Florida.[1]

To appreciate the change in the CRO industry it is interesting to compare survey results about a decade apart on research trends and involvements of CROs. Barnett Associates, Inc. conducted a survey of companies using CROs in 1989 for the Associates of Clinical Pharmacology.[6] The purpose of this survey was to determine key trends in pharmaceutical research over the following decade (the 1990s). A survey instrument was sent to "opinion leaders" in 26 companies and responses were received from 17. One of the eight trends reported was

> CROs will be increasingly involved in all aspects of the clinical research process, including managing clinical research projects and monitoring study sites for the industry.

Participants were asked to describe their past, current, and anticipated use of CROs for handling of complete development programs, as well as for components of the programs. Only six out of the 17 responding companies contracted full clinical development programs to CROs, and that accounted for only 5 to 15% of their development programs. Some of the smaller companies reported much more extensive use of CROs for this purpose. The sample, however, was heavily skewed toward the larger companies (14 out of the 17 respondents were among the largest 30 pharmaceutical companies); therefore, this could not necessarily be cited as a representative trend among smaller companies.

Of the 17 responding companies, 10 reported using CROs for the selection of investigators through writing of final study reports for about 8% of their studies. Only six of these companies, however, reported using CROs for these services 3 years earlier for only about 5% of their studies. A definite trend towards increased use of CROs for monitoring of individual studies was also indicated. In addition, the survey that 12 out of 17 respondents currently use CROs to monitor 5 to 10% of their studies, and 5 projected the use of CROs to monitor up to 17% of their studies 3 years later, increasing up to 25% 5 to 7 years later.

More recently, the Tufts Center for the Study of Drug Development conducted three surveys between 1998 and 2003 "to characterize CRO demographics, CRO interactions with sponsors and other outsourcing entities, expansion and contraction in sponsor demand for CRO services, and the response of CROs to the factors shaping the transformation of the R&D environment."[7] Among the findings reported by authors Christopher-Paul Milne, and Cherie Paquette, A.B. of the Tufts Center for the Study of Drug Development, the following well illustrate the establishment of CROs as critical participants in clinical research in the last decade.

1. With the globalization, multinational availability of CRO services is increasing. This follows the trend of the financial and IT sectors and also has been facilitated by the International Conference on Harmonisation (ICH) and the expansion of international trade, communication and travel. Asia and Australia appear to be the growth targets.

2. Patient recruitment is becoming more difficult and accounts for a significant portion of clinical development delays and R&D budget resources. "As academic medical centers (AMCs) have waned as the partner-of-choice of sponsors for conducting clinical trials, CROs have become conduits to patients and investigators that were formally the natural preserve of the AMCs. CRO methods for recruitment are resource-intensive and dependent on personal contact and relationship building, — something that CROs are more willing and better positioned to do than the pharmaceutical firms (or biotech, for different reasons). The CRO cog in the R&D wheel is kept in place by their continued access to patients, which now necessitates global reach. The hands-on methods used by CROs for recruitment are well-suited to non-traditional countries where the technology infrastructure is variable, recruitment service providers are not consistently available, and cultural taboos or even regulatory restrictions may limit media or Internet advertising... as obstacles for recruitment through hospitals and private practices are likely to increase in the US and Europe with the implementation of the Heath Insurance Portability & Accountability Act (HIPAA) regulations and the European Clinical Trials Directive, access to patients will drive further globalization of CRO services."[7]

3. From a regulatory perspective, while the Clinical Trial Directive is predicted to have a large eventual impact on submissions, processes and clinical research in the European Union, no final perspective emerged out by

the implementation date, i.e., May 1, 2004 because of nonuniform timelines in implementation across the member states. In contrast, in the U.S.A., the impact of the FDA Modernization Act (FDAMA) of 1997 and PDUFA III are clearer. These contained provisions intended to encourage conducting pediatric as well as pharmaco-economic studies, development of medicines for serious and life-threatening diseases (the fast-track provisions), submission of efficacy supplements, harmonization of regulatory requirements and the fulfillment of postmarketing commitments (PMCs). These have directly and indirectly given rise to an increase in demand for related CRO services, especially in the areas of pediatric research (although this has declined since the temporary demise of the pediatric rule in late 2002), supplemental studies, bio-availability, postmarketing studies, and studies in serious and life-threatening diseases. The demand for pharmaco-economic studies which showed an initial increase, decreased in recent years. Also, there has been higher than expected demand for preclinical and early clinical development services, as well as for postmarketing services.

According to the Tufts researchers, "CROs have shown themselves to be highly adaptable and have increased their value to sponsors by serving as reservoirs of specialized skills and resources in a highly unsettled R&D environment. Access to patients and the provision of global services will help to maintain CRO viability in the short-term. Long-term goals should include managing the CRO-sponsor relationship to maximize resource utilization and minimize cost and delay, acquiring new competencies ahead of the demand curve, and addressing sponsor concerns about staff turnover, company stability, and competing demands for resources."[7]

In another recent trend, the FDA has adopted a more consultative approach with sponsors in the postFDAMA era, which has led to increased demand for consultative services, including protocol design, representation at FDA meetings (preIND, preNDA, End of Ph II), clinical development planning and expert advisory services. In addition to the proliferation of niche providers of such services, the impact is also evident in some larger CROs (such as Parexel, Quintiles and PRA International) providing consultative services.

Another development has been the increase in demand for Data Monitoring Committee (DMC) work for larger morbidity and mortality trials, stemming in part from increased awareness of the need for DMCs, which was also reflected in the 2001 FDA draft guidance on that subject. This work tends to involve CRO statisticians in particular, performing either the role of Independent Statistician reporting to the DMC or, more rarely, that of Voting Statistician on the DMC. It is now quite common for CROs to be involved in the former role and also as the Data Analysis Center for the DMC, performing unblinded analyses independently of the trial project team to avoid biasing the trial. Voting membership has a more limited role among CROs, partly because of the level of experience required, but some CROs (e.g., PRA International) also perform this function as a matter of routine.

IV. WHY DO PHARMACEUTICAL COMPANIES USE CROs?

The time required to bring a new product to market has been the basic reason for the pharmaceutical companies to outsource clinical development and related activities to CROs as against mobilizing internal resources to do it. The time required to bring a new product to market is quite long relative to its patent life but the pressure of competition makes it extremely important to get a new product to market as quickly as possible even before any other company with similar product does it. Saving a few months or even days can result in million of dollars in additional revenue. If a company does not have trained staff available when a new pharmaceutical entity reaches the clinical development stage, valuable time could be lost before the necessary resources could be acquired and deployed. Addition of resources for the clinical development has to match with the company's research activities and the creation of increased capacity for the clinical development should not be proved to be redundant at any time. The use of CROs with relevant experience and resources therefore becomes the obvious choice to avoid the delays. This strategy also avoids a commitment to resources for which the need may soon disappear. Used in this way, CROs become a shared resource among many companies. This helps smoothening out the peaks in the workload for individual companies caused by fluctuating number of compounds at the development stage.

Another reason why pharmaceutical companies may turn to CROs is that CROs have minimum mobilization time and are often able to focus resources more quickly on a new project than pharmaceutical companies can. This can be attributed, at least in part, to the fewer levels of decision making authorities in CROs.

CROs can play an even more important role for new companies or start-up companies that have compounds at the development stage with no drug development capabilities. CROs provide these companies with a way to begin development of new pharmaceutical entities immediately without having to wait until they can develop the capabilities internally. Such companies would find it even more difficult to build the resources internally than companies that already have some clinical development staff but who would require additional personnel to undertake a new project. The start-up companies lack the basic infrastructure and the expertise necessary to assemble such resources quickly. This is the situation, for example, with many emerging biotech companies.

A pharmaceutical company may also use a CRO because of a special expertise the CRO has acquired. The CRO may have recent valuable experience in an area where the pharmaceutical company does not have. (The DMC work discussed already provides an example.) CROs can pass on the benefit of their experience gained from different clients on similar projects and while addressing a new project, the CROs can evolve the best combination of the different approaches they encountered.

The trend toward internationalization of drug development already noted in the previous section provides a final reason why pharmaceutical companies turn to CROs for assistance. The high cost and the lengthy time required to develop a new drug are compelling reasons to use data from studies undertaken in other countries when applying for registration within a given country. More uniform regulatory requirements and increased acceptance of data from other countries by regulatory authorities have made this much more feasible than it used to be in the past. Companies with international operations have moved, or are moving, to standard procedures depending on the country of operation in order to meet the goal of international drug development. For companies without an international presence, CROs provide means for accomplishing this goal. These companies can pursue development in different countries through CROs that have established operations in the target countries. Many CROs have created international operations specifically to meet the increased demand for international drug development.

V. THE ROLE OF THE STATISTICIAN IN CRO ACTIVITIES

The role of the statistician in CRO activities depends on whether the statistician works for the CRO or the sponsoring company. It also depends on the type of company contracting the services of the CRO and the amount of responsibility they are willing to transfer to the CRO. If the sponsor has no statistician, as might be the case for a start-up company, the statistician for the CRO would assume the full responsibility associated with the analysis and reporting function for a clinical trial or clinical development program. In this case, the CRO statistician's function would be essentially the same as that of a statistician working for the sponsoring company. Various aspects of this function are addressed in other chapters of this book and will not be dwelt on here. Consultative, design and regulatory interaction functions have become increasingly common statistical outsourcing requests in recent years.

The above would also hold if the sponsoring company assigned full responsibility for a program to the CRO. Such a complete transfer of responsibility, although increasingly common, is not the norm. Attention must then be given to the issues interaction between the company statistician and the CRO statistician to accomplish the objectives of the program effectively. This issue, along with related aspects of the interaction between the sponsor and the CRO, will be the focus of the remainder of this chapter.

When a study or program is contracted to a CRO, the freedom given to the CRO's statistician to control the statistical aspects of the program must be made clear. This is especially important if the only portion of the studies that constitute a development program are contracted to the CRO. In such cases, care must be taken to ensure that the statistical approach is consistent among studies. For example, the choice between parametric and nonparametric analysis may appear arbitrary for one study, while in another the choice seems to be obvious. Similarly, the choice between the Cochran–Mantel–Haenszel procedure and some other categorical data analysis such as a log-linear model analysis may be primarily a matter of preference. Consistency among studies should then dictate which analytic approach is used in the primary analysis. The primary project statistician for the sponsoring company must, in such cases, assume a major role in coordinating the analyses between the sponsor and the CRO. The statistical approach, conventions to be followed, and formats to be used must be determined and communicated to everyone involved. This does not mean, however, that the statistician of the sponsoring company should necessarily dictate the approach. Selection of the best approach should be a joint effort between the sponsor and CRO statisticians who are involved in the analysis. The key to the success of the project is good communication by both parties throughout the process.

In the early stage of the project, good communication regarding analysis and reporting issues is especially important. It is, in fact, desirable to have as much information as possible during the resource planning phase of the project. This will allow for a more realistic estimate of the work to be done. The sponsoring company's statistician can help facilitate this by making sure that the specifications for the project clearly delineate any special analysis and reporting considerations. Although the statistician may not be responsible for developing the project description, she or he should still be involved in preparing the specifications for the analysis and reporting. Sample reports and examples of tabular displays in the desired format can be quite helpful in communicating such requirements and have become a standard part of industry Statistical Analysis Plans (SAPs). Additional background information, including findings and data problems from similar studies, can also help prevent time from being spent ineffectively during the analysis process. Failure to establish realistic expectations and clear specifications for the services required can lead to a poor working relationship and unfulfilled objectives.

In the situation discussed above, it is clear that the primary project statistician for the sponsoring company must use strong project management skills in coordinating the analysis and reporting. Although this is also true when the project is handled entirely within the company, additional considerations are necessary when a CRO is used for some studies. It must be recognized that the CRO statisticians are not part of the *statistical culture* of the sponsoring company. Thus, they may not be accustomed to the same conventions and ways of doing things as those within the company. Failure to communicate this kind of information early in the process can lead to misunderstandings and to infructuous and expensive iterations in the analysis and reporting process. These, in turn, can lead to unwarranted delays in completion of the project.

The statistician for the CRO can also help facilitate the kind of interaction between the sponsor and the CRO that is essential to a successful joint development program. Preparing detailed analysis plans and submitting those to the sponsor for approval prior to performing the analysis and preparing the reports for a project will ensure mutual understanding with regards to its content and approach. The plans should indicate specific tabular summaries to be included and the formats for presentation. Such measures, by providing a focused plan of attack for the statistician and statistical programmers to follow, can substantially increase the efficiency of the analysis and reporting process.

A complete development program is contracted to the CRO with the intention of transferring the full responsibility for coordinating the analysis and reporting function. If, however, the sponsoring company has a strong internal statistical group, some interaction between the sponsor and CRO statisticians is still important. A certain *statistical culture* is likely to exist within the company which may have an impact on the statistical approach that is used and the conventions those are followed in presenting the data. Reviewers of the report will have certain expectations and may wish to retain a certain amount of control over what is done. It is incumbent upon the CRO statistician to be aware of these issues and to address them early in the program. As in the case of a joint development program, detailed analysis plans approved by the sponsor can enhance understanding and reduce the number of iterations required to complete the analyses and reports.

The purely statistical aspects of the work are the same and require the same basic knowledge and training no matter whether a statistician works for a pharmaceutical company or a CRO. Clearly, however, it is beneficial for a CRO statistician to have previous experience for a pharmaceutical company. Such experience provides a greater understanding of the needs of the pharmaceutical companies and the analysis and reporting processes within the organization. Similarly, many pharmaceutical and biotech companies now consider CRO background to be a substantial asset in a prospective statistician, as CROs often provide broad experience across many protocols as well as standards and cultures of diverse clientele. Joint clinical development programs between CROs and pharmaceutical companies demand additional skill for strong communication and project management. These are required on both sides if the analysis and reporting function are to be effectively accomplished through the joint efforts of two independent organizations.

REFERENCES

1. Small CROs Rise to the Global Challenge, CenterWatch, June 2004.
2. Pink Sheet, December 2003.
3. Schaub, W., Searching for a CRO—can the Internet help?, *Appl. Clin. Trial.*, 12(4), 45–48, 2003.
4. Pace of CRO Acquisitions Accelerates, *CenterWatch*, 9(7), 1–8, 2002.
5. Smith, N., The strains of pharming it out, *Scrip Mag.*, July/August, 32–33, 2002.
6. Barnett, S.T., Hilsinger, R., Harwood, F., and Ballard, R., Clinical research practices for the 1990s: results of a survey conducted for the Associates of Clinical Pharmacology, *J. Clin. Res. Pharmacoepidemiol.*, 4, 7–23, 1990. Code of Federal Regulations. *Title 21: Food and Drugs*, U.S. Government Printing Office, Washington, DC, Part 312, p. 63, 1991.
7. Milne, C.-P. and Paquette, C., Meeting the challenge of the evolving R&D paradigm: what role for CROs? *Am. Pharm. Outsour.*, 2004, http://americanpharmaceuticaloutsourcing.com/article = 32

19 Global Harmonization of Drug Development — A Clinical Statistics Perspective

*Peter H. van Ewijk, Bernhard Huitfeldt,
and Jia-Yeong Tsay*

CONTENTS

I. INTRODUCTION

The swelling costs for drug development combined with increasing price pressure on drugs imply that the home market has become too small for many pharmaceutical companies. One solution to this problem has been to expand the markets and globalize the business. The process of globalization started in the U.S.A. and Europe in the 1970s, but has accelerated since the 1990s. This process has been further facilitated by the recent opening up of the former Soviet Union with its satellite states and through the open policy of China.

In the pharmaceutical industry, globalization may involve multinational research, development, marketing application, manufacturing, and sales of new drugs in different parts of the world. One underlying driver of globalization is competition. When globalization took hold, competition got tougher.[1] The pharmaceutical industry is a particularly highly competitive industry in addition to its being highly regulated. Continuous research and development to feed the pipeline of new compounds is a way of staying ahead of competitors and may even become a matter of survival for many pharmaceutical companies. In consequence, a global pharmaceutical company has to evaluate its strategy of global resource allocation and its efficient use to optimize productivity and enhance its ability to compete.

Statistics is a field that makes an important contribution to drug development from early discovery to the commercialization of a product. In particular, the clinical trial phases engage statisticians in the design, conduct, analysis, and interpretation of data, in which both scientific and operational contributions are provided. This chapter will focus on the global harmonization of drug development in the international pharmaceutical industry from the clinical statistics perspective. We will discuss the current trends of the pharmaceutical industry with regard to globalization, its alignment to the current trends, what opportunities and possible downside we may face, and give our conclusions on the bottom line of global harmonization in the drug development process.

II. CURRENT TRENDS

A. ECONOMIC ENVIRONMENT

The development of a new drug is a very lengthy and costly process. In 1991, DiMasi et al.[2] found that from synthesis of a new chemical entity (NCE) in the lab to the final approval for marketing as a new drug, it would typically take more than a decade and cost $231 million. The trend of high cost in pharmaceutical research and development has continued to climb at a much higher rate than inflation during the last decade[3] and in the 2000s the development cost of a new drug has escalated to $802 million dollars.[4] This is also evident from the Center for Medicine Research (CMR) data as illustrated in the following graph (Figure 19.1).

Sales and R&D expenditure follow parallel upward curves, whereas development time is flat and number of new drugs decreases by about 40%. These two opposite trends imply that it costs increasingly more to develop a new drug and also that it is more and more difficult to successfully develop a new drug for marketing. This indicates that each drug that reaches the market needs to generate higher revenues to compensate for the increased costs.

Next to the increase in development cost, we see pressure from governments all over the world to limit the costs for healthcare, including treatment with pharmaceuticals. Therefore, the health economic documentation of a new drug becomes more and more important for the industry, primarily for justifying prices and reimbursements.

Another challenge presented to the pharmaceutical industry is that the patents of many major drugs expire in the mid 2000s, including the blockbusters of Merck's Zocor and Pfizer's Norvasc, for example. As a consequence, pharmacists are encouraged to use generics, prices for drugs are forced down, and some drugs are no longer reimbursed. All trends tend to put pressure on the margin and force companies to lower their costs and broaden their markets

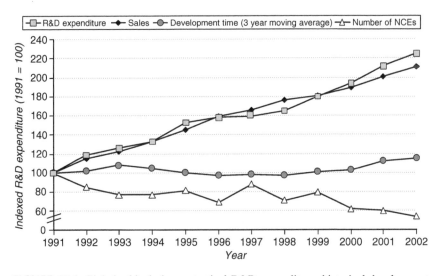

FIGURE 19.1 Global ethical pharmaceutical R&D expenditure, historical development time, NCE, output and sales 1991–2002. (Source: From CMR International 2003 R&D Compendium, March 2003. With permission.)

to increase sales. These trends prescribe a difficult time for the pharmaceutical industry in the mid 2000s.

On the other hand, the pharmaceutical market has continued to grow, though at a slower rate. For example, from November 2002 to October 2003, the world pharma annual sales still went up by 7% to $307 billion at constant exchange rates as reported by Scrip.[5] For the U.S.A., it went up 10% to $159.4 billion, with income from sales more than the rest of the world combined. It is expected that this trend will continue in the next decade, because the baby boomers will increase demand of drugs not only to treat diseases, but also to improve their quality of life.

B. SPREADING RISKS AND SYNERGY EFFECTS

With the trends of increasing costs to discover and develop new drugs and bring them to the market, pharmaceutical companies have to develop their business strategies to countervail these challenges. The common strategies are, for examples, merger, partnering, outsourcing (onshore and offshore), cosourcing, copromotion, cross-licensing, reengineering, and global harmonization of relevant processes and systems, as part of corporate strategy to enhance productivity and profitability and reduce the time to an optimal market share.

Merger is certainly a convenient way to compensate for the shortage of pipeline or to synergize expertise and resources. The merger trend in the pharmaceutical industry seems to be getting heated. In the five years from 1998 to 2003, Johnson & Johnson bought 34 companies and used its marketing power to turn some of their products into blockbusters, e.g., the arthritis drug, Remicade, from Centocor as reported by Arner and Weintraub.[6] Certainly, there are some more famous mega-mergers, e.g., Pfizer with Warner Lambert and Pharmacia, Ciba-Geigy with Sandoz, Glaxo with Burroughs Wellcome and SmithKline Beecham, Hoechst Roussel with Marion Merrell Dow and Rhone-Poulenc Rorer to become Aventis that was merged into Sanofi-Aventis, Astra with Zeneca, among others. Each of the aforementioned companies may have been the result of several mergers in the past as illustrated in the case of Sanofi-Aventis. In general, these mergers often aim at complementing the product portfolio for higher revenue and eliminate duplicate resources to reduce costs. Reducing the time to a good market share, spreading the risk and the other trends mentioned above, mean for the clinical statistician a much higher possibility of exposure to the outside world. The actual scenarios range from new colleagues in a merger setting to cooperation in a partnership or CRO setting.

Another trend in the pharmaceutical industry is to increase the development activities in lower cost countries, so called offshoring. Recruitment of patients for clinical trials in these countries is rapidly increasing. Some companies have even set up clinical development centers or data management centers in lower cost countries as the high tech industry did.[7]

C. COOPERATION AMONG REGULATORY AUTHORITIES, INDUSTRY, AND MEDICAL ORGANIZATIONS

Countries in the industrialized world recognized at different times in different regions that it was important to have an independent evaluation of medicinal products before they are allowed on the market, because some of them experienced tragic incidences (e.g., Elixir Sulfanilamide disaster and Thalidomide tragedy) of using medicinal products in their countries in the early to mid 20th century. During the 1960s and 1970s, those developed countries had experienced a rapid increase of laws, regulations, and guidelines for reporting and evaluating the data on safety, quality, and efficacy of new medicinal products. In the meantime, the pharmaceutical industry started expanding internationally to new global markets. Although the regulatory authorities in different countries required similar scientific data to evaluate the safety, quality, and efficacy of new medicinal products, the detailed technical requirements in different countries or regions were so different that the industry found it necessary to duplicate many expensive and time consuming studies in animals or humans in order to market new drugs in different markets. These diverging regulatory requirements resulted in escalation of R&D costs, more expensive health care to the public, and delayed availability of safe and efficacious drugs to patients in need.

In the 1980s, countries in the European Community started seeking harmonization of regulatory requirements. Their success in the regulatory harmonization prompted discussion on expanding the harmonization to other parts of the industrialized world. During that period, there were several bilateral discussions among regulatory authorities of Europe, Japan, and the U.S., i.e., the European Agency for the Evaluation of Medicinal Products (EMEA), the Ministry of Health, Labor and Welfare (MHLW), and the Food and Drug Administration (FDA), respectively, on possibilities of harmonization among their regions. In the meantime, the authorities approached the International Federation of Pharmaceutical Manufacturers' Associations (IFPMA) to discuss a joint regulatory-industry initiative on international harmonization and the International Conference on Harmonization (ICH) was conceived. In April 1990, the European Federation of Pharmaceutical Industries and Associations (EFPIA) hosted a meeting in Brussels, at which ICH was officially born.

Under ICH Guidelines,[8] sponsors of new drug applications now will be able to submit dossier or NDA documents to Europe and the U.S. using the Common Technical Documents structure. More or less the same data of same studies from different parts of the world in the same format can be used for most parts of the submission, and to Japan with some additional data from "Bridging Studies" as described in ICH-E5 Guideline. ICH has developed many other guidelines pertinent for clinical statistics, including ICH-E3 (The structure and content of a clinical study report), ICH-E9 (Statistical principles for clinical trials), and ICH-E10 (The choice of control in clinical trials) that provide good statistical guidelines for trial design, analysis, and presentation of results. Following ICH guidelines as accepted by EU, U.S., and Japan for new drug development, the pharmaceutical industry will be able to reduce a considerable amount of costs and to reduce the development time to register their drugs in different markets.

In the implementation of the above ICH guidelines, it was recognized by the European central regulatory body, EMEA, that they needed to be complemented in a number of areas to be fully effective. Therefore, EMEA initiated the development of a number of so called "Points to Consider" documents with the aim to facilitate the review of submissions and at the same time guide the pharmaceutical industry of the expected application of the ICH guidelines. These documents cover topics such as meta-analysis of clinical trials, handling of missing data, and multiplicity.[9] Examples of other cooperative efforts that have resulted in global standards are the Medical Dictionary for Regulatory Activities (MedDRA) for coding of adverse events and ICD-10 for classifications of diseases, which will be gradually replaced by MedDRA.

D. INCREASING COOPERATION AMONG COMPANIES

Among pharmaceutical companies, the cooperation is increasing, particularly with regard to political and regulatory issues. The Pharmaceutical Research and Manufacturers of America (PhRMA) is an organization representing "the country's leading research-based pharmaceutical and biotechnology companies, which are devoted to inventing medicines that allow patients to live longer, healthier, and more productive lives." Through PhRMA, its members pursue their cooperation to voice their interests and concerns to the government bodies like Congress or FDA about health care policies or pharmaceutical industry regulations. They frequently use their influence to lobby law-makers on drug related policy that may have profound effects on the pharmaceutical industry. Within the pharmaceutical industry, leaders of biostatistics and data management have plenty of opportunities to make their share of contribution through the Biostatistics and Data Management Technical Group (BDMTG) in the PhRMA. For instance, the BDMTG has established task forces to study specific issues and convey the issues and possible solutions to the FDA's attention. In the meantime, through their interaction with the FDA, they develop a partnership with the regulatory agency for the process of new drug development. In Europe the PhRMA equivalent is the EFPIA. There are no formal relations between EFPIA and the statistics community in Europe, except for some occasional contacts in relation to review of guidance documents.

In order to achieve further cooperation among companies to enhance efficiency to collect, process, and report data and information of clinical trials, the Clinical Data Interchange Standards Consortium (CDISC) was formed. The CDISC is an open, multidisciplinary, nonprofit organization committed to the development of industry standards to support the electronic acquisition, exchange, submission, and archiving of clinical trials data and metadata for medical and biopharmaceutical product development. Its impact will be dependent on the acceptance of the outcome among industries and its recognition by regulatory bodies. The FDA has been engaged in developing CDISC as submission data standards, which will be compatible with a greater scope of more general health data standards, called HL7, which was accepted by the U.S. Department of Health and Human Services. The impact of CDISC on the pharmaceutical industry and other regulatory bodies could be profound. Further details on CDISC can be seen at the website of http://www.cdisc.org/standards/index.html.

E. BUILDING A STRONG PROFESSIONAL COMMUNITY

The pharmaceutical industry requires highly sophisticated research and development. Statistics is an indispensable and integral part of R&D. Every year the Drug Information Association (DIA) has held numerous workshops on various topics about pharmaceutical R&D, including many statistics-related ones. Through DIA, statisticians in this industry have great opportunity to interact and develop a strong professional group within DIA. The American Statistical Association (ASA) established a Biopharmaceutical Section to provide a forum for statisticians working on pharmaceutical problems. The members of this section are very active in the ASA and have strong common interest to exchange their experiences, ideas, and regulatory information. It is interesting to note that in each annual joint statistical meetings, the sessions sponsored by the Biopharmaceutical Section always show very high attendance. Another statistical association that has regular activities in the biopharmaceutical area is the International Chinese Statistical Association (ICSA). Since 1990, the ICSA has regularly sponsored symposia on the themes of biopharmaceutical statistics.

In Europe, the European Federation of Statisticians in the Pharmaceutical Industry (EFSPI) is the leading statistical body with professional activities focused on the pharmaceutical industry. The objectives of the EFSPI are: "To promote professional standards of statistics and the standing of the statistical profession in matters pertinent to the European pharmaceutical industry; To offer a collective expert input on statistical matters to national and international authorities and organizations; To exchange information on and harmonize attitudes to the practice of statistics in the European pharmaceutical industry and within the member groups." Its members come from various European countries and its impact on the development of pharmaceutical statistics is well recognized. The largest national group within EFSPI is Statisticians in the Pharmaceutical Industry (PSI), which is based in the U.K. but with members from all over Europe.

F. IMPLICATION OF CURRENT TRENDS ON CLINICAL STATISTICS

Current trends of globalization in the pharmaceutical industry present challenges and opportunities to clinical statisticians. These trends concern an organization's outsourcing strategies, definition of common roles and responsi-bilities across the company, recruitment, training and education of staff, and finally the development of a globally harmonized process for the statistical work including sharing of resources and best practices. Other aspects concern global clinical development plans and the issue of bridging data from one region to another.

As mentioned earlier, drug development is a very lengthy and costly process. A clinical statistician can contribute to the process in many ways. For example, in the global drug development, harmonized statistical processes within a company can increase the efficiency in statistical work and reduce the chance of errors in statistical programming and data analyses, and thus shorten the development time. Efficient clinical trial design can reduce study costs and increase trial sensitivity to enhance the chance of a positive study. Presentation of more precise and accurate clinical data to regulatory agencies can be more convincing and will raise the chance of drug approval. Clinical statistics plays a critical role in these examples. In general, according to DiMasi,[4] clinical phases of a new drug development is most costly ($467 million in mean cost) and time consuming (72.1 months in mean time). The potential impact of clinical statistics on clinical development can be quite large. For instance, if statisticians can increase the success rates of drugs moving through clinical trials from currently estimated 21.5% to 33% by more efficient design, the average development costs can be reduced by $242 million for a drug, as calculated by DiMasi.[4]

G. AVAILABILITY OF ADVANCED TECHNOLOGY ALLOWING METHODOLOGY IN MODELING AND SIMULATION

Rapid increase of computer power and advanced technology turned drug discovery and research to a new era. Progress in genomics, including the complete sequencing of all human genes, enables many pharmaceutical companies to understand better the relationship of a disease and some relevant genes. Similarly, through the progress in proteomics, lab scientists try to understand the influence of protein on certain diseases. Many traditional animal studies became obsolete in drug discovery since the Genomics Revolution. Even some early clinical trials can be simulated in computer, so called *in silico*. Some major pharmaceutical companies can test their hypotheses on virtual patients in computer. They can also analyze relationship of genes or proteins to some diseases. With the help of advanced technology and computer power, the pharmaceutical companies can not only minimize the discovery waste, but also reduce clinical development time. Statisticians can play an important role as shown in Chapter Q.

H. INCREASED EXPOSURE TO PUBLIC SCRUTINY

Governments and regulatory agencies in the different regions and countries have been following the pharmaceutical industry for decades with ever-increasing attention. Clinical statisticians are used to guidelines and demands from the authorities and Institutional Review Boards. Meetings with the FDA on design of programs and studies to discuss the type and format of data for a file or to defend a dossier are quite common experiences for project statisticians. Safety in studies in life-threatening disease is nowadays routinely followed by Data Monitoring Committees (DMCs). These committees operate independently of the sponsor and are formed by experts from outside the pharmaceutical industry. One of the members is a statistician. The DMC has a big influence on the study because this committee can advise whether to stop or continue a study. The sponsor's statistician influences defining the roles and responsibilities of the DMC and plays an important role in the provision of the data. Many times statisticians are heavily involved in discussions on blinding issues. Next to the Data Monitoring Committee, there is a Steering Committee in many large studies. The steering committee is a new influential stakeholder, e.g., during protocol development. For a clinical statistician the existence of DMCs and steering committees means more interactions with the outside world.

A more recent development is the growing influence of external scientific world and public opinion. In addition to those committees around a study, academia and scientific bodies can influence clinical development. This ranges from the role of the investigators in clinical studies, ownership of data of studies to publications of the results. Statisticians in all companies share the value of carrying out their analyses in an unbiased way and publishing the results objectively. This role, however, is not always recognized by public opinion or the scientific community. In a joint editorial, Davidoff et al.[10] plead for more awareness of sponsor relationship and scientific integrity. They proposed to strengthen the role of the investigators: "We encourage investigators to use the revised ICMJE requirements on publication ethics to guide the negotiation of research contracts. Those contracts should give researchers a substantial say in trial design, access to the raw data, responsibility for data analysis and interpretation, and the right to publish." This proposal was not strictly implemented as such, but it stresses the importance to keep the quality and integrity of the studies, analyses, and reports at the highest level. It also encourages statisticians in their independent role and statistical ethics.

Another highly influential factor is formed by large-scale outcome studies. For instance, the Women's Health Initiative (WHI) trial of estrogen plus progestin in healthy postmenopausal women[11] resulted in a profound impact on the clinical practice in hormone replacement therapy. Another example with similar impact in the clinical practice in prevention of cardiovascular events was the ALLHAT study.[12,13] Discussions on the design and results of these high-profile studies take place in the public arena. In this manner clinical statisticians and their methodology become exposed to a much broader scrutiny.

III. INDUSTRY ALIGNMENT TO CURRENT TRENDS

As was described above, many global harmonization initiatives are pursued in different domains of clinical drug development involving the scientific community in general, regulatory agencies, and the international pharmaceutical industry in particular. In addition, internal industry demand for increased efficiency and cross-country cooperation drives the work for change towards increased global harmonization. For companies that have developed through organic growth or local acquisitions, this harmonization could be more naturally incorporated into the development of the company. However, for companies that are mergers of companies of different origins this puts additional strain on the process of global harmonization in terms of organization, processes, and human resources.

A. ORGANIZATION

The balance between a project-dominated and a function-dominated organization varies across companies and over time within a company. However, in most companies the clinical statisticians belong to one functional organization and are assigned to projects as needs arise. For nonclinical statisticians the picture is more scattered — in some companies these are organized together with the clinical statisticians, in others they are separately organized or directly employed by the nonclinical functions they are supporting.

For larger companies operating from different sites, each site usually has a group of statisticians. The reporting line for these statisticians is either to a local clinical function, possibly with a coordinating global skills leader, or directly to a global head of statistics. The latter model seems to dominate in larger international companies. It gives the statistics function a more pronounced global leadership and responsibility.

In most companies statistical programming and sometimes data management also belong to one and the same skills center enabling a close cooperation concerning operational matters and skills and capability development.

B. OUTSOURCING

Contract Research Organizations (CROs) are frequently used within the pharmaceutical industry for outsourcing of data management, monitoring, and sometimes also statistical work. The use of CROs for statistical work is more likely when a complete study from protocol to report is outsourced. Otherwise, the statistical design and statistical analysis are usually regarded as strategic elements of a clinical study and are therefore usually performed by inhouse experts. As a result of the globalization of drug development, the pharmaceutical industry is starting to build alliances with large global CROs for these activities. This will create benefits from large-scale agreements and promote consistent and efficient cooperation across countries and projects. There is little evidence yet of the use of resources in lower cost countries for statistical work. Planning, analysis, and reporting of clinical trials are usually done in close cooperation with the rest of the development team and cannot easily be done from long distance. Areas where there might be potential for use of such resources are for programming of descriptive statistical output and macros. Further detailed discussion on CROs can be seen in Chapter T.

C. ROLES AND RESPONSIBILITIES

The structure of statistical work in clinical drug development is rather well established in the pharmaceutical industry. Roles like Study Statistician and Project Statistician exist in most companies with small variations in responsibility. The former role is responsible for an individual study, the latter role for a whole project involving many studies from all phases. The Project Statistician usually also has a leadership role in relation to the Study Statisticians in the project. Higher level statistical roles may also exist such as Global Project Statistician with global responsibility for all projects formed around different indications or pharmaceutical formulations of a drug. Some companies have also appointed Statistical Experts for a whole Therapeutic Area. Other roles may exist, for example, Research Statistician with primary focus on methods development or with responsibility for certain capability areas, such as modeling and simulation or Bayesian methodology.

For an efficient and transparent cooperation across sites and countries it is important that these roles are given similar definitions. This should be easier to accomplish than trying to harmonize job titles, which appear to be more dependent on the local environment.

D. RECRUITMENT, TRAINING, AND EDUCATION

Statisticians in the pharmaceutical industry have the privilege of belonging to a strong professional community. Many in the U.S.A. and Europe have a broadly similar academic background with usually a M.Sc. or a Ph.D. in statistics or mathematical statistics. However, "Statistician" is not generally a profession protected by public authorization, even though certification schemes are in place in some countries, for example, United Kingdom, The Netherlands, Germany, and Spain. Therefore, a person could in principle be a statistician without any formal training at all. In Europe there is a large variation in educational programs that could lead to a statistical degree, and more or less statistics can be combined with many different subjects. An EFSPI Working Party[14] made an attempt to define the criteria for a "Qualified Statistician," which could be used as a reference for an appropriate background of a statistician in the international pharmaceutical industry.

The pharmaceutical statistical science has developed into a rather homogenous discipline through the decisive influence from the U.S. regulatory agency, and more recently also from the European regulators, and from some strong academic institutions in the U.S.A. and United Kingdom. This has created a favorable breeding ground for international recruitment of statisticians to the pharmaceutical industry and for secondment of individuals between groups at different sites. The same statistical language is spoken in most places.

However, the development of methodology has created a number of subspecialities, for example, in bioequivalence, sequential designs, interim analysis, and multiplicity. A global company is in a better position to develop the necessary critical mass for exploiting these new opportunities and to share experience and expert knowledge across sites and projects within the company.

Statistical work in a pharmaceutical industry is mostly about application of statistical methodology in medical and biological research. Therefore, understanding of the medical and biological aspects of the research is essential apart from being an expert in the possibilities and limitations of statistical methodology. In particular, the Global Project Statisticians also face other challenges in a global environment, for example, they must lead teams of statisticians from many countries, handle regulatory interactions across the world regarding statistical issues, and balance contending wills expressed by strong investigators from different parts of the world.

E. Harmonization of Processes

From a statistical point of view the clinical development of a drug represents the conducting of a series of clinical studies each containing a more or less fixed sequence of events. This includes the development of a study protocol and case report forms, data capture, cleaning and validation of data, the creation of a study database, statistical analysis, interpretation and reporting of study results, and finally a publication in most of the cases as depicted in Figure 19.2.

In all of these activities the study statistician is either accountable or a major contributor. Within this framework the actual carrying through of these activities can be done in a number of ways using different templates and standards, different division of labor on functions and roles, and using different tools. It is a general aspiration for a global company to harmonize these processes across different sites and projects. By doing so multiple different working practices,

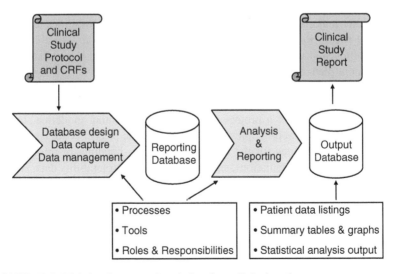

FIGURE 19.2 High-level process description for a clinical study.

supporting technologies and tools can be eliminated and more efficient cooperation could be established within all parts of the company. This will also facilitate simplification and streamlining of generic core activities so statistical experts could focus their time and talents on value-added activities in studies, data and reports. See for example a report from the Pharmacia experience by Mc Glynn.[15]

F.   GLOBAL CLINICAL DEVELOPMENT PLANS

It is now common that large international companies already from the outset plan for a global development of a new drug. The series of clinical studies to be performed then need to cover variations in incidence and prevalence of the disease between countries, different medical practices, different control treatments, and different regulatory standards. For example, the requirement for placebo-controlled studies and the possibilities to actually perform such studies in different countries is going to be a major challenge for the future and is something that must be accounted for early in the clinical development plan as reported by Huitfeldt et al.[16]

Current standards of confirmatory therapeutic and outcome studies necessitate that the conducting of large multinational clinical studies will involve thousands of patients. Pharmaceutical companies with a broad international presence can set up such large-scale studies much easier than smaller local companies through the engagement of their local marketing companies and the collaboration with international cooperative groups. These studies do present special statistical challenges for the design, conduct, analysis, and interpretation. Statisticians will necessarily play an essential role in such studies, not least in the sample size calculation, which becomes particular critical both with respect to the costs and feasibility.

Another major statistical challenge is to plan for the possibilities to use data from one region for registration in another region. Therefore, for a successful global submission the bridging strategies should be part of the global clinical development plan. See Section III.G below.

For a large clinical program involving many countries it will be fruitful to have a far reaching coordination and harmonization of the statistical approaches, possibly documented in a project wide statistical planning guideline. In such a document the general principles to be adopted by the project could be outlined, including common rules for the analysis of studies, handling of missing data, definition of analysis populations, analysis of safety and tolerability data, and also approaches to any meta-analyses to be performed for the integrated summaries of efficacy and safety including templates for cross-study data presentations. These approaches should then satisfy the highest scientific standards and regulatory requirements (usually with FDA as the objective) to ensure a successful worldwide registration.

It is also important to develop a common technical environment for all statisticians involved in a project regardless of location. Such an environment could include standard variable definitions and rules for derived variables, common coding conventions and dictionaries, common data cleaning and validation procedures, a unified definition of the database structure, standard access of data from a reporting database or a clinical data warehouse, common structure for organizing analysis datasets, programs, and outputs. In addition, it is very useful to develop a set of validated and documented programs (macros) easily accessible to produce standard output, e.g., patient data listings, patient demographics, safety data, and medical history. In order to accomplish this wish-list one has to invest a lot of resources, but this investment is profitable in the long run and can release energy and power to the essential scientific issues.

G. STATISTICAL ASPECTS ON BRIDGING

Most global development programs have a core consisting of a major registration package for the U.S./Europe supplemented by global and/or local programs for market development and support. For Japan and other Asian countries this core package cannot be used as such without being supplemented by additional studies, so called bridging studies. The purpose of these is to support the extrapolation of the conclusions from clinical trials performed in one region to another region, usually from the Western to Asian countries by linking the two regions with regard to some key characteristics. These key characteristics could be based on pharmacokinetic or pharmacodynamic variables but also on clinical efficacy and/or safety variables. Regions can differ in a number of aspects such as genetic, demographic, nutritional, or medical practice. From a statistical point of view bridging studies pose a number of challenges including nonrandomized comparisons, assessment of equivalence or nonequivalence, and sample size. Because of the nonrandomized nature of bridging studies, the collection of appropriate covariates becomes particularly important in order to evaluate any nonequivalence by adjusting for such covariates. The sample size in a bridging study is a balance between feasibility and a formal approach based on a power analysis. It is also a balance between regulatory requirements and the need for the company to ensure an effective and safe treatment for the new region. A more regulated bridging has been possible by the ICH guideline "Ethnic factors in the acceptability of foreign data."[8] Further statistical aspects of bridging can be found in Liu and Chow[17] and Chapter 20.

IV. THE OTHER SIDE OF THE COIN AND HR PERSPECTIVES

The previous section may have given the impression that harmonization and globalization only have advantages. Everyone who has been involved in these processes, however, will agree that these trends seem unavoidable though not necessarily always advantageous and/or easy to handle in all aspects. This section will focus on the other side of the coin.

A. ORGANIZATION

As described earlier, most companies have some sort of matrix organization in which in general the statisticians belong to a functional organization and are assigned to projects. This is a complex structure that inherently brings ambiguities in decision making. Decision lines can be long and many stakeholders are involved. The decision power is further diluted when different sites in different countries or even different continents are involved in global projects. In the end this can lead to decisions being taken "too late" or by managers who are "too far" from the work floor.

B. ROLES AND RESPONSIBILITIES

Although the role of a Project Statistician does not seem to change greatly when moving into a global arena, the need for communicational, social, and political skills becomes even more prominent. One must be able to handle different cultures, different ways of communication, and company politics. Managing, or maybe better "influencing," people from a long distance, both in geographical and cultural meaning, can be quite a challenge. Project Statisticians therefore, should be highly communicative and comfortable with video- and tele-conferencing, and use E-mail in a proper way. The cultural background influences the way of communication. Statisticians working on a global scale, so called Global Project Statisticians in some companies, should be able to understand the "real" message, regardless of the exact words of the message.

Of course, company politics is not a new phenomenon. However, Global Project Statisticians will have a much wider internal interaction than in the past and thus will more likely be confronted with company politics. This global focus makes life for statisticians much more challenging, interesting, and rewarding. So, from a dull number cruncher who would never leave his room far away, the statistician has changed into a player on the global scene. Statisticians travel all over the world and expatriate statisticians are no longer an exception.

C. RECRUITMENT, TRAINING, AND EDUCATION

With these social, cultural, and political skills becoming more and more important in the global collaboration, one can wonder whether the technical, statistical background still should be the main driver when appointing new leaders in the statistical arena. However, strong strategic thinking is expected from these persons. Therefore, the Global Project Statisticians and managers in the statistical departments should have a strong training in statistics. This is indeed the usual background of statisticians in the pharmaceutical industry. Already at recruitment the social and communicational skills form an important aspect in the choice. Furthermore, training and career development are very much focused on the social, political, and leadership skills.

D. Cultural Aspects

In spite of the professional concordance that exists among statisticians involved in clinical drug development, this cannot conceal some major differences that exist between companies and between countries regarding cultural matters. These cultural differences make cross-country cooperation sometimes difficult and rather challenging. They could concern not only different native languages, but also differences in management styles, performance assessment, common values, etc. These aspects of globalization are not specific to statisticians, but cannot be ignored in the belief that the strong professional solidarity could smooth over such differences.

Cultural or political differences can also cause the regulatory authorities or governments to set different requirements, which can complicate the work of a statistician. One example is the requirement about part of the demographic data that need to be assembled, namely race and ethnic origin (see, e.g., the FDA's draft guideline). The classification required can easily be implemented in the U.S., but is difficult to handle or even illegal in some other countries. A statistician will ask for a consistent classification over all sites in a study and project. If this does not happen, one can easily end up with overlapping classes, causing the disposition of subjects to become incomprehensible and the programming of tables highly complicated.

E. Balance between Harmonization, Standardization, and Flexibility

As indicated above, harmonization of processes will aim to increase the efficiency and free resources for value-added statistical activities. However, there is a balance between harmonization and standardization and flexibility. Global harmonization in general brings a quite strict system of standard procedures, with a major part laid down in operating procedures, standards and computer applications. Maintaining the standards can become a major effort. Or worse, there is a clear danger that the standards become a goal in themself.

In this setting, changing the standards gets very complicated due to the many stakeholders and interdependencies. For instance, changing the protocol numbering system, which for statisticians is hardly relevant, can be an enormous challenge since so many departments use these numbers, ranging from controllers and financial people to clinical monitors in the field. These standards and the difficulty of changing them can seriously decrease the flexibility and become counterproductive.

Many companies therefore have a hierarchy of standards: the core or company standards refer to all activities, like the Adverse Event form. The level below the company standards is of the therapeutic area standards, followed by the project standards. In most companies the statistical standards within a project are maintained by the Global Project Statistician. This seems to be the right balance between short decision lines and flexibility versus efficiency, predictability of output, and smooth interfacing. Next, more flexibility is brought into the early phases of clinical development. For phase I studies in general, less strict standards are used. A similar attitude is seen with regard to early phase II activities.

The danger of too rigid standards can even be truer for the IT-applications and -systems. Especially, if no sensible split up is made, in independent modules with a limited number of interdependencies, it is very likely that the systems become so complicated that no one can oversee the whole and the effect of changes can only be sorted out by trial and error. A good example of an activity with many interdependencies and stakeholders is the randomization. The procedures and systems for randomization form a fundamental basis for the clinical studies as every statistician knows. Many parties, often in quite different parts of a pharmaceutical company, are involved or rely upon the randomization system. During development of such a system, pressure will be high to adapt the system to the wishes and standards of the different departments. Management should be very keen to keep the scope of the system limited and the interfaces simple.

Other situations where different standards will collapse, are partnering, merging, or take over. During take over it is likely that the standards of the company taking over are imposed upon the other. This brings a big shocking effect. People may interpret this forced change as a statement of low performance in the past. This of course is not true: there are many ways to do a job, with negligible differences in final output. Next, this change will bring a feeling of discomfort, since one has to get accustomed to the new standards and find the ways to go. A statistician going from one company to another will have a similar experience.

F. GLOBALIZATION AND THE INDIVIDUAL

The overload of SOPs, guidelines (who really knows all ICH-guidelines?) and other standards can make a statistician new to the industry wonder what kind of world the person has entered. For the "senior" employees this may look like a well defined and well structured environment in which it is clear to see what your degrees of freedom are. A newcomer can be highly uncertain of what he/she is allowed to decide upon personally, and where to go if one wants to know personal authority in changing the standards. So, this might lead to lack of ownership and critical attitude. This will lower motivation and probably will negatively impact the quality of the work.

The high degree of regulation can seriously lower the drive for innovation and become a denominational factor for more experienced statisticians. People will be inclined to follow the routes that others have already taken, or that they have taken themselves in the past, and are less willing to take risks and follow other routes. Even if one really sees opportunities and is willing to take another course, it can take enormous perseverance to change the course of the company, like a small individual trying to change the course of a huge ship. This is detrimental to innovation and flexibility. Statisticians should realize that the standards are there to help them and free their time for highly value added activities, which will increase productivity in the end.

Therefore, management should strive for a good mix of people: innovators, who will keep looking for other routes and will challenge standards, and builders, who can form the backbone of the company and will keep the processes, applications, and systems going and modify where needed.

G. Harmonization, Regulatory Authorities, and Governments

Despite the ICH-initiatives and the globalization trend in societies, still there are strong differences between countries, which impact the job of a statistician. Noninferiority, just to name one subject, is treated differently by the FDA and the EMEA (see Huitfeldt et al.[16]). The position on placebo-controlled studies is also far from unanimous over the globe. Even if the regulatory authorities would be able to come to a complete harmonization of their requirements, cultural differences will remain a contributor to differences in results and final decisions on the dossier. Balant and Balant-Gorgia[18] give an interesting overview of cultural aspects that can contribute to the drug response.

V. SUMMARY AND CONCLUSIONS

Drug development is increasingly expensive. There is a pressure on prices from regulators and customers; fewer and fewer new drugs reach the market, and companies encounter increasing competition as never before. These trends result in continuing attempts to expand the markets and globalize the business by the pharmaceutical industry in order to save costs and increase revenues through spreading of risks and seeking synergy of effects from mergers and partnerships. This is facilitated by the technical and scientific development, which supports the global aspirations by the industry through increasing cooperations between regulatory authorities, industry, and medical organizations.

Clinical statistics is an important contributor through all phases of the clinical development and the current trends of globalization present many challenges and opportunities. This affects organization, outsourcing, roles and responsibilities, recruitment, training and education of staff, and processes for the statistical work. Other aspects of globalization relate to the clinical development plan including the statistical aspects of bridging, and the need for global standards and a common technical environment.

Clinical statistics is not only affected by these trends but should also take responsibility to lead the technical and statistical aspects of this development in terms of implementing standards, controlling for variability, sensible analyses and interpretation of multinational studies and programs, etc.

The downside of this development is the risk for large unwieldy organizations with decision-makers far away from the shop floor. A too far reaching standardization is difficult to pursue and maintain and has a tendency to conserve old thinking and prevent innovation and flexibility to flourish. Working in an international environment puts additional strains on communication, social and language skills, and adaptation to different cultural environments.

Globalization of the pharmaceutical industry seems to prevail and even be further reinforced. Clinical biostatistics is heavily affected by this development but can also make significant contributions to the capitalization of the opportunities created thereby. Much of the standardization and harmonization that follow globalization of the industry can, if sensibly implemented, allow the clinical statisticians to focus on the added value of their scientific and operational contributions.

REFERENCES

1. Soros, G., *George Soros on Globalization*, New York, Public Affairs, pp. 149–180, 2002.
2. DiMasi, J.A., Hansen, R.W., Grabowski, H.G., and Lasagna, L., Cost of innovation in the pharmaceutical industry, *J. Health Econ.*, 10, 107–142, 1991.
3. Barrett, A., Carey, J., and Arndt, M., Feeding the drug pipeline, *Business Week*, 78, May 12, 2003.
4. DiMasi, J.A., Hansen, R.W., and Grabowski, H.G., The price of innovation: new estimates of drug development costs, *J. Health Econ.*, 22, 151–185, 2003.
5. Scrip — World Pharmaceutical News, S00827726 — Scrip, filed December 23, 2003, PJB Publications Ltd, December 29, 2003.
6. Arner, F. and Weintraub, A., Can J&J tough out its drought? *Business Week*, 84 January 26, 2004.
7. Robison, M. and Kalakota, R., *Offshore Outsourcing: Business Models, ROI and Best Practices*, Mivar Press, Alpharetta, GA, pp. 73–100, 2004.
8. ICH — International Conference on Harmonization (see website: http://www.ich.org).
9. EMEA — the European Agency for the Evaluation of Medicinal Products (see website: http://www.emea.eu.int).
10. Davidoff, F., DeAngelis, C.D., Drazen, J.M., et al., Sponsorship, authorship, and accountability, *J. Am. Med. Assoc.*, 286, 1232–1234, 2001, Editorial.
11. Writing Group for the Women's Health Initiative Investigators, Risks and benefits of estrogen plus progestin in healthy postmenopausal women, *J. Am. Med. Assoc.*, 288, 321–333, 2002.
12. The ALLHAT Officers and Coordinators for the ALLHAT Collaborating Research Group, Major outcomes in high-risk hypertensive patients randomized to angiotensin-converting enzyme inhibitor or calcium channel blocker vs. diuretic: the antihypertensive and lipid-lowering treatment to prevent heart attack trial (ALLHAT), *J. Am. Med. Assoc.*, 288, 2981–2997, 2002.
13. Cardiovascular outcomes using doxazosin vs. chlorthalidone for the treatment of hypertension in older adults with and without glucose disorder: a report from the ALLHAT Study, *J. Clin. Hypertens.*, 6, 116–125, 2004.

14. EFSPI Working Party, Qualified statisticians in the European pharmaceutical industry, *Drug Info. J.*, 33, 407–415, 1999.
15. McGlynn, B., Built for speed, *Scrip Mag.*, May, 23–25, 2003.
16. Huitfeldt, B., Danielson, L., Ebbutt, A., and Schmidt, K., Choice of control in clinical trials — issues and implications of ICH-E10, *Drug Info. J.*, 35, 1147–1156, 2001.
17. Liu, J. and Chow, S.-C., Bridging studies in clinical trials, *J. Biopharm. Stat.*, 12, 359–368, 2002.
18. Balant, L.P. and Balant-Gorgia, E.A., Culture difference: implications on drug therapy and global drug development, *Int. J. Clin. Pharm. Ther.*, 38, 47–52, 2000.

20 Bridging Strategies in Global Drug Development

Mamoru Narukawa and Masahiro Takeuchi

CONTENTS

I. INTRODUCTION

Research and development (R&D) of a pharmaceutical product requires considerable time as well as a large amount of resources (human, money, etc.). It is said[1] that it takes around 15 years from the start of research on a compound of future pharmaceutical product to its registration as a new drug, and that the success rate is one out of some 12,000. Against this background, many of the pharmaceutical companies are working hard to develop global strategies to promote efficiency as well as concentration of pharmaceutical research and

345

development. Merger and acquisition (M&A) has been on the sharp increase especially in the U.S. and European countries against the backdrop of liberalization of trade and investment — the pharmaceutical industry is no exception. Many major pharmaceutical companies have been making strong efforts to expand business overseas.

The activities of the International Conference on Harmonization (ICH) must have added great momentum to such globalization of the pharmaceutical industry and new drug development. Out of many guidelines adopted at the ICH, the guideline on "Ethnic factors in the acceptability of foreign clinical data" has been exerting great influence on the strategy of new drug development in the world.[2,3] This guideline has been put to practical use since 1998, and several issues to be considered in successfully implementing it have been pointed out.

This chapter presents the historical background and the current status of international harmonization concerning new drug development, focusing on the handling of foreign clinical data, and discusses some statistical issues to be considered to promote the use of foreign clinical data for new drug registration.

II. GLOBALIZATION OF PHARMACEUTICAL INDUSTRY AND NEW DRUG DEVELOPMENT

Table 20.1 shows the pharmaceutical sales by region in 2003.[4] The pharmaceutical industry will be one of the few growth industries that will lead the world economy in the future. It is expected that the world market in pharmaceuticals will grow steadily for the foreseeable future. It should be noted that almost all the ten top selling products are marketed worldwide.

Striving to secure the scale of R&D cost, to supplement the pipeline of future new drugs, and to expand the sales force in the circumstances where the steep

TABLE 20.1
Pharmaceutical Sales by Region in 2003

Region	Sales ($ billion)	% Global Sales
North America	229.5	49
European Union	115.4	25
Rest of Europe	14.3	3
Japan	52.4	11
Asia, Africa, and Australia	37.3	8
Latin America	17.4	4
TOTAL	466.3	100

IMS World Review 2004. www.ims-global.com

surge of R&D expenditure is anticipated in this biotechnology age, about half of the top 20 pharmaceutical companies have experienced merger or acquisition during these ten years. Although some doubt has been raised as to just getting bigger and bigger,[5] this trend is expected to continue. Actually, almost all of the top companies have been doing business such as research and sales of pharmaceuticals globally, and some new drugs that were developed simultaneously in the world have already been marketed in European countries, Japan, and the U.S. There has been a recognized need to find ways to reduce development time, to reduce duplication of efforts and wastage of clinical and animal resources, and thereby, to reduce costs for new drug development. The biotechnology revolution makes the situation even more urgent.

III. INTERNATIONAL HARMONIZATION OF PHARMACEUTICAL REGULATION AND ICH

From the viewpoint of saving resources as well as providing new drugs to patients sooner, there will be a great impact if pharmaceutical companies can utilize data for new drug registration that were collected in foreign countries, without conducting additional domestic studies. Based on this kind of idea, when utilizing foreign data including data from clinical studies, expectation of expanding the range and depth had been increasing, reflecting the recent globalization of new drug development. In addition to the globalization and consolidation in the industry, governments in charge of pharmaceutical regulation found a need to increase communication with each other, and thus formed bilateral and multilateral efforts for this purpose.

The International Conference on Harmonisation of Technical Requirements for Registration of Pharmaceuticals for Human Use is a joint regulatory-industry initiative on international harmonization with the aim to provide availability of new drugs to patients sooner through harmonizing technical requirements of new drug registration in Europe, Japan, and the United States. This is done by promoting mutual acceptance of new drug registration data, and by avoiding duplication of clinical and animal studies without compromising the regulatory obligations of securing safety and effectiveness. It was established in 1990 as a joint regulatory-industry effort to improve, through harmonization, the efficiency of the process for developing and registering good quality, safe and effective new drugs in the world. A variety of topics, mainly in the three areas, i.e., quality (chemical and pharmaceutical quality assurance), safety (*in vitro* and *in vivo* nonclinical studies), and efficacy (clinical studies) were chosen, and have been discussed toward establishing harmonized guidelines. Its general process is to identify and then reduce differences in technical requirements for new drug development among regulatory agencies. Agreement has been made on more than 50 topics, and harmonized guidelines have been implemented in the three regions.

IV. ICH E-5 GUIDELINE

A. History

When a substantial body of clinical data, including those of Phase III confirmatory studies, has been gathered in certain regions, global drug development would be accelerated if the evidence of efficacy and safety could be extrapolated to another region without repeating clinical studies on the same scale in the new region. This is the principal concept for utilizing foreign clinical data.

Historically, it was recognized widely in the three regions (European countries, Japan, and the United States) that ethnic and regional differences that could influence the evaluation of new drugs are unavoidable barriers in accepting foreign clinical data. Each region established its regulation in the 1980s concerning the conditions for registration of new drugs based on foreign clinical data. Although emphasizing the importance of the quality of the clinical studies conducted in foreign countries, each region showed the policy that foreign clinical data would be acceptable as long as it was applicable to the domestic population and its medical practice, which had been serving in practice as an impediment to the use of foreign clinical data.[6,7]

The former policy on the handling of foreign clinical data in Japan was published by the Ministry of Health and Welfare (MHW) in 1985.[7] It was based on the research conducted by MHW that pointed out the following issues to be considered in the use of foreign clinical data:

(a) Racial difference between Japanese and Caucasians/Whites/Blacks, and the difference of environment and medical practice between Japan and other countries.
(b) Credibility and quality of foreign clinical data.

As a result, MHW declared that, although foreign clinical data with credibility and quality could be used as new drug registration data, the following three types of studies, in principle, should be conducted in Japan: (a) pharmacokinetic studies, (b) dose-response studies, and (c) well-controlled studies to demonstrate the drug's efficacy and safety. It was a time when no guidelines on good clinical practice (GCP) had been established, nor had new drug development been globalized. Under these circumstances, the research report emphasized the difference of pharmacokinetics, efficacy and safety between Japanese and other populations.

The issue "ethnic factors to be considered in the acceptability of foreign clinical data," which was proposed by Japan, was adopted as a formal topic (Topic E-5) at the ICH meeting in 1992. After that, the Expert Working Group of this topic continued to work extensively, and the draft guideline was agreed on in March of 1997, which was released for comments afterwards. The guideline was finalized in February of 1998, and was implemented in the three regions in 1998.[2] This ICH guideline recommends regulatory and development strategies to permit clinical data collected in one region to be used for the support of drug registration in another region while allowing for the influence of ethnic factors.

B. ETHNIC FACTORS

A critical issue in utilizing foreign clinical data is the role of ethnic factors, i.e., the difference in efficacy and safety between populations. The word "ethnicity" originates from the Greek word "ethnos" meaning nation or people. Ethnic factors are factors that relate to race or to a large ethnic population classified based on common characteristics and customs. The ICH guideline clarifies ethnic factors related to drug evaluation and classifies them into two categories, i.e., intrinsic ethnic factors and extrinsic ethnic factors. It discusses their potential influence on efficacy, safety, and dose/dosage regimens of a new drug, as well as the methods to evaluate their influence. While examples of intrinsic ethnic factors include genetic polymorphism and sensitivity of receptors, medical practice and clinical trial methodology are examples of extrinsic ethnic factors.

Intrinsic ethnic factors are factors associated with the drug's recipient. The difference of pharmacokinetic profiles due to genetic polymorphism of a metabolic enzyme is one of the typical examples of the effect of intrinsic factors. It is reported that there exist rapid acetylators and slow acetylators for certain drugs such as isoniazid (anti tuberculosis),[8] and the ratios of rapid/slow are different among races. Their plasma concentration curves often show a great difference, and it would lead to the difference of clinical response and safety among races. The differences of responses to β-blockers and ACE inhibitors between Whites and Blacks are reported as examples of pharmacodynamic difference among races.[9,10]

On the other hand, extrinsic ethnic factors are associated with culture and environment of the regions/populations. Examples of extrinsic ethnic factors are the difference of diagnosis criteria, intervention including concomitant medication, and endpoints/evaluation method in clinical studies among regions. The existence of extrinsic ethnic factors and the degree of their influence is hard to evaluate precisely. Nevertheless, if diagnostic methods or criteria for a certain disease are different among regions, the target population of clinical studies or treatment could be different among them. Also it can be supposed that the degree of apparent effect of a certain drug differs due to the difference of concomitant medications to the disease among regions, which could lead to a considerable difference in the evaluation of the drug's benefit/risk. Actually, there are some drugs of which the recommended dosages are different greatly among regions, and the difference seems to have no relation to the degree of deficiency of the drugs' metabolizing enzymes among the races.[11]

It is reported that higher incidence of vasospastic response in the early post Acute Myocardial Infarction (AMI) phase is observed in Japanese compared with Caucasians.[12] Although the causes have not been clarified so far, this has resulted in the difference of medication for the prevention of recurrence of ischemic heart diseases between the populations: calcium antagonists are predominantly prescribed for Japanese and β-blockers for Caucasians. The ICH guideline emphasizes that the influence of such intrinsic and extrinsic ethnic factors should be ascertained in considering the use of foreign clinical data.

C. Bridging Study

A bridging study is a clinical study conducted in a new region to evaluate the possibility of building a bridge between the original and the new region, in other words, to evaluate the applicability of clinical data collected in the original (foreign) region to the new (domestic) population. The ICH guideline classifies the bridging study into the following three types: (a) no need for clinical bridging study (pharmacokinetic studies serve as bridging studies), (b) controlled pharmacodynamic studies, and (c) controlled clinical studies.

When "similarity" is shown as a result of the bridging study, and the foreign clinical data are judged to be applicable to the population in the new region, the foreign clinical data package becomes acceptable as a basis for registration of the new drug in the new region. Regretfully, the ICH guideline does not describe practical approaches as to what kind of a bridging study should be planned and conducted under a specific situation. Also, it does not describe practical criteria as to the judgment of similarity of the study results, which affects the sample size of the bridging study.

A simpler bridging study would be better as far as pharmaceutical companies are concerned. On the contrary, from the viewpoint of regulatory agencies, it is often difficult to evaluate the influence of ethnic factors including extrinsic ones by evaluating only pharmacokinetic data that are collected under rather experimental circumstances and provide little information on clinical evaluation. The experience of judgment on the approvability of new drugs based on foreign clinical data is another important factor.

The necessity and the content of a bridging study cannot be decided mechanically, because the situations are unique to the factors such as the characteristics of the drug under investigation, its targeted disease, and the experience of the regulatory body. Importantly, we should continue to accumulate our experience and endeavor to improve the environment for enabling a more simple bridging study by adopting surrogate/pharmacodynamic endpoints and shorter study period leading to the realization of the spirit of ICH.

V. STATISTICAL ISSUES IN EVALUATING THE ACCEPTABILITY OF FOREIGN CLINICAL DATA

A. Pharmacokinetic Study

Although our ultimate goal in the judgment of usability of foreign clinical data is to confirm the similarity of clinical response (efficacy and safety) to the drug between populations in different regions, it would be of great help if we can identify the existence as well as the degree of the influence of intrinsic ethnic factors on pharmacokinetic profiles.

Comparison of pharmacokinetic profiles between the populations in the original (foreign) region and the new region is an essential step in considering the use of foreign clinical data. When we evaluate the similarity of pharmacokinetic profiles between populations, it would be a usual way to select some pharmacokinetic parameters of interest and compare them between the populations. The parameters need to be linked to the knowledge about the relationship between the pharmacokinetic profiles and the pharmacodynamic response. Several different approaches have been applied for the calculation of average pharmacokinetic parameters, including the naïve averaged data approach, the standard two-stage approach, and the simultaneous approach (mixed-effects model). Each method has its pros and cons, and it is important that the obtained results are robust in order to make a correct comparison. The strictness of comparison should depend on the degree of evidence for the similarity of clinical efficacy and safety between the populations.

Recently the mixed-effects approach has been often used in new drug development because it offers the possibility of gaining integrated information on pharmacokinetics from relatively sparse data obtained from study subjects. In the analysis of population pharmacokinetics, nonlinear mixed-effects models are usually used, and the maximum likelihood method is generally employed for the estimation of population pharmacokinetic parameters. Because of the statistical complexity, careful attention must be paid to some statistical issues in order to obtain reliable and robust results.

Because pharmacokinetic models are nonlinear in individual-specific pharmacokinetic parameters, log likelihood functions in population pharmacokinetic modeling involve a multiple integral that has no closed-form solutions. One of the remedies is to approximate the nonlinear model by using the first order Taylor expansion around the mean value 0 of the interindividual variation. This approximation converts a nonlinear form in individual and random effects to a linear form. However, during this process, the second (which corresponds to interindividual variation) and further terms are ignored indicating that there is no variation among subjects.[13] This may introduce bias if the above condition does not hold. Also, as already pointed out, this approach gives biased estimates for population means and variances of pharmacokinetic parameters when the parameters are highly correlated within a subject.[14]

In addition, although it is one of the merits for nonlinear mixed-effects model that we can use all the data obtained in the study including those of patients who have dropped out from the study, we need to pay attention to the handling of missing data.[15] We may face the situation that there is a difference in pharmacokinetic profiles between the patients who have completed the study and those who have dropped out, and we cannot validate the model to describe the difference.

B. EVALUATION OF EFFICACY

Evaluation of efficacy in the bridging study has two aspects to be considered: design issues and statistical issues. In conducting a bridging study, securing the quality and credibility of the data is essential. At the same time, comparability of the data is an important factor from the viewpoint of study design, because the evaluation of extrapolatability is examined based on the similarity between the data obtained from the bridging study and the corresponding foreign clinical data. The evaluation can be done more easily and precisely if the designs of the studies are similar. As for the endpoints used in the study, validity (reflecting clinically relevant effects properly), inter/intra-rater reliability, and objectivity are required. Also we should pay attention not only to the difference of entry criteria but also to the actual demographic data of the patients participating in the study.[16]

As for statistical issues, we should bear in mind that the ICH guideline does not require "same" efficacy but only "similar" efficacy for the data from both regions. Estimation of the efficacy becomes critical in the evaluation of the similarity of the data between populations. This is different from the regular statistical practice of the evaluation in new drug application, viz., hypothesis test. The challenge is that the estimated efficacy from a small bridging study must be robust. Several approaches to examining the similarity have been proposed.[17–19] Another issue is the sample size calculation of the bridging study without specification of type I and II errors. It is preposterous in a spirit of ICH if a bridging study requires a sample size equal to that in the original study. Further research is required regarding the definition of "similarity" and the associated sample size calculation.

C. Evaluation of Safety

In considering the use of foreign clinical data for new drug registration, the issue of the drug's safety is apt to take a back seat to the issue of efficacy. Actually, the ICH guideline does not spare a lot of pages for the discussion on the extra-polatability of safety data to the new region.

In the first place, efficacy and safety are inseparable in dealing with pharmaceuticals, and the issue of safety should not be belittled. We cannot deny the possibility that the safety profiles of the drug differ among regions/populations because of the influence of ethnic factors such as the difference of medical practices among regions. In general, however, it requires a much larger database (sample size, duration of treatment) for the evaluation of safety of a new drug compared with the case for the efficacy. Therefore it would be a practical and reasonable approach to leave the further safety evaluation to the postmarketing surveillance if we find no major concern for its safety after assessing the safety database composed of foreign clinical studies and the bridging study for efficacy.

The postmarketing safety study comes to play a very important part in the process of new drug development and evaluation. As for new drugs that are approved mainly based on foreign clinical data without having enough domestic safety information, more attention should be paid to their postmarketing surveillance especially during the period just after the launch on the market. The case for gefitinib (a drug for patients with advanced nonsmall cell lung cancer) and severe acute interstitial pneumonia in Japan reminds us of this lesson.[20] The method of postmarketing safety study, including the number of patients and the duration of exposure to the drug, should be investigated from a statistical viewpoint based on the character of each drug.

Owing to the adoption of the ICH guideline, new drugs that have been approved with safety database mainly composed of foreign clinical studies are expected to be more common in the near future. In such cases, fortunately, fairly large amounts of safety data obtained from such foreign clinical studies are often available before initiating postmarketing safety studies in the new region. How we plan and conduct postmarketing safety studies effectively as well as efficiently by best utilizing such information is our challenge.[21] We would like to encourage further discussions on the issue of safety evaluation from the viewpoint of utilizing foreign clinical data for new drug registration.

VI. CONCLUSIONS AND EXPECTATION FOR GLOBAL DRUG DEVELOPMENT

When we consider the use of foreign clinical data, we fall in a dilemma between the two ideas that are both the key words of the ICH activity:

(a) Reduce the resources for new drug development, and provide safe and effective new drugs for patients sooner.
(b) Should not compromise on securing the safety and efficacy of new drugs.

Thus, regulatory agencies face a challenge when they make a judgment about the safety and efficacy of new drugs for their citizens based on data gathered in a different region. Many years have passed since the implementation of the ICH guideline, and each regulatory agency has been accumulating its experience on evaluating foreign clinical data. In Japan, more than ten new drugs have been registered mainly based on foreign clinical data, and a lot of promising products are under development according to the principle of the guideline.

Most parts of the ICH guideline are written on the assumption that the foreign clinical data have been already collected and the sponsor conducts a bridging study afterward (retrospective approach). However, in order to make a new drug available to the patients sooner, worldwide simultaneous development is preferable. Conduct of the international multi-center collaborative study is one of the solutions, by which we can establish the efficacy and safety of the new drug; at the same time we can evaluate the influence of ethnic factors among different populations. Although they are a kind of large simple trial and are not studies for obtaining regulatory registration, some successfully conducted multinational clinical studies have been reported, where many centers in Asia, Europe, and North America participated.[22,23]

Because of the fast-paced development in biotechnology, the way of looking at intrinsic ethnic factors has been changing. Schwartz[24] pointed out that some articles dealing with the effects of racial/ethnic factors on drugs' efficacy and safety offer "no plausible biologic justification for making such distinctions," and that "race is a social construct, not a scientific classification." With the advance of human genomic analysis, the intrinsic ethnic factors are expected to take account in due time of the issue of genetic factors.

Concerning extrinsic ethnic factors, the great efforts of ICH for the establishment of a number of harmonized guidelines have resulted in the harmonization of design and methods of clinical studies, and the influence of extrinsic ethnic factors related to the methodology and conduct of clinical studies have been becoming a legacy. On the other hand, as for the extrinsic ethnic factors related to medical practice in general, the overall trend seems to be moving toward global harmonization (see Chapter 19 for relevant information), but we need further to accumulate our experience and to evaluate it.

The situation surrounding the issue of ethnic factors has been changing rapidly in some fields and gradually in others from the time when the ICH guideline was established in 1998. The strategy of new drug development in the worldwide market has been changing as well. But it should be kept in mind that the points we presented in the previous sections will remain valid for the near future. We expect continued rigorous discussion on these issues.

ACKNOWLEDGMENTS

The authors express their gratitude to distinguished Professor James H. Ware at Harvard School of Public Health for his valuable comments and encouragement.

REFERENCES

1. Japan Pharmaceutical Manufacturers Association, JPMA DATABOOK, www.jpma.co.jp, January 2004.
2. ICH Secretariat, ICH Harmonized Tripartite Guideline: ethnic factors in the acceptability of foreign clinical data, Geneva, 1998.
3. Narukawa, M., New policy on the utilization of foreign clinical data and our future task, *Jpn. J. Clin. Pharmacol. Ther.*, 31(2), 229–236, 2000, in Japanese.
4. IMS HEALTH, IMS World Review, 2004.
5. Bigger isn't always better, *Nature*, 418(6896), 353–354, 2002.
6. Food and Drug Administration, Department of Health and Human Services, 21 Code of Federal Regulations 314.60 Foreign data, U.S. National Archives and Records Administration.
7. Ministry of Health and Welfare, The handling of clinical study data conducted in foreign countries, No. 660 notified by the Director General of Pharmaceutical Affairs Bureau on June 29, 1985; Japan Ministry of Health and Welfare: Tokyo, 1985.
8. Wood, A.J.J. and Zou, H.H., Ethnic differences in drug disposition and responsiveness, *Clin. Pharmacokinet.*, 20, 350–373, 1991.
9. Johnson, J.A., Racial differences in lymphocyte beta-receptor sensitivity to propranolol, *Life Sci.*, 53, 297–304, 1993.
10. Exner, D.V., Dries, D.L., Domanski, M.J., and Cohn, J.N., Lesser response to angiotensin-converting-enzyme inhibitor therapy in black as compared with

white patients with left ventricular dysfunction, *NEJM*, 344(18), 1351–1357, 2001.

11. Yasuhara, H., Ethnic factors which influence drug evaluation, *Folia. Pharmacol. Jpn.*, 104, 67–78, 1994, in Japanese.

12. Pristipino, C., Beltrame, J.F., Finocchiaro, M.L., Hattori, R., Fujita, M., Mongiardo, R., Cianflone, D., Sanna, T., Sasayama, S., and Maseri, A., Major racial differences in coronary constrictor response between Japanese and Caucasians with recent myocardial infarction, *Circulation*, 101, 1102–1108, 2000.

13. Yafune, A., Takeuchi, M., and Narukawa, M., Statistical issues regarding the first-order approximation in nonlinear mixed effects models, *Jpn. J. Clin. Pharmacol. Ther.*, 31(6), 705–713, 2000, in Japanese.

14. Steimer, J., Mallet, A., Golmard, J., and Boisvieux, J., Alternative approaches to estimation of population pharmacokinetics parameters: comparison with the nonlinear mixed-effect model, *Drug Metab. Rev.*, 15, 265–292, 1984.

15. Laird, N.M., Missing data in longitudinal studies, *Stat. Med.*, 7, 305–315, 1988.

16. Takeuchi, M., Statistical issues on bridging studies, In *Bridging Strategies: Extrapolating Clinical Data to New Regions for New Drug Development*, *Proceedings of the First Kitasato University-Harvard School of Public Health Symposium*, Lagakos, S.W. and Takeuchi, M., eds., Digital Press, Tokyo, pp. 123–130, 2001, October 5–6.

17. Ware, J.M., The challenge of bridging, In *Bridging Strategies: Extrapolating Clinical Data to New Regions for New Drug Development*, *Proceedings of the First Kitasato University-Harvard School of Public Health Symposium 2000*, Lagakos, S.W. and Takeuchi, M., eds., Digital Press, Tokyo, pp. 105–121, 2001, October 5–6.

18. Shih, W.J., Clinical trials for drug registrations in Asian-Pacific countries: proposal for a new paradigm from a statistical perspective, *Control Clin. Trials*, 22, 357–366, 2001.

19. Chow, S.C., Shao, J., and Hu, O.Y.P., Assessing Sensitivity and Similarity in Bridging Studies, *J. Biopharm. Stat.*, 12(3), 385–400, 2002.

20. Inoue, A., Saijo, Y., Maemondo, M., Gomi, K., Tokue, Y., Kimura, Y., Ebina, M., Kikuchi, T., Moriya, T., and Nukiwa, T., Severe acute interstitial pneumonia and gefitinib, *Lancet*, 361(9352), 137 2003.

21. Narukawa, M., Yafune, A., and Takeuchi, M., Observation of time-dependent adverse events and the influence of drop-out thereon in long-term safety studies — simulation study under the current practice of post-marketing safety evaluation in Japan, *J. Biopharm. Stat.*, 14(2), 403–414, 2004.

22. Brenner, B.M., Cooper, M.E., Zeeuw, D.D. et al. Effects of losartan on renal and cardiovascular outcomes in patients with type 2 diabetes and nephropathy, *NEJM*, 345(12), 861–869, 2001.

23. PROGRESS Collaborative Group, Randomized trial of a perindopril-based blood-pressure-lowering regimen among 6105 individuals with previous stroke and transient ischaemic attack, *Lancet*, 358, 1033–1041, 2001.

24. Schwartz, R.S., Racial profiling in medical research, *NEJM*, 344(18), 1392–1393, 2001.

21 Design and Analysis Strategies for Clinical Pharmacokinetic Trials

Lianng Yuh and Yusong Chen

CONTENTS

I. INTRODUCTION

One of the steps necessary for characterizing a new drug dosage form is to conduct an *in vivo* bioavailability study. The Food and Drug Administration (FDA) requires that pharmaceutical companies perform these studies in order to produce a new drug application (NDA) or an abbreviated new drug application (ANDA). Specific details related to the requirements for an NDA are presented in the Federal Register (January 7, 1977)[1] while Cabana and Douglas[2] give bioavailability guidelines for investigational new drug application (IND) development.

Bioavailability, as defined by Metzler,[3] "includes the study of the factors which influence and determine the amount of active drug which gets from the administered dose to the site of pharmacologic action as well as the rate at which it gets there." Since it is often difficult or impossible to measure drug at its site of action, drug concentrations in the systemic circulation (blood, plasma or serum) are used as a surrogate. The object of bioavailability study is to quantify the relative amount and rate of absorption of the administered drug which reaches the general circulation intact. It may be noted that the FDA has defined bioavailability as "the rate of ingredient and extent to which it is absorbed."

There are a number of types of biopharmaceutic studies those involve measurement of bioavailability of one or more dosage forms, viz.:

Absolute bioavailability: These studies involve a comparison of a nonparenteral dosage form (e.g., an oral form) relative to an IV (intravenous) solution.

Relative bioavailability or bioequivalence: These studies are used to determine if the rate and extent of a test formulation are equivalent to those of a reference formulation. These studies are discussed in details in this chapter.

ADME (Absorption, Distribution, Metabolism, Excretion): These studies are run to determine the pharmacokinetics and metabolic profile of a dosage form.

Dose proportionality: These studies are conducted to determine the correlation between increase in doses of a drug and its bioavailability.

In course of development of a drug, many other special studies, such as, determination of the effects of renal impairment, food, and concomitant medications on the bioavailability of the drug, are conducted.

Factors influencing the estimate of the bioavailability of a dosage form are numerous but essentially fall into two categories. The first is made up of physical characteristics of the dosage form and includes such items as tablet compression force, particle size, solubility, and dissolution rate. The second category contains certain design factors which can affect the drug level profile. For example, the choice and spacing of the sampling times must be carefully chosen so that the drug concentration can be accurately determined. The choice of sampling times also affects the precision of estimates of the pharmacokinetic parameters. The amount of physical activity permitted during a study and whether or not a subject fasted prior to administration of medication are the other design factors having marked effects on drug levels. However, even under controlled conditions blood and urine concentrations often differ markedly, even for subjects with similar ages, heights, weights, general health, and other demographic factors (Gibaldi,[4] Chapter 7).

To establish the bioavailability of a dosage form, a multidisciplinary approach to design and analysis of these studies is mandatory. To determine which of the factors need to be controlled, whether patients or healthy volunteers should be studied, and what statistical design will yield the required information, a statistician's input to the planning is a must. The purpose of this chapter is to provide some insight into the choice of design and method of statistical analysis of single-dose *in vivo* bioavailability studies.

II. BIOAVAILABILITY OF A SINGLE FORMULATION

A. COMPARTMENTAL MODELS

For determination of the pharmacokinetic properties of a drug it is frequently useful to represent the body as a system of interconnected compartments. The compartments are more of a conceptual device useful for analyzing drug concentration data than having only limited physiological meaning. The commonly used compartmental models are the one-compartment (Figure 21.1) and the two-compartment types (Figure 21.2).

In Figure 21.1 the entire body is viewed as a single-compartment with K_a representing the rate of absorption of drug into the system and K_e, the rate of elimination of drug from the system. Gibaldi and Perrier[5] point out that viewing the body as a one-compartment model does not mean that the concentration of drug throughout the body tissues at any given time is same, rather the model does assume that the changes of drug concentrations in plasma quantitatively reflect

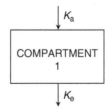

FIGURE 21.1 One-compartment model.

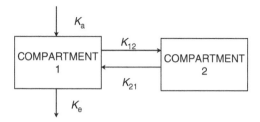

FIGURE 21.2 Two-compartment model.

drug concentration changes in the tissues. A system of two compartments is shown in Figure 21.2. Typically the first compartment is taken to represent blood plasma and the second compartment the peripheral tissues. The constants K_{12} and K_{21} represent transfer rates of drug between plasma and tissue, and K_e denotes the elimination rate of the drug.

Input of drug into the model is usually assumed to be zero or first order, depending on the route of administration, while elimination from the compartments and transfer between compartments are assumed to be of first order. By zero order input, we mean the input rate of drug to be constant; first order input and elimination implies the input and elimination rates to be proportional, respectively, to the amount of drug at the absorption site and to the amount of drug in the compartment through which the drug is eliminated. The above assumptions regarding rates of input, transfer, and elimination require that the equation relating the concentration of drug to time can be rewritten as a sum of exponentials. For example, the equation corresponding to the concentration of drug in the single-compartment model (Figure 21.1) is as follows:

$$C(t_i) = \frac{FD}{V} \frac{K_a}{K_a - K_e} (e^{-K_e t_i} - e^{-K_a t_i}) \qquad (21.1)$$

where

$C(t_i)$ = concentration of drug in the compartment at time t_i
F = fraction of the dose that is absorbed
D = dose of drug
V = apparent volume of distribution of the drug
K_a = absorption rate constant
K_e = elimination rate constant

Note that for suitable choices of a_j and λ_j, the right-hand side of Equation 21.1 can be written as

$$\sum a_j e^{-\lambda_j t_j}$$

Equation 21.1 is appropriate when the drug is administered orally. If the drug is administered through IV injection or some other route of administration and the body is viewed as a single compartment, then Equation 21.1 would no longer be appropriate. Wagner[6] discussed the one-compartment and various multicompartment models and provides equations for the concentration of drug in the various compartments following several different routes of administration.

B. PARAMETER ESTIMATION

1. Individual Modeling

Table 21.1 displays concentrations of drug A in whole blood for one subject following a single oral solution of 260 mg. The first step in the analysis of such data is identification of the underlying model, usually based on information obtained from a preliminary study or from reported published data. If such additional data are not available, fitting the sequence of concentrations to the equations generated by both the one-compartment and two-compartment systems should be attempted. Computer programs utilizing nonlinear least-squares algorithms are usually employed to obtain best-fitting estimates of the pharmacokinetic parameters (e.g., K_a, K_e) for a particular model. The criterion of goodness of fit is usually taken to be minimization of the quantity

$$\sum_{i=1}^{n} (Y_i - \hat{Y}_i)^2 \tag{21.2}$$

where Y_i is the observed concentration at time t_i, $\hat{Y}_i$ is the concentration predicted by the fitted model at time t_i, and n is the number of samples collected from the subject. Hence we attempt to find the set of estimates of the pharmacokinetic parameters that minimizes the residual sum of squares.

TABLE 21.1
Concentration of Drug A in Whole Blood

Sampling Time (h)	Concentration (ng/ml)
0.5	0.70
1.0	1.11
2.0	1.36
3.0	1.17
4.0	0.99
6.0	0.71
8.0	0.50
10.0	0.31
14.0	0.14
18.0	0.06
24.0	0.20

Several problems make the fitting procedure difficult. First, because the algorithm employs iterative techniques, they usually require initial estimates of the parameters. In addition, if one considers the residual sum of squares (Equation 21.2) as a $p+1$ dimensional surface (where $p = $ number of parameters), it is easy to envision other problems. This surface may have many peaks and valleys causing the program to converge to a local and not to a global minimum. Additionally, the minimum may occur at a nearly flat spot on the surface, implying that there is a wide range of parameter values which give approximately the same value of Equation 21.2. Fortunately, these difficulties can often be overcome if one has available initial estimates of the parameters that are fairly close to the true values. One method to obtain initial estimates is discussed in Appendix A.

Example. As an illustration of the model-fitting technique, the data presented in Table 21.1 were fit to Equation 21.1 using the program WinNonLin.[7] In this particular example, F was unknown, so the parameters to be estimated were K_a, K_e, and V/F. A portion of the output from the program is presented in Tables 21.2 and 21.3. The model fits the data fairly well, at least as evidenced by the residuals.

There are several factors that must be considered in assessing the adequacy of the model. In particular, one should always make a careful comparison of the observed and predicted concentrations. Examination of the concentration time profile may reveal a delay in the start of absorption at *zero* or *near zero* concentrations at the first sampling time(s). This indicates the need for a lag time in the model. Equation 21.1 with a lag time incorporated into the model can be written as

$$C(t_i) = \frac{FD}{V} \frac{K_a}{K_a - K_e} [e^{-K_e(t_i - L)} - e^{-K_a(t_i - L)}] \qquad (21.3)$$

A lag time dose not improve the fit with this data set, but may considerably improve the fit with other data sets.

TABLE 21.2
WinNonLin Nonlinear Estimation Program

Parameter	Estimate	Standard Error	95% Confidence Interval		
Volume/F	0.519007	0.013550	0.487760	0.550253	Univariate
			0.470458	0.567556	Planar
K_a	1.019687	0.054103	0.894925	1.144449	Univariate
			0.825838	1.213536	Planar
K_e	0.202623	0.005682	0.189520	0.215727	Univariate
			0.182264	0.222983	Planar

TABLE 21.3
WinNonLin Nonlinear Estimation Program. Summary of Nonlinear Estimation

X	Observed Y	Calculated Y	Residual	Weight	SE − Y	Standardized Residual
0.5	0.7000	0.7287	− 0.0287	0.1841	0.0197	− 1.4983
1.0	1.1100	1.0962	0.0138	0.1161	0.0216	0.5087
2.0	1.3600	1.2905	0.0695	0.0947	0.0182	2.0568
3.0	1.1700	1.1965	− 0.0265	0.1101	0.0190	− 0.8789
4.0	0.9900	1.0285	− 0.0385	0.1301	0.0181	− 1.4092
6.0	0.7100	0.7076	0.0024	0.1815	0.0128	0.0962
8.0	0.5000	0.4747	0.0253	0.2577	0.0096	1.1940
10.0	0.3100	0.3169	− 0.0069	0.4156	0.0084	− 0.4241
14.0	0.1400	0.1409	− 0.0009	0.9203	0.0064	− 0.0899
18.0	0.0600	0.0627	− 0.0027	2.1474	0.0042	− 0.3869
24.0	0.0200	0.0186	0.0014	6.4423	0.0018	0.3321

Corrected sum of squared observations = 2.25042
Weighted corrected sum of squared observations = 0.728326
Sum of squared residuals = 0.872375×10^{-2}
Sum of weighted squared residuals = 0.111569×10^{-2}
$S = 0.118094^{-1}$ with 8 degrees of freedom
Correlation (observed, predicted) = 0.9981
AIC (Akaike Information Criteria) = − 68.78113
SBC (Schwarz's Bayesian Criteria) = − 67.58745
AUC (0 to last time) computed by trapezoidal rule = 9.46750

For this example, the weight for each observation was taken as WT = $1/y$. The weights were than normalized so that the sum of the weights equals the number of observations, 11.

In assessing the validity of the parameter estimates, the widths of the confidence limits need to be considered. Two types of limits can be seen to be available per Table 21.2. The univariate limits are calculated in the usual way as the parameter estimate ($\pm$) the appropriate t statistic multiplied by the standard error of the parameter estimate. The planar limits are derived from an estimated 95% joint confidence region for the parameters and will always be wider than the univariate limits. From the width of the confidence limits reported in Table 21.2, it can be concluded that there are variety of estimated parameters that yield equivalently good fits of Equation 21.1 to the data.

In addition, it should always be checked to see if there are systematic deviations from the fitted model. This is easily done by inspection of the residual values in Table 21.3. For example, if the model overestimates larger concentrations and underestimates smaller concentrations, then one should try weighting the observed concentrations, the Y values, by $1/E(Y)$ or $1/\sqrt{E(Y)}$. Other weighting schemes may help remove other biases. If weights are used, the criteria for "best" fit would be to use those estimated parameters that minimize

$$\sum_{i=1}^{n} W_i (Y_i - \hat{Y}_i)^2$$

where W_i is the weight assigned to the ith concentration. An excellent review of this topic was presented by Peck et al.[8]

An examination of the residual values can also help identify outliers or aberrant observations. Least-squares procedures are very sensitive to outliers and the presence of one in the data set can cause sizable bias in the parameter estimates. To combat this problem Rodda et al.[9] have developed a nonparametric procedure which lessens the effect that an aberrant observation has upon the estimates of the parameters. Their procedure, known as Ordered Simultaneous Estimation Procedure (OSEP), performed quite well relative to least-squares procedures on simulated data sets containing several different types of outliers. The OSEP procedure is recommended when the true model is known and outliers are known to exist.

Giltinan and Ruppert[10] have demonstrated the use of the generalized least-squares estimator (GLS) in pharmacokinetic modeling. Sheiner et al.[11] applied extended least squares (ELS) to obtain the regression and variance parameters simultaneously. ELS is equivalent to the maximum likelihood estimator (ML) using the normal likelihood function. The advantages and the disadvantages of the ELS method have been discussed extensively by Jobson and Fuller,[12] Carroll and Ruppert[13] and van Houwelingen[14] in the statistical literature, and by Finney[15] in the pharmacokinetic literature. Beal and Sheiner[16] have compared GLS and the modified extended iteratively reweighted least-squares estimators (MEIRLS). Their results indicated that these two estimators have similar efficiencies and both are superior to ELS. The approach using Bayes' theorem was discussed by Katz et al.[17] and Racine-Poon.[18]

2. Population Modeling

It has been explained how the estimates of pharmacokinetic parameters based on data obtained from a single subject are derived. In a multisubject trial, the distribution of the parameter values in the population is usually estimated. As Steimer et al.[19] indicated, there are two types of data from the multisubject studies, e.g., experimental data and observational data. The experimental studies involve healthy volunteers. Such studies are well designed with balanced and less variable data. The results of the studies provide the estimates of basic pharmacokinetic parameters and information for adjusting the individual dosage regimens.

Population studies, which are unbalanced and more variable than the experimental studies, involve the collection of observational data from the treated patients in the efficacy trials. The results of the observational studies can be used for pharmacokinetic screening and postmarketing surveillance. Reference is drawn to Whiting et al.[20] and Grasela et al.[21] for more discussion of the applications of these data.

Many procedures have been developed for population modeling with the basic assumption, that the subjects have a common pharmacokinetic model. Certainly, the Naive-Pooled-Data and Naive-Averaging-of-Data approach are biased and not efficient.[19,22,23] Another approach is called the "Two-Stage Method." In the first stage of this method, individual data are fitted to obtain the individual parameter estimate using the methods suggested in Section II.B. The final population parameter estimate is obtained using the combined individual estimates. To apply this method, each subject needs sufficient data to derive a reasonable individual estimate. The simple two-stage method does not consider the variability associated with each individual estimate. It often underestimates the variabilities associated with the population parameters. A modified two-stage method was proposed by Prevost,[24] which incorporated both inter- and intra-subject variabilities in the model. The two-stage method approach using Bayes' theorem was discussed by Katz and D'Argenio,[25] Racine-Poon,[18] and Racine-Poon and Smith.[26] A comprehensive review of different analytical strategies and applications was provided by Yuh et al.[27]

Weiner and Jordan[28] have investigated a procedure that fits all subjects simultaneously allowing the pharmacokinetic parameters to be functions of known physiological factors. Particularly, V, the apparent volume of distribution, is frequently related to body weight or body surface area. This can be of particular importance if the estimates of pharmacokinetic parameters are used to predict drug levels at steady state. Sheiner and Beal[29-31] proposed a nonlinear mixed effects model (NONMEM) using ELS with the first order approximation to pool the individual data to obtain a population estimate and the individual estimates simultaneously. A computationally intensive procedure using the nonparametric ML was derived by Mallet.[32] Steimer et al.[19] and Katz[23] have reviewed these procedures. The nonlinear mixed affects model approach is preferred for the observational data because the lack of the quality of the individual data. Linstrom and Bates[33] have developed a new computing algorithm using the NONMEM approach while Gelfand et al.[34] proposed a full Bayesian procedure using Gibb's sampler. Since it is difficult to define the criteria for evaluating different procedures, it has not been determined which of the above methods is best in any given situation. ELS is the procedure with a commercial computer package based on NONMEM.[35] Starting with version 8, SAS introduced PROC NLMIXED[36] for nonlinear mixed modeling. It has similar functionality as NONMEM's $PRED for models that can be specified on one's own, however, it has nothing comparable to PREDPP, which is a subroutine of NONMEM software specialized to the kinds of predictions in pharmacokinetic data analysis. PROC NLMIXED has options for exact maximum likelihood estimation using quadrature-based methods in addition to first order approximation methods such as those in NONMEM. PKBugs[37] is an efficient and user-friendly interface for specifying complex population pharmacokinetic models within WinBUGS software,[38] which is a Bayesian modeling framework that can be used to analyze pharmacokinetic data. PKBugs makes Markov Chain Monte Carlo (MCMC)[39, 40] techniques available to practitioners in the field of population pharmacokinetics (PK) via a short-hand notation for data entry as in NONMEM. It is recommended that the analyst analyzes the data using several of the above methods before drawing any definitive conclusion.

III. COMPARATIVE BIOAVAILABILITY STUDIES

A. Introduction

Thus far assessing the bioavailability of a single formulation has been dealt with, frequently, though, it is necessary to conduct comparative bioavailability studies. For example, one of the requirements for producing an ANDA is to compare the bioavailability of the new generic formulation to a standard or reference formulation and changes in manufacturing practice may necessitate conducting a comparative bioavailability study.

In this section guidelines regarding the choice of criteria for comparison of two dosage forms have been provided and the designs as well as analyses most commonly used in relative bioavailability trials have been discussed. Other pharmacokinetic studies such as food effect, age effect and dose proportionality studies can be assessed using similar principles. Following FDA's Bioequivalence Public Hearing, the statistical decision criteria for solid dosage formulation bioequivalence studies were clearly defined.[41]

B. Choice of the Criteria for Comparison

Prior to discussion of the design and analysis of relative bioavailability studies, several choices of the bioavailability criteria for comparing the two dosage forms will be first discussed. In practice it is customary to choose several criteria, each related to specific aspects of the drug concentration profiles, with which the formulations are compared. The choices depend on the type of bioavailability study conducted. For example, the criteria for comparing the timed-release capsule with an immediate-release tablet may differ from those for comparing a single formulation of drug manufactured at different locations. The following are the criteria commonly used as a basis for comparing two formulations. For a given study, the investigator chooses one or more of these variables as a basis for comparing the two dosage formulations.

1. Area under the Concentration Curve

Area under the concentration curve (AUC), the integral of concentration of the drug over time, measures the total amount of drug absorbed. AUC is probably the commonly used variable for comparing two formulations. For a given profile, this quantity is usually calculated from the sequence of plasma concentrations by the trapezoidal rule

$$\text{AUC}_{o-t} = \sum_{i=2}^{N} \frac{C(t_i) + C(t_{i-1})}{2}(t_i - t_{i-1}) \qquad (21.4)$$

where $t_0 = 0$ and N is the number of samples those were taken after administration of the dosage form. Equation 21.4 should be used as an estimate of total absorption only if $C(t_N)$ is zero or near-zero. Otherwise, the bioavailability of the formulation could be seriously underestimated. If $C(t_N)$ is somewhat greater than zero, then the AUC should be extrapolated to infinite time by adding the term $C(t_N)/\lambda$ to the value of Equation 21.4. In the additional term, λ represents the terminal rate constant. However, it is preferred to report AUC(0: last quantifiable concentration) if λ cannot be precisely estimated.

2. Peak Concentration (C_{max})

Peak concentration is usually calculated as the maximum observed $C(t_i)$. Although in actuality, the peak concentration will most likely be higher and occur at some time point other than one of the sampling times, the approximation is usually adequate for comparative purposes.

3. Time to Peak Concentration (T_{max})

Time to peak concentration is usually taken to be the time at which the maximum concentration was observed. T_{max} and C_{max} are used jointly to measure the rate of absorption.

4. Cumulative Percentage of Drug Recovered ($A_c^{\%}$)

It is applicable to urine data and the cumulative percentage of drug recovered is calculated as the cumulative amount recovered in some time interval (e.g., 24 h) divided by the initial dose. As with AUC, $A_c^{\%}$ can be extrapolated to infinity as well.[6]

5. Estimated Absorption Rate (K_a)

It is sometimes desirable to compare two formulations on the basis of their estimated absorption rates. For example, suppose that in order to lengthen the period of time through which a tablet retains its potency, a pharmaceutical firm begins to manufacture the tablets with a new protective coating. It would then be of interest to compare the absorption rate of the coated tablets with that of the uncoated ones. As discussed in Section III.B, first it is necessary to be able to identify the underlying pharmacokinetic model in order to estimate K_a.

6. Elimination Half-Life

The elimination half-life of a drug, $t_{1/2}$, can be estimated by dividing 0.693 by the absolute value of the slope of the terminal linear phase of the concentration profile when plotted on semi-log scale. For the model displayed in Figure 21.1, $t_{1/2} = 0.693/K_e$.

7. Concentration Profiles

Instead of comparing formulations on the basis of univariate values derived from the sequence of blood levels, the entire concentration profiles can be compared using a multivariate method such as profile analysis (Ref. 42, pp. 205–216). This can help distinguishing between two formulations those differ in onset and duration but are equivalent in terms of AUC.

One inherent problem in the statistical evaluation of these data is that the parameters (1–6) are estimated rather than measured directly. Often, the standard errors of the estimates are quite heterogeneous across subjects and that may invalidate the assumptions underlying an analysis of variance.

Many of the variables discussed above can be estimated in an alternative manner, by taking an appropriate function of the estimated pharmacokinetic parameters. For example, by integrating Equation 21.1 from zero to infinity, one can show that the estimate of AUC is $FD/\hat{V}\hat{K}$. Other expressions can be derived for peak concentration and time-to-peak concentration. This method of estimation is not to be recommended unless the underlying pharmacokinetic model can be identified and the parameters be accurately estimated. Because of problems associated with model misspecification, regulatory agencies prefer calculation of parameters by the above methods rather than from fitted parameters.

For bioequivalence studies, AUC and C_{max} are the primary response variables. T_{max} is not considered to be a primary response variable due to its highly discrete nature.[43] Pharmacokinetic constants, elimination half-life, and the concentration–time profile are also considered as secondary variables. For urine samples, the cumulative percentages of drug recovered are often used as the primary response variables. If a multiple dose study is conducted, the minimum plasma concentration (C_{min}) and the fluctuation index $[(C_{max} - C_{min})/C_{avg}]$, both of which are measured under steady-state conditions, are also parameters of interest.[41]

C. Designing a Comparative Bioavailability Study

It is well known that the inter-subject variability is larger than the intra-subject in the bioavailability of most of the drug formulations. As a result, designs that enable each subject to serve as his or her own control are most frequently employed in comparative bioavailability studies except for drugs with an extremely long half-life or toxicity problems. Such designs have an advantage over other designs because the former, the comparison of formulations is free from subject-to-subject variation. One example of such a design, viz., the two-period crossover design, is presented in Table 21.4.[44] It may be noted that each subject received each of the two formulations according to one of two

TABLE 21.4
A Two-Period Crossover Design

Sequence	Period	
	1	2
1	A	B
2	B	A

predetermined sequences. Between each dose period there is a wash-out period of sufficient length to ensure that the first drug has been eliminated from the subject's system. The wash-out period should be at least five times the terminal half-life of the drug.

The design presented in Table 21.4 can easily be extended to compare more than two formulations. These larger crossover designs are usually constructed so that the allocation of formulations to periods forms a Latin square design. One such design for comparing four formulations is presented in Table 21.5.

In a 2×2 crossover design, the carry over effect is confounded with the formulation, sequence, and period effect unless the Balaam design (crossover design with extra periods, Table 21.6) is utilized. Using this type of design, it is possible to only estimate the within-subject variability but the formulation by subject interaction[45-47] can also be assessed.

Westlake[48] has discussed the use of balanced incomplete block designs for comparative bioavailability studies involving a large number of treatments. Yuh and Ruberg[49] have presented several balanced and unbalanced crossover designs using an oversampling technique for a drug to drug interaction study (Table 21.7).

D. SAMPLING TIMES

The next step in designing the study is to determine the number and spacing of collection times for the plasma or urine samples. There are several guidelines that can be helpful in selecting the times for drawing samples.

TABLE 21.5
A Four-Period Crossover Design

Sequence	Period			
	1	2	3	4
1	A	B	C	D
2	B	D	A	C
3	C	A	D	B
4	D	C	B	A

TABLE 21.6
An Extra-Period Crossover Design

Sequence	Period		
	1	**2**	**3**
1	A	B	A
2	B	A	B

A control urine or plasma sample should always be taken just prior to administration of drug. This ensures that subject has no residual amounts of drug in his or her system from previous study days and that the subject has not inadvertently ingested the drug with some concurrent medication or food. The remaining samples should be taken at times sufficient to determine the profiles of the concentration curves. For orally administered drugs, samples should be taken most frequently during the absorption phase when the profile is most rapidly changing and less frequently during the elimination phase.

If pharmacokinetic parameters are to be estimated from the data, the total number of samples should be sufficiently large so that there are enough degrees of freedom to estimate σ^2 (e.g., ≥ 6) to allow for a reasonable test of the adequacy of the compartmental model. In addition, the plasma or urine concentrations should have returned to near-zero levels by the time the last sample is taken. For more discussion about optimal sampling design, we refer to the papers by D'Argenio,[50] DiStefano,[51,52] Landaw,[53] Katz and D'Argenio,[25] and Drusano et al.[54]

Once the appropriate design has been determined for the bioavailability study, the final step is to determine the number of subjects to be included in the study. Since it is closely related to the method of data analyses, the sample size calculation will be discussed in the next section.

TABLE 21.7
Incomplete Partially Balanced Crossover Design

Sequence	Period			
	1	**2**	**3**	**4**
1	A	E	C	D
2	B	F	D	E
3	C	G	E	F
4	D	A	F	G
5	E	B	G	A
6	F	C	A	B
7	G	D	B	C'

Having discussed various considerations in design comparative trials and the choice of the criteria for comparison, the following paragraphs will discuss the analysis of such data.

IV. ANALYSIS OF COMPARATIVE BIOAVAILABILITY STUDIES

A. ANALYSIS OF VARIANCE MODEL

Before performing an analysis of the data it should be first ensured that the concentrations of drug in the predosing samples are at or near the lower limit of quantitation. If other than trace amounts are measured in these control samples, then it is recommended to analyze only the first-period data. In this case, the investigator should notice that there is only half data available for the analysis and the comparison is inter-subject instead of intra-subject. The analysis would then proceed along the lines of a oneway analysis of variance. For the remainder of the discussion it will now be assumed that, at most, trace amounts of drug are measured in the control samples.

Because the control samples can be used to check on the existence of residual effects, the data analysis can be proceeded with the model without residual effect (Equation 21.5), to allow for testing of equality of sequence, treatment, and period effects:

$$Y_{ijk} = \mu + \psi_i + \zeta_{ij} + \pi_k + \varphi_l + \varepsilon_{ijk} \tag{21.5}$$

where

Y_{ijk} = univariate response [log-transformed (AUC), peak concentration, etc.] for the jth subject within the ith sequence at period k
μ = overall mean
Ψ_i = effect of the ith sequence
ζ_{ij} = effect of the jth subject within the ith sequence
π_k = effect of the kth period
φ_l = effect of the lth formulation
ε_{ijk} = random error

The analysis of variance for more complicated crossover designs is discussed in Ref 55. In addition, Westlake[48] as well as Yuh and Ruberg[49] have discussed the analysis of the balanced and partially balanced incomplete crossover designs.

Example. A study was undertaken to compare the relative bioavailabilities of two batches of drug B in terms of the 0 to 24 h AUC (Table 21.8). This study involved a two-period crossover design with 12 subjects randomly allocated to each of the two sequences. The log-transformed AUC was analyzed using

TABLE 21.8
Area under the Curve (0–24 h)

	Period 1		Period 2	
Subject	Formulation	AUC (μg h/ml) (0–24 h)	Formulation	AUC (μg h/ml) (0–24 h)
1	2	1697.45	1	1636.21
2	1	800.54	2	636.29
3	2	1050.98	1	615.61
4	1	1049.72	2	1013.16
5	2	936.53	1	113.20
6	1	1504.35	2	1094.96
7	2	1277.87	1	1603.63
8	2	1548.28	1	1411.44
9	2	964.41	1	129.55
10	1	1458.60	2	1341.08
11	1	1602.51	2	1470.85
12	1	688.35	2	576.33
13	1	1841.53	2	1312.68
14	1	1259.93	2	1037.75
15	1	1227.14	2	931.89
16	2	1339.08	1	1241.25
17	2	931.91	1	613.14
18	2	1136.23	1	547.66
19	2	1534.56	1	823.46
20	2	794.44	1	952.24
21	1	1538.59	2	1131.16
22	1	874.06	2	1133.22
23	2	1478.62	1	1385.12
24	1	1328.58	2	1131.90

an ANOVA model, with fixed effects for sequence, period, formulation, and random effect for subject, nested within the sequence. The least-squared mean of the difference and its 90% confidence interval were calculated from the fitted model, the least-squared mean of the difference and its 90% CI were then anti-log-transformed to obtain the estimate of the ratio and its 90% confidence interval. The least-squared means of each formulation and their 95% confidence intervals were calculated in a similar manner.

Figure 21.3 is the scatter plot for the log-AUC of formulation 1 vs. formulation 2. The plot suggests there are two outliers, subjects 5 and 9. Therefore, the data were analyzed with or without these subjects. The results are reported in Table 21.9. Usually the results from the analysis including the outliers should be reported, while the analysis excluding outliers serves only for the purpose of sensitivity assessment.

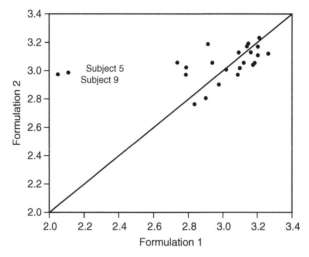

FIGURE 21.3 Scatter plot of log-AUC (formulation 1 vs. formulation 2).

TABLE 21.9
Analysis of AUC Data

Source	df	Sum of squares of log-AUC	F	p-value
Sequences	1	0.027	0.295	0.5919
Subjects (sequence)	22	2.018	—	—
Periods	1	0.427	9.198	0.0061
Formulations	1	0.018	0.392	0.5381
Error	22	1.022	—	—

	Geometric mean of AUC	C.I.
Summary of Results		
Formulation 1	925.76	(748.69, 1012.51)*
Formulation 2	1012.51	(818.84, 1251.70)*
Ratio (1 vs. 2)	91.4%	(71.5%, 116.9%)**
Summary of Results without Subjects 5 and 9		
Formulation 1	1111.48	(982.88, 1256.61)*
Formulation 2	1135.53	(1004.15, 1284.10)*
Ratio (1 vs. 2)	100.6%	(88.7%, 108.0%)**

*95% confidence interval; **90% confidence interval.

B. The Power Approach

Because the objective of the bioavailability studies is to show that the test formulation is equivalent to the reference formulation, the FDA used a decision criterion which is based on the power of the test, to detect a 20% difference between the reference and test treatment means. This rule stated that the two formulations are bioequivalent, if the *p*-value for the formulation effect is greater than a prespecified level of significance and the power of the test to detect a 20% difference between the reference and test means, is greater than or equal to 80%. This rule is no longer used by the FDA and other agencies as the primary criterion for assessment of bioequivalence.

C. Confidence Interval Approach

The development of the bioequivalence of two formulations discussed in Section IV.A was based on the classical theory of hypothesis testing. Traditionally, this methodology has been applied in those situations where it is desired to show that a significant difference exists in the effects of two treatments; usually, though, this is not the objective of a comparative bioavailability study. Instead, it is usually desired to assess the difference in the relative bioavailabilities of the two formulations in terms of some univariate measure such as AUC, and determine if the difference is within acceptable limits. It would thus seem that a confidence interval approach might be more appropriate in some instances. Westlake,[56] Metzler,[3] Shirley,[57] and O'Quigley and Baudoin[58] have discussed this approach in the context of comparative bioavailability trials.

In general, the 90% confidence interval for the ratio in formulation means is computed as follows:

$$\left\{ \left[\frac{\bar{X}_T - \bar{X}_R}{\bar{X}_R} \pm \frac{t_{\nu, 0.975} S_d}{\bar{X}_R} \right] + 1 \right\} \times 100\% \qquad (21.6)$$

where

$\bar{X}_i$ = mean observed response with formulation i, i = T,R (where T and R denote the test and reference formulations)
S_d = standard error of the difference in formulation means using the error mean square obtained from the analysis of variance
ν = degrees of freedom for error.

Substituting the appropriate values into Equation 21.6 we obtain (84.7%, 112.6%) as the 90% confidence interval for the ratio in formulation means. Thus, these two formulations are considered bioequivalent if we use ± 20% as the acceptable limits. Also, the end points of this percent-scaled confidence interval are obtained by treating the reference mean as a constant. The correct (exact) confidence interval for the ratio of the means can be obtained using Fieller's theorem.[59,60] Note that this asymmetric exact confidence interval is usually somewhat wider than the approximate confidence interval.

Westlake[61] has also modified the confidence interval approach and developed a confidence interval symmetric about the origin. Mantel[62] indicated that these symmetric confidence intervals do not show the location of the sample value and they are always longer than the traditional confidence interval. However, as Westlake mentioned, the symmetric interval is used merely as a decision making tool. It is noted that the confidence coefficient for the Westlake interval is always greater than $1 - \alpha$. Again, since the sample mean is used as a constant, Westlake's symmetric confidence interval is only an approximation. The exact symmetric confidence interval has been derived by Mandallaz and Mau.[63] We refer to Steinijans and Diletti,[64] Kirkwood,[65] and Metzler[66] for additional discussions of the use of the symmetric confidence interval.

D. Bayesian Approach

Rodda and Davis[67] first suggested that bioequivalence could be assessed using Bayesian analysis. They computed the posterior probability — the observed relative bioavailability is within the acceptable limits. Selwyn et al.[68] have also proposed a Bayesian procedure using a more complex statistical model. Rodda and Davis' rule is equivalent to Westlake's while the decision rule based on Mandallaz and Mau's confidence interval is equivalent to that using the Bayesian procedure proposed by Selwyn and Hall.[69] Gelfand et al.[34] suggested a Bayes procedure using Gibb's sampler to evaluate bioavailability or bioequivalence studies.

Example. For the example in Section II.B, if Y_{ik} ($i = 1$ to 24, $k = 1,2$) are the AUC of subject i in period k, we may specify a Bayesian model as follows:

$$Y_{ik} \sim \text{log-Normal}(m_{ik}, \sigma_1^2)$$

$$m_{ik} = \mu + [(2\text{-sequence}_i)(2 - k) + (\text{sequence}_i - 1)(k - 1)]\varphi + (2 - k)\pi + \delta_i$$

$$\delta_i \sim \text{Normal}(0, \sigma_2^2)$$

$$\mu, \pi, \varphi \sim \text{Normal}(0, 1^{-6})$$

$$1/\sigma_1^2, 1/\sigma_2^2 \sim \text{Gamma}(0.001, 0.001)$$

After running WinBUGS 1.4,[38] we obtained the mean (standard deviation) ratio of formulation, 0.92 (0.14), the 95% creditable interval, (0.71, 1.11), and the probability the ratios fall into (0.8, 1.25) 0.78.

E. Anderson and Hauck's Procedure

Because of the nature of equivalence trials, an alternative hypothesis that the difference of the two formulation means will fall within a prespecified interval has to be setup. This concept was discussed originally by Lehmann[70] and Bondy.[71] Anderson and Hauck[72] have adopted this idea using the following pair of hypotheses:

$$H_0 : \mu_T - \mu_R \leq \log(0.8) \text{ or } \mu_T - \mu_R \geq \log(1.25)$$

$$H_1 : \log(0.8) < \mu_T - \mu_R < \log(1.25)$$

where μ_T and μ_R are the expectations of the log-transformed pharmacokinetic parameters. Note that the null hypothesis states that the two formulation means are *not* equivalent while the alternative hypothesis states those to be equivalent. The test statistic they consider is

$$T = \frac{\bar{X}_T - \bar{X}_R - 1/2[\log(0.8) - \log(1.25)]}{S(1/n_T + 1/n_R)}$$

where the X's and n's are the sample means (in the logarithmic scale) and sample sizes, respectively, and S is the standard deviation (square root of MSE) obtained from the analysis of variance model. As they discussed, the distribution of T is generally unknown. Thus, the exact critical value cannot be found. However, the Student's t distribution can be used as an adequate approximation. A similar approach was used by Rocke.[73] It is noted that there is a small probability that the null hypothesis will be rejected even when the difference of the two means is not within the acceptable limits.

F. TWO ONE-SIDED TESTS PROCEDURE

Schuirmann[74] proposed a procedure that consists of two pairs of testing hypotheses:

$$H_{01} : \mu_T - \mu_R \leq \log(0.8)$$

$$H_{11} : \mu_T - \mu_R > \log(0.8)$$

and

$$H_{02} : \mu_T - \mu_R \leq \log(1.25)$$

$$H_{12} : \mu_T - \mu_R > \log(1.25)$$

where μ_T and μ_R are the expectations of the log-transformed pharmacokinetic parameters. It may be noted that this procedure was originally developed based on the untransformed values.

This procedure decomposes the interval hypotheses H_0 and H_1 into two sets of onesided hypotheses. This two one-sided tests procedure will conclude equivalence of two formulation means if and only if both H_{01} and H_{02} are rejected at a chosen nominal level of significance (e.g., 0.05). The design rule based on the two one-sided tests procedure ($\alpha = 0.05$) is equivalent to the rule, based on the traditional 90% confidence interval.

In the same paper, Schuirmann also compared the rejection regions and the probability characteristics of his procedure to the power approach and showed that the two one-sided tests procedure is superior to the power approach in general.

Metzler[66] performed a simulation study to evaluate the power of different decision rules — two one-sided tests procedure (traditional confidence interval), Westlake's symmetric confidence interval (Rodda and Davis' procedure), Mandallaz and Mau's approach, and Anderson and Hauck's procedure. He defined the power of a decision rule for bioequivalence to be the probability of rejecting bioequivalence of a test formulation given the true relative bioavailability. Based on the probability of rejection curve, Westlake's rule is similar to the Anderson and Hauck's procedure if the coefficient of variation is less than 20%. The probability of rejection is close to 0.90 for all rules except the one based on the two one-sided tests procedure. To make this rule alike others, a larger value (viz., $2 \times \alpha$) should be used. If the coefficient of variation is greater than or equal to 30%, only the rule by Mandallaz and Mau is different from others.

Example. For the example in Section II.B, the log-transformed AUC was analyzed using an ANOVA model with fixed effects for sequence, period, formulation, and random effect for subject nested within the sequence. The least-squared mean of the difference and its 90% confidence interval were calculated from the fitted model; the least-squared mean of the difference and its 90% CI were then antilog-transformed to obtain the estimate of the ratio and its 90% confidence interval. The least-squared means of each formulation and their 95% confidence intervals were calculated in a similar manner.

The results are reported in Table 21.10.

G. Individual and Population Bioequivalence

Thus far, the so-called average bioequivalence has been discussed, which concerns only the similarity of the mean values between the innovator drug product and its generic copies in terms of AUC and C_{max}. Theoretically, this may

TABLE 21.10
Analysis of AUC Data

	Geometric Mean of AUC	C.I.
Summary of Results		
Formulation 1	925.76	(748.69, 1012.51)*
Formulation 2	1012.51	(818.84, 1251.70)*
Ratio (1 vs. 2)	91.4%	(71.5%, 116.9%)**
Summary of Results without Subjects 5 and 9		
Formulation 1	1111.48	(982.88, 1256.61)*
Formulation 2	1135.53	(1004.15, 1284.10)*
Ratio (1 vs. 2)	100.6%	(88.7%, 108.0%)**

*95% confidence interval; **90% confidence interval.

not be sufficient because the bioavailability is a random variable; the similarity of the mean values does not guarantee the similarity of the distribution. In addition to the mean values, the variances of AUC and C_{max} should be taken into consideration as well. If a bioequivalence criterion takes the mean values of AUC and C_{max} as well as the variances of AUC and C_{max} into account, then the bioequivalence defined by this criterion is called population bioequivalence. The equivalence of the distributions of AUC and C_{max} between formulations does not guarantee the similarity of the equivalences among individual patients. In others words, the subject by formulation interaction should be taken into consideration as well, while discussing bioequivalence. If a bioequivalence criterion takes into account not only the mean values and variances but also the subject by formulation interaction, then the bioequivalence defined by this criterion is called individual bioequivalence.

The variability of pharmacokinetic parameters can be divided into three components: difference in average bioavailabilities, variance of the subject-by-formulation interaction, and difference in intra-subject variabilities. Accordingly, bioequivalence criteria should be able to control all these three components. Criteria can either be set for each individual characteristic separately which are called disaggregate criteria, or a single criterion rule which controls all three characteristics simultaneously, which is called aggregate criteria. According to the distribution measures, both population and individual bioequivalence criteria can be grouped as either moment-based or probability-based criteria.

The early attempt for individual bioequivalence was reflected in a FDA-proposed rule of the late 1970s which used the individual ratios. This rule states that two formulations are equivalent if and only if at least 75% of these individual ratios are between the 75 and 125% limits. As an example, the data reported in Table 21.11 is considered. It may be noted that six out of 18 (33%) of the subjects had a bioavailability on formulation one within 25% of that of formulation two. Clearly, these two formulations are not bioequivalent if the 75/75 rule is applied. As Westlake[75] pointed out, the underlying principle of this 75/75 rule is similar to the construction of the tolerance interval. Haynes[76] performed a simulation study to investigate the 75/75 rule and showed that there is a greater probability to accept the test formulation if the coefficients of variations for the test and reference formulations are identical and smaller, respectively. In addition, a test formulation compared to a reference formulation with equal variability had less chance of acceptance than the case when the reference formulation has smaller variability.

However, if the individual ratio is the parameter of clinical interest, a confidence interval for the central tendency of these individual ratios[77,78] should be constructed. Yuh also indicated that the individual bioequivalence is similar to the percentage change from baseline in the conventional efficacy trials. This parameter is more difficult to analyze because it is a ratio of two random variables. That is, the ratios are not normally distributed even if the original random variables are normally distributed. Thus, the sample median or a robust estimator should be used to assess the central tendency of these

TABLE 21.11
Listing of Individual Ratios (%)

Subject	AUC Reference (2)	AUC Test (1)	Ratio (Formulation 1/Formulation 2) (%)
1	1735	3340	193
2	2594	2613	101
3	2526	1138	45
4	2344	2738	117
5	938	1287	137
6	1022	1284	126
7	1339	1930	144
8	2463	2120	86
9	2779	1613	58
10	2256	3052	135
11	1438	2549	177
12	1833	1310	71
13	3852	2254	59
14	1262	1964	156
15	4108	1755	43
16	1864	2302	124
17	1829	1682	92
18	2059	1851	90
Median			109
(Min/Max)			(43, 193)

ratios.[78] Anderson and Hauck[79] also discussed a procedure for treating the individual ratio as a binary response.

Yuh[80] proposed to assess bioequivalence using the concordance correlation. The concordance correlation measures a combination of the formulation — mean and variability differences and the linear correlation between the formulations. Note that the concordance correlation is equal to one if two formulations have identical means and variabilities and the linear correlation is equal to one.

Various moment-based criteria have been proposed.[79, 81–83] In 1997, FDA[82] proposed the following criterion for population bioequivalence

$$(\mu_T - \mu_R)^2 + (\sigma_{TT}^2 - \sigma_{TR}^2) - \theta_P \max(\sigma_{TR}^2, \sigma_{T0}^2) < 0$$

where

μ_T = population average response of the log-transformed measure for the test formulation

μ_R = population average response of the log-transformed measure for the reference formulation

σ_{TT}^2 = total variance of the test formulation

σ_{TR}^2 = total variance of the reference formulation

σ_{T0}^2 = specified constant total variance
θ_P = bioequivalence limit

and the criterion for individual bioequivalence

$$(\mu_T - \mu_R)^2 + \sigma_D^2 + (\sigma_{WT}^2 - \sigma_{WR}^2) - \theta_I \max(\sigma_{WR}^2, \sigma_{W0}^2) < 0$$

where

μ_T = population average response of the log-transformed measure for the test formulation
μ_R = population average response of the log-transformed measure for the reference formulation
σ_D^2 = subject-by-formulation interaction variance component
σ_{WT}^2 = within-subject variance of the test formulation
σ_{WR}^2 = within-subject variance of the reference formulation
σ_{W0}^2 = specified constant total variance
θ_I = bioequivalence limit.

To test for population or individual bioequivalence between the test and the reference formulations, the estimates of the left-hand side and their upper confidence limits need to be calculated. If the upper limit is less than zero, the test formulation is bioequivalent to the reference formulation in the chosen sense. WinNonLin software has the functionality to perform these tests.

Conventional nonreplicated designs, such as the two by two crossover design, can be used for average and population bioequivalence comparisons. Replicated crossover designs are required because individual bioequivalence relies on the estimated within-subject, within-formulation variation, and the correlation between formulations.

The FDA proposed criteria for population and individual bioequivalence described above employ aggregate statistics which combines information related to the differences in bioavailability among formulation means and the differences in bioavailability variation of formulations (between and within subjects), and the correlation between formulations. Given the initial model and assumptions, the mathematical theory is very interesting. However, a number of practical and technical challenges should be addressed. The clinical relevance of a subject by formulation interaction as measured by σ_D^2 has not been demonstrated. To date, no association between clinical failure and this interaction has been illustrated. As a consequence of the aggregate criteria, a numerical trade-off occurs between various terms, e.g., a substantive difference in means can be compensated by a decrease in within-subject variance in the test formulation relative to the reference formulation. The proposed criteria do not mandate a hierarchical testing process (i.e., the order of the means, the variances, and σ_D^2). In other words, a successful demonstration of individual bioequivalence does not imply population or average bioequivalence. It is recognized that the individual bioequivalence approach tries to address to the "switchability" issue between two test products. In 2003, the FDA, deleted the individual bioequivalence approach from the draft guidance[84] and recommended sponsors to continue usage of the average bioavailability approach as the primary method.

Statistical methods to evaluate population and individual bioequivalence trials remain to be scientifically challenging and interesting. Carrasco and Jover[85] introduced the structural equation model (SEM) for assessing individual bioequivalence. Dragalin et al.[86] used the Kullback–Leibler divergence (KLD) as a measure of discrepancy between the distributions of two formulations, which declares bioequivalence of two formulations if the upper bound of a level-α confidence interval for the KLD is less than a predefined regulatory criterion. This new methodology overcomes some disadvantages of the corresponding measures recommended by FDA. In particular the KLD: (i) possesses the natural hierarchical property (IBE $\Rightarrow$ PBE $\Rightarrow$ ABE); (ii) satisfies the properties of a true distance metric; (iii) is invariant to monotonic transformations of the data; (iv) generalizes easily to the multivariate case where equivalence on more than one parameter (for example, AUC, C_{max} and T_{max}) is of interest, and (v) is applicable to a wide range of distributions of the response variable (for example, those in the exponential family). A review of different statistical approaches was provided by Chow and Liu in order to understand the theories behind various methods.[87]

H. Choosing the Sample Size

One component of a bioavailability study is to determine the number of subjects to be included in the study. Here the sample size estimation strategy using the average bioequivalence criterion and the two one-sided t-tests procedure have been demonstrated. Suppose the log-transformed pharmacokinetic data are to be analyzed. If significance level is assumed to be α, the probability of the type II error be β, the expected difference of the log-transformed pharmacokinetic data be θ, the equivalence margin be δ, and the standard deviation of the log-transformed pharmacokinetic data be σ, then one way to calculate the sample size is given as follows:

$$n = \text{int}\left\{2\frac{[t_{\alpha}(n) + t_{\beta/2}(n)]^2}{\min\{(\delta - \theta)^2, (-\delta - \theta)^2\}}\sigma^2\right\} + 1$$

Because the number of subjects, n, on the right hand side is unknown, the calculation will be iterative, starting with an initial value, n_0, n_1 is calculated; n_{m+1} is calculated from n_m; the process is continued till n is unchangeable. For a parallel design the if σ is the total standard deviation, then the n is the number of subjects for each group. For a crossover design, if σ is the intra-subject standard deviation, then n is the total number of subjects (because each subject will give a pair of data points).

When designing a crossover study there is no intra-subject standard deviation available, which can be then calculated from the inter-subject standard deviation as $\sigma_{intra} = \sqrt{(1 - \rho)}\sigma$, where ρ is the intra-subject correlation coefficient, which is oftentimes assumed to be 0.5.

I. OTHER TOPICS

Other approaches include the transformation and nonparametric methods. There are several reasons one may perform a logarithmic transformation of the pharmacokinetic parameters. Both Westlake[88] and Rodda[47] gave a good discussion of the rationale for performing the transformation. An Advisory Committee to FDA recommended a logarithmic transformation of pharmacokinetic data. However, our experience shows that the distribution of the difference in formulations is usually symmetric if the subject effect is removed (as in the analysis of a crossover study). It should be noted that the acceptable lower (upper) limit under an anti-logarithmic transformation is 80% (125%) and the power calculation is different from that using the raw data.

If the underlying distribution is not normally distributed or there are potential outliers, nonparametric methods may be utilized to assess bioequivalence. Several nonparametric methods have been proposed for the crossover studies.[89–92] These methods except for Hodges–Lehman methods are useful for testing hypotheses; however, such methods may not be appropriate for the purpose of estimation because, clinically, it is difficult to interpret the confidence interval on the rank scale.

If studies involve more than two treatments, multiple confidence intervals for each pharmacokinetic parameter will be constructed and adjustments for these multiple comparisons should be made. However, most classical procedures are developed to adjust Type I error which may widen the confidence interval. Little work has been done to address the issue of adjustment of multiple confidence intervals.

If a crossover study design is used, a logical approach will utilize the within-subject comparisons and the individual ratio is also a parameter of interest. It may be noted that if the logarithmic transformation is performed, the individual ratios have to be implicitly analyzed. Replicated designs can be important because these can provide a good estimate for inter- and intra-subject variability, respectively. These designs can also adjust for carry over effects. Clearly, there are many unanswered questions and more research needs to be done in the future.

ACKNOWLEDGMENTS

This chapter is based on a previous version co-authored by Daniel Weiner and Lianng Yuh. We would like to acknowledge Dr. Weiner's significant contributions to the previous edition. We also would like to express our appreciation to Dr. Bruce Birmingham for his valuable comments.

APPENDIX A. PEELING TECHNIQUE FOR OBTAINING STARTING VALUES

The importance of good starting values in obtaining the best estimates of the parameters has been previously discussed. In this section, one method of obtaining initial estimates is discussed. The method will be illustrated by estimating the parameters in Equation 21.1 for the simulated data presented in Table 21.12. The first step is to plot the data on semi logarithmic paper, as in Figure 21.4. It may be noted that in Equation 21.1 if it is assumed that $K_a > K_e$ (which is true for most drugs), then for large enough t, the second exponential term is near-zero. Let $T(t_i)$ denote the equation of this terminal phase. Then

$$T(t_i) = \frac{FD}{V} \frac{K_a}{K_a - K_e} e^{-K_e t_i} \qquad \text{(A21.1)}$$

Taking logarithms to base 10 of both sides we obtain

$$\log T(t_i) = \log\left(\frac{FD}{V} \frac{K_a}{K_a - K_e}\right) - \frac{K_e t_i}{2.303} \qquad \text{(A21.2)}$$

Thus, if a line is drawn through those points lying on the terminal linear portion of the curve on semilog scale, it would have slope of $-K_e/2.303$ and would intercept

$$\log\left(\frac{FD}{V} \frac{K_a}{K_a - K_e}\right)$$

The constant 2.303 is the reciprocal of the log to base 10 of e. Although working with logarithms to base 10 may be somewhat unusual since the underlying

---

TABLE 21.12
Simulated Data

Time	Concentration	Extrapolated Concentration Using $T(t_i)$	Residual Concentration $R(t_i)$
0.5	35.43	80.60	45.17
1.0	45.47	66.29	20.82
1.5	45.33	54.52	9.19
2.0	40.85	44.84	3.99
2.5	35.25		
3.0	29.68		
5.0	13.78		
7.0	6.19		
9.0	2.78		
11.0	1.27		

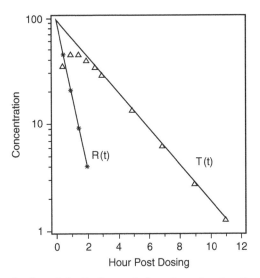

FIGURE 21.4 Application of the Peeling technique for estimating the pharmacokinetic parameter in a one-compartment model.

pharmacokinetic models can be written as sums of exponentials, it is the conventional methodology of practitioners in this area and its use will be adopted here. In Figure 21.4 it has been seen that the last six points fall nearly in a straight line. Selecting the first and last of these six values, the slope can be estimated by

$$\frac{\log T(11) - \log T(2.5)}{11 - 2.5} = 0.17$$

Thus $K_e = -0.17(-2.303) = 0.39$ and the estimated intercept from Figure 21.4 is $\log(98)$. We have then that

$$T(t_j) = \log(98) - 0.17t_i \tag{A21.3}$$

If Equation 21.1 is subtracted from Equation A21.1 and call the result $R(t_i)$, we have

$$R(t_i) = \frac{FD}{V} \frac{K_a}{K_a - K_e} e^{-K_a t_i} \tag{A21.4}$$

Again, taking logs of both sides of Equation A21.4, it is noted that $\log R(t_i)$ is linear with slope $-K_a/2.303$ and intercept

$$\log\left(\frac{FD}{V} \frac{K_a}{K_a - K_e}\right)$$

To obtain an estimate of K_a Equation A21.3 is first used to obtain extrapolated concentrations for those four points not in the terminal linear portion of the curve.

These values are recorded in the third column of Table 21.11. Then $R(t_i)$, $i = 1, 2, 3, 4$, are obtained by subtracting column three from column two. The slope of log $R(t_i)$ can easily be found to be -0.69; thus $K_a = -0.69(-2.303) = 1.59$. Using the intercept of either log $T(t_i)$ or log $R(t_i)$ (they should be equal), one can estimate either V or V/F depending on whether or not F is a known quantity. If the two intercepts did not coincide, the implication is that a lag time is needed in the model.

The true values used in simulating the data were $K_a = 1.50$ and $K_e = 0.40$ with $a = 0.01$. Although the estimated values were very close to the true values of the parameters in this example, this will not always be the case. It is sometimes difficult to determine which points to include as lying on the terminal linear portion of the curve. This is especially the case when K_a and K_e are nearly equal. Wagner[6] (pp. 59–63) illustrates the use of the peeling technique for more complicated models.

As is evidenced by the discussions in Sections II and III, model identification can be quite difficult. Even if the model can be assumed to be known, it may be difficult to obtain precise estimates of the pharmacokinetic parameters. Alternative models are available if estimates of the pharmacokinetic parameters are not needed. For example, splines and polynomial models often give good fits to drug concentration data. Usually, though, estimates of the pharmacokinetic parameters are needed to predict blood levels after multiple dosing (Ref. 6, pp. 144–147).

REFERENCES

1. Federal Register, Vol. 42. No. 5, Book 1, pp. 1624–1653, January 7, 1977.
2. Cabana, B.E. and Douglas, J.F., Bioavailability: Pharmacokinetic Guidelines for IND Development. Paper presented at *15th Annual International Pharmaceutical Conference, Austin, TX*, February 23–27, 1976.
3. Metzler, C.M., Bioavailability: a problem in equivalence, *Biometrics*, 30, 309–317, 1974.
4. Gibaldi, M., *Biopharmaceutics and Clinical Pharmacokinetics*, Lea & Febriger, Philadelphia, 1977.
5. Gibaldi, M. and Perrier, D., *Pharmacokinetics*, Marcel Dekker, New York, 1982.
6. Wagner, J.G., *Fundamentals of Clinical Pharmacokinetics*, Drug Intelligence, Hamilton, IL, 1975.
7. WinNonLin. *User's Manual*, Pharsight Corporation, Mountain View, CA, 2002.
8. Peck, C.P., Beal, S.L., Sheiner, L.B., and Nichols, A.I., ELS nonlinear regression: a possible solution to the choice of weights problem in analysis of individual pharmacokinetic data, *J. Pharmacokinet. Biopharm.*, 12, 545–558, 1984.
9. Rodda, B.E., Sampson, C.B., and Smith, D.W., The onecompartment open model: some statistical aspects of parameter estimation, *Appl. Stat.*, 24, 309–318, 1975.
10. Giltinan, D.M. and Ruppert, D., Fitting heteroscedastic regression models to individual pharmacokinetic data using standard statistical software, *J. Pharmacokinet. Biopharm.*, 17, 601–614, 1989.

11. Sheiner, L.B., Rosenberg, B., and Melmon, K.L., Modeling of individual pharmacokinetics for computer-aided drug dosage, *Comput. Biomed. Res.*, 5, 441–459, 1972.

12. Jobson, J.D. and Fuller, W.A., Least squares estimation when the covariance matrix and parameter vector are functionally related, *J. Am. Stat. Assoc.*, 75, 176–181, 1980.

13. Carroll, R.J. and Ruppert, D., A comparison between maximum likelihood and generalized least-squares in a heteroscedastic linear model, *J. Am. Stat. Assoc.*, 77, 878–882, 1982.

14. van Houwelingen, J.C., Use and abuse of variance models in regression, *Biometrics*, 43, 1073–1081, 1988.

15. Finney, D.J., Models, formulations and statistics, In *Variability in Drug Therapy*, Rowland, M., Sheiner, L.B., and Steiner, J.-L., eds., Raven Press, New York, pp. 11–123, 1985.

16. Beal, S.L. and Sheiner, L.B., Heteroscedastic nonlinear regression, *Technometrics*, 30, 327–337, 1988.

17. Katz, D., Azen, S.P., and Schumitzky, A., Bayesian approach to the analysis of nonlinear models, *Biometrics*, 37, 137–142, 1981.

18. Racine-Poon, A., Bayesian approach to nonlinear random effect models, *Biometrics*, 41, 1015–1023, 1985.

19. Steimer, J., Mallet, A., and Mentre, F., Estimating individual pharmacokinetic variability, In *Variability in Drug Therapy*, Rowland, M., Sheiner, L.B., and Steiner, J., eds., Raven Press, New York, pp. 65–111, 1985.

20. Whiting, B., Kelman, A.W., and Grevel, J., Population pharmacokinetics — theory on clinical application, *Clin. Pharmacokinet.*, 11, 387–401, 1986.

21. Grasela, T.H., Antal, E.J., Ereshefsky, L., Wells, B.G., Evans, R.L., and Smith, R.B., An evaluation of population pharmacokinetics in therapeutic trials. Part II. Detection of a drug–drug interaction, *Clin. Pharmacol. Ther.*, 42, 433–441, 1987.

22. Rodda, B.E., Sampson, C.B., and Smith, D.W., The onecompartment open model: some statistical aspects of parameter estimation. Abstract 2057, *Biometrics*, 28, 1180, 1972.

23. Katz, D., Population density estimation, *Prog. Food Nutr. Sci.*, 1, 325–338, 1988.

24. Prevost, G., Estimation of Normal Probability Density Function from Samples Measured with Nonnegligible and Nonconstant Dispersion. Internal report 6-77, Adersa-Gerbios, 2 avenue de ler Mai, F-91120 Palaiseau, 1977.

25. Katz, D. and D'Argenio, D., Experimental design for estimating integrals by numeric quadrature, with applications to pharmacokinetic studies, *Biometrics*, 39, 621–628, 1983.

26. Racine-Poon, A. and Smith, A.F.M., Population models, In *Statistical Methodology in the Pharmaceutical Sciences*, Berry, D.A., ed., Marcel Dekker, New York, pp. 139–162, 1989.

27. Yuh, L., Beal, S., Davidian, M., et al., Population pharmacokinetic/pharmacodynamic methodology and applications, *Biometrics*, 50, 566–575, 1994.

28. Weiner, D.L. and Jordan, D.C., Incorporating Subject Variability into Pharmacokinetics Models. Paper Presented at *Midwest Biopharmaceutical Statistics Workshop, Muncie, IN*, May 23–24, 1978.

29. Sheiner, L.B. and Beal, S.L., Evaluation of methods of estimating pharmacokinetic parameters: I. Michaelis–Menten model: routine clinical pharmacokinetic data, *J. Pharmacokinet. Biopharm.*, 8, 553–571, 1980.

30. Sheiner, L.B. and Beal, S.L., Evaluation of methods of estimating pharmacokinetic parameters: II. Bioexponential model and experimental pharmacokinetic data, *J. Pharmacokinet. Biopharm.*, 9, 635–651, 1981.
31. Sheiner, L.B. and Beal, S.L., Evaluation of methods for estimating population pharmacokinetic parameters. III. Monoexponential model: routine clinical pharmacokinetic data, *J. Pharmacokinet. Biopharm.*, 11, 303–319, 1983.
32. Mallet, A., A maximum likelihood estimation method for random coefficient regression models, *Biometrika*, 73, 645–656, 1986.
33. Linstrom, M.J. and Bates, D.M., Nonlinear mixed effects models for repeated measures data, *Biometrics*, 46, 673–687, 1990.
34. Gelfand, A.E., Hills, S.E., Racine-Poon, A., and Smith, A.F.M., Illustration of Bayesian inference in normal data models using Gibbs sampling, *J. Am. Stat. Assoc.*, 85, 972–985, 1990.
35. Beal, S.L. and Sheiner, L.B., *NONMEM User's Guide, parts I–VII*, NONMEM Project Group, San Francisco, 1992.
36. SAS Institute Inc., SAS OnlineDoc 9.1.3, SAS, Cary, NC, 2004.
37. Lunn, D., *pkBugs User Guide*, Version 1.1, Imperial College School of Medicine, London, 1999.
38. Spiegelhalter, D., Thomas, A., Best, N., and Lunn, D., *WinBUGS User Manual*, Version 1.4, MRC Biostatistics Unit, Institute of Public Health, Cambridge, UK, 2003.
39. Bennett, J.E., Racine-Poon, A., and Wakefield, J.C., MCMC for nonlinear hierarchical models, In *Markov Chain Monte Carlo in Practice*, Gilks, W.R., Richardson, S., and Spiegelhalter, D.J., eds., Chapman & Hall, London, pp. 339–357, 1996.
40. Best, N.G., Tan, K.K.C., Gilks, W.R., and Spiegelhalter, D.J., Estimation of population pharmacokinetics using the Gibbs sampler, *J. Pharmacokinet. Biopharm.*, 23, 407–424, 1995.
41. FDA. *Report by the Bioequivalence Task Force on Recommendations from the Bioequivalence Hearing Conducted by the FDA*, Bioequivalence Task Force, FDA, Washington, D.C., 1988.
42. Morrison, D.F., *Multivariate Statistical Methods*, McGraw-Hill, New York, 1976.
43. Chen, M. and Jackson, J., The role of metabolites in bioequivalency assessment. I. Linear pharmacokinetics without first-pass effect, *Pharm. Res.*, 8, 25–32, 1991.
44. Jones, B. and Kenward, M.G., *Design and Analysis of Crossover Trials*, Chapman & Hall, New York, 1989.
45. Hwang, S., Huber, P.B., Nesney, M., and Kwan, K.C., Bioequivalence and interchangeability, *J. Pharm. Sci.*, 67, IV 1978.
46. Ekbohm, G. and Melander, H., The subject-by-formulation interaction as a criterion of interchangeability of drugs, *Biometrics*, 45, 1249–1254, 1989.
47. Rodda, B.E., Bioavailability: design and analysis in statistical methodology, In *The Pharmaceutical Sciences*, Berry, D.A., ed., Marcel Dekker, New York, pp. 57–81.
48. Westlake, W.J., The use of balanced incomplete block designs in comparative bioavailability trials, *Biometrics*, 30, 319–329, 1974.
49. Yuh, L. and Ruberg, S.J., Latin square designs in a comparative bioavailability study, *Drug Inf. J.*, 24, 289–297, 1990.
50. D'Argenio, D.Z., Optimal sampling times for pharmacokinetic experiments, *J. Pharmacokinetic. Biopharm.*, 9, 739–755, 1981.

51. DiStefano, J.J. III, Optimized blood sampling protocols and sequential design of kinetic experiments, *Am. J. Physiol.*, 240, 259–265, 1981.

52. DiStefano, J.J. III, Algorithms, software and sequential optimal sampling schedule designs for pharmacokinetics and physiologic experiments, *Math. Comput. Simul.*, XXIV, 531–534, 1982.

53. Landaw, E.M., Optimal multicompartmental sampling designs for parameter estimation: practical aspects of the identification problem, *Math. Comput. Simul.*, XXIV, 525–530, 1982.

54. Drusano, G.L., Forrest, A., Snyder, M.J., Reed, M.D., and Blumer, J.L., An evaluation of optimal sampling strategy and adaptive study design, *Clin. Pharmacol. Ther.*, 44, 232–238, 1988.

55. Winer, B.J., *Statistical Principles in Experimental Design*, McGraw-Hill, New York, 1971.

56. Westlake, W.J., Use of confidence intervals in analysis of comparative bioavailability trials, *J. Pharm. Sci.*, 61(8), 1340–1341, 1972.

57. Shirley, E., The use of confidence intervals in biopharmaceutics, *J. Pharm. Pharmacol.*, 28, 312–313, 1976.

58. O'Quigley, J. and Baudoin, C., General approaches to the problems of equivalence, *Statistician*, 37, 51–58, 1988.

59. Locke, C.S., An exact confidence interval from untransformed data for the ratio of two formulation means, *J. Pharmacokinet. Biopharm.*, 12, 649–655, 1984.

60. Schuirmann, D.J., Confidence Intervals for the Ratio of Two Means from a Crossover Study. *Proceedings of 1989 Biopharmaceutical Section of the American Statistical Association*, American Statistical Association, pp. 121–126, 1990.

61. Westlake, W.J., Symmetric confidence intervals for bioequivalence trials, *Biometrics*, 32, 741–744, 1976.

62. Mantel, N., Do we want confidence intervals symmetrical about the null value? *Biometrics*, 33, 759–760, 1977.

63. Mandallaz, D. and Mau, J., Comparison of different methods for decision making in bioequivalence assessment, *Biometrics*, 37, 213–222, 1981.

64. Steinijans, V.W. and Diletti, E., Statistical analysis of bioavailability studies: parametric and nonparametric confidence intervals, *Eur. J. Clin. Pharmacol.*, 24, 127–136, 1983.

65. Kirkwood, T.B.L., Bioequivalence testing — a need to rethink, *Biometrics*, 37, 589 1981.

66. Metzler, C.M., Statistical methods for deciding bioequivalence of formulations, In *Oral Sustained Release Formulation: Design and Evaluation*, Yacobi, A. and Halperin-Walega, E., eds., Pergamon Press, New York, 1988.

67. Rodda, B.E. and Davis, R.L., Determine the probability of an important difference in bioavailability, *Clin. Pharmacol. Ther.*, 28, 247–252, 1980.

68. Selwyn, M.R., Dempster, A.P., and Hall, N.R., A Bayesian approach to bioequivalence for the two by two changeover design, *Biometrics*, 37, 11–21, 1981.

69. Selwyn, M.R. and Hall, N.R., On Bayesian methods for bioequivalence, *Biometrics*, 40, 1103–1108, 1992.

70. Lehmann, E.L., *Testing Statistical Hypotheses*, Wiley, New York, 1959.

71. Bondy, W.H., A test of an experimental hypothesis of negligible difference between means, *Am. Stat.*, 23, 28–30, 1969.

72. Anderson, S. and Hauck, W.W., A new procedure for testing equivalence in comparative bioavailability and other clinical trials, *Commun. Stat.*, A12, 2663–2692, 1983.
73. Rocke, D.M., On testing for bioequivalence, *Biometrics*, 40, 225–230, 1984.
74. Schuirmann, D.J., A comparison of two onesided tests procedure and the power approach for assessing the equivalence of average bioavailability, *J. Pharmacokinet. Biopharm.*, 15, 657–680, 1987.
75. Westlake, W.J., Statistical aspects of comparative bioavailability trials, *Biometrics*, 35, 273–280, 1979.
76. Haynes, J.D., Statistical simulation study of new proposed uniformity requirement for bioavailability studies, *J. Pharm. Sci.*, 70, 673–675, 1981.
77. Yuh, L., On Robust Estimation in Bioavailability/Bioequivalence Studies, *Proceedings of Bio International 1989, Toronto, Canada*, 162–165, 1990.
78. Yuh, L., Robust procedures in comparative bioavailability studies, *Drug Inf. J.*, 24, 741–751, 1990.
79. Anderson, S. and Hauck, W.W., Consideration of individual bioequivalence, *J. Pharmacokinet. Biopharm.*, 18, 259–273, 1990.
80. Yuh, L., On assessing bioequivalency using the concordance correlation coefficient, *Proceedings of Bio-International 1992, Bad Homburg, Germany*, pp. 283–288, 1993.
81. Anderson, S. and Hauck, W.W., Consideration of individual bioequivalence, *J. Pharmacokinet. Biopharm.*, 18, 259–273, 1992.
82. FDA, *In vivo Bioequivalence Studies Based on Population and Individual Bioequivalence Approaches*, 1997.
83. Sheiner, L.B., Bioequivalence revisited, *Stat. Med.*, 11, 1777–1778, 1992.
84. FDA, *Bioavailability and Bioequivalence Studies for Orally Administered Drug Products — General Considerations*, 2003.
85. Carrasco, J.L. and Jover, L., Assessing individual bioequivalence using the structural equation model, *Stat. Med.*, 22, 901–912, 2003.
86. Dragalin, V., Fedorov, V., Patterson, S., and Jones, B., KLD for evaluating bioequivalence, *Stat. Med.*, 22, 913–930, 2003.
87. Chow, S.C. and Liu, J.P., *Design and analysis of bioavailability and bioequivalence studies*, Marcel Dekker, New York, 2000.
88. Westlake, W.J., Bioavailability and bioequivalence of pharmaceutical formulations, In *Biopharmaceutical Statistics for Drug Development*, Peace, K.E., ed., Marcel Dekker, New York, pp. 329–352, 1988.
89. Koch, G.G., The use of nonparametric methods in the statistical analysis of twoperiod changeover design, *Biometrics*, 28, 577–584, 1972.
90. Hauschke, D., Steinjans, V.W., and Diletti, E., A distribution-free procedure for the statistical analysis of bioequivalence studies, *Int. J. Clin. Pharmacol. Ther. Toxicol.*, 28, 72–78, 1990.
91. Pabst, G. and Jaeger, H., Review of methods and criteria for the evaluation of bioequivalence studies, *Eur. J. Clin. Pharmacol.*, 38, 5–10, 1990.
92. Ltauschke, D., Steinjans, V.W., and Diletti, E., A distribution-free procedure for the statistical analysis of bioequivalence studies, *Int. J. Clin. Pharmacol. Ther. Toxicol.*, 28, 72–78, 1990.

22 Stability Studies of Pharmaceuticals

Yi Tsong, Chi-wan Chen, Wen Jen Chen,
Roswitha Kelly, Daphne T. Lin, and Karl K. Lin

CONTENTS

I. INTRODUCTION

The stability of a drug substance or drug product is the capacity of that substance or product to remain within the established acceptance criteria to ensure its identity, strength, quality, and purity within a specified period of time. Regulatory agencies require that adequate testing be performed by an applicant to demonstrate the stability of the drug substance or product in support of the approval for a marketing registration application. The purpose of stability testing is to provide evidence on how the quality of a drug substance or product varies with time under the influence of a variety of environmental factors, such as temperature, humidity, and light. This assessment is used to establish the recommended storage conditions and a retest period for the drug substance or a shelf-life for the drug product.

A retest period is the period of time during which a drug substance is expected to remain within its acceptance criterion and, therefore, can be used without testing in the manufacture of a given drug product, provided that the drug substance has been stored under the defined conditions. A shelf-life (also referred to as expiration dating period) is the period of time during which a drug product is expected to remain within the approved acceptance criteria, provided that the drug product has been stored under the conditions defined on the container label.

The International Conference on Harmonization (ICH) of Technical Requirements for Registration of Pharmaceuticals for Human Use has in recent years issued a series of guidelines on the design and conduct of stability studies of pharmaceuticals, and on the evaluation of stability data derived from such studies. ICH Q1A (R2) *Stability Testing 11/21/2003 of New Drug Substances and Products*[1] defines the core stability data package that is sufficient to support the registration of a new drug application in the tripartite regions of the European Union, Japan, and the United States. Q1A(R2) recommends that at least three primary batches of the drug substance and product be tested for stability at prescribed storage conditions and time points. ICH Q1D *Bracketing and Matrixing Designs for Stability Testing of New Drug Substances and Products*[2] provides guidance on reduced designs for stability studies. It outlines the circumstances under which a bracketing or matrixing design can be used. Bracketing is a reduced design where only samples of the extremes of a factor are tested at all time points. Matrixing is a reduced design where a selected subset of the total number of possible samples from all factor combinations would be tested at a specified time point. ICH Q1E *Stability Data Evaluation*[3] describes the principles of stability data evaluation and various approaches to the statistical analysis of stability data in establishing a retest period for the drug substance or a shelf-life for the drug product, which would satisfy regulatory requirements.

Although these guidelines have provided harmonized guidance in the three ICH regions on the designs, conduct, and data analysis of stability studies to support a drug application registration, the discussion on statistical detail is limited.

In this chapter, the discussion will focus on the statistical aspects of stability studies in general. In Section II, various statistical designs suitable for stability studies will be discussed, including full and fractional factorials. In Section III, statistical analyses for simple and complex stability studies will be discussed in detail. Alternative statistical analyses based on the mixed-effects model and on an equivalence approach will be presented in Section IV.

II. DESIGNS OF STABILITY STUDY

The main application of statistics to stability studies is in the estimation of the shelf-life for the product. Historically, this has been a simple problem of linear regression, where the shelf-life was determined by the earliest intersection of one of the 95% confidence bands around the regression line constructed from the long-term data of a single batch or from the combined data of several batches.[4-6] In an effort to save cost and resources, several complicated designs have been proposed.[7-11] These include fractional factorial designs and other strategies. However, their applicability to a given case needs to be cautiously evaluated.

In the simplest case, a sufficient number of container units from a batch are put on long-term storage in a controlled environment (e.g., 25°C/60%RH), and samples are taken from the chamber at predetermined time points, namely, at 0, 3, 6, 9, 12, 18, 24, 36, 48, etc., months, and tested for appropriate physical, chemical, biological, and microbiological attributes. The concentration of time points during the first year provides an early warning system to unexpected loss in stability. To support the marketing application of a drug product, the stability of a minimum of three batches needs to be evaluated. The minimum of three batches is a compromise between cost and statistical requirements for estimating between-batch variability. In the data analysis it can be determined whether data from the batches can be combined, when it would usually lead to a longer shelf-life estimate.

Many products are supplied in several strengths and different container closure systems, e.g., bottle, blister pack, and various container sizes and fills. In the traditional design, at least three batches of each configuration of strength and container size need to be put on stability for the estimation of the shelf-life of the combination. This leads to either independent designs for individual strength/ container combinations or one overall factorial design in which the effects of batch, strength, container, etc., on the stability of the dosage form are investigated. If the assumption of equal variances across the various combinations of factors holds, the potential advantage of the full factorial over separate regression models lies in the common error term and the potential pooling of data across design factors. Combining the data will lead to a higher precision in the error variance estimation when the model used is correct. If the data can be pooled across design factors, a common and usually longer shelf-life may be applied to all product configurations. However, a full factorial design can be costly.

In an effort to save resources and time, several types of reductions from the full factorial design have been proposed, most notably bracketing and matrixing. However, not each product is amenable to these approaches. For example, bracketing or matrixing can be applied to various strengths of a tablet dosage form only if they come from basically the same granulation or have closely related formulations. For more detailed prerequisites, ICH Q1D should be consulted.

Bracketing is an approach in which only the extreme configurations of strength and container are studied. The basic assumption is that the configurations of strength and container studied are no more stable than those not studied. Care needs to be taken that the numeric extremes (e.g., highest strength versus lowest strength, largest bottle versus smallest bottle) are not automatically assumed to represent the most and least stable configurations.[12,13] Surface area to headspace ratios in a container or other similar assessment of product vulnerability to moisture, oxygen, and light need to be evaluated in determining which configurations represent the extremes. A bracketing design can be considered as separate studies (of the extreme configurations) or as one study, and the data obtained should be analyzed accordingly. Table 22.1 gives an example of a bracketing design.

TABLE 22.1
Example of a Bracketing Design

Strength		50 mg			75 mg			100 mg		
Batch		1	2	3	1	2	3	1	2	3
Container size	15 ml	T	T	T				T	T	T
	100 ml									
	500 ml	T	T	T				T	T	T

Key: T = Sample tested

Matrixing is a design of a stability schedule, in which only a fraction of the samples are tested at a specified time point. Statistically, it is a fractional factorial approach. All configurations of the design factors, e.g., strength and container size, are considered in one factorial design, but only a fraction of all possible factor combinations is tested at any specified time points. Subsets of factor combinations vary across time points. Certain prerequisites, such as common granulation, etc., need to be met before a multiple factor analysis approach can be considered. For further information, ICH Q1D should be consulted. As it is assumed that the stability of the samples tested represents the stability of all samples, matrixing over factors with different expected stability patterns (such as, different container closure systems or different storage conditions) is not acceptable. The simplest matrixing approach involves reducing the testing schedule of each batch (see Table 22.2). For regulatory purposes, certain time points (e.g., 0, 12, 24 months) are required on all batches, others may be matrixed. A much greater reduction in

TABLE 22.2
Examples of Matrixing Designs on Time Points for a Product with wo Strengths

Strength	Time point (months)	One-Half Reduction								One-Third Reduction							
		0	3	6	9	12	18	24	36	0	3	6	9	12	18	24	36
S1	Batch 1	T	T		T	T		T	T	T	T		T	T		T	T
	Batch 2	T	T		T	T	T		T	T	T	T		T	T		T
	Batch 3	T		T		T	T		T	T		T	T	T	T	T	T
S2	Batch 1	T		T		T			T	T		T	T	T	T	T	T
	Batch 2	T	T		T	T	T		T	T	T	T		T	T		T
	Batch 3	T		T		T		T	T	T	T	T		T	T		T

Key: T = Sample tested

TABLE 22.3
Examples of Factor and Time Matrixing Designs for a Product with Three Strengths and Three Container Sizes

	Strength								
	S1			S2			S3		
Container size	A	B	C	A	B	C	A	B	C
Batch 1	T1	T2		T2		T1		T1	T2
Batch 2		T3	T1	T3	T1		T1		T3
Batch 3	T3		T2		T2	T3	T2	T3	

Key:

Time-point (months)	0	3	6	9	12	18	24	36
T1	T		T	T	T	T	T	T
T2	T	T		T	T		T	T
T3	T	T	T		T	T		T

S1, S2, and S3 are different strengths. A, B, and C are different container sizes. T = Sample tested

cost and resources occurs when design factors as well as time points are matrixed (see Table 22.3). The savings of a matrixed design over a full design are obvious. Care must be taken to ensure that the matrixing design results in a valid fractional factorial design which can be statistically analyzed. However, because of the reduced amount of data collected, certain terms of the model may become nonestimable and the study may instead have to be analyzed using separate models on disjoint subsets. Therefore, an applicant assumes the risk of possibly estimating a shorter shelf-life than had a full model been employed.

In rare occasions, bracketing and matrixing can be combined into a single design.

The above mentioned discussions on the use of bracketing and matrixing designs cover the basic regulatory needs. There are more detailed design criteria discussed in the literature. Nordbrock[10] suggested choosing between designs based on the power of detecting differences in slopes of desired factors. Nordbrock uses the term "matrixing" and "fractional factorial-type designs" for bracketing and matrixing, respectively. He listed ten different designs starting with a complete factorial and designs with combinations of reduced time points and various reduced factors. Though some aspects of his approach (e.g., including different container closure systems or considering different storage conditions in one design) may be controversial, he recommended choosing the most powerful design among designs that are acceptable and of equal sample size, to increase savings in cost and resources. Ju and Chow[14] on the other hand recommended that the precision of the shelf-life estimate should determine which design to use.

For a fixed sample size, they proposed the design with the best precision for estimating shelf-life. For a fixed, desired precision, the design with the smallest sample size is considered the best choice. DeWoody and Raghavarao[15] developed a method for choosing the time vectors such that the design is optimal in terms of maximum information per unit cost. Although the full factorial provides maximum information, it is also the most costly design. For a fixed (reduced) number of time points, the design with the largest information per unit cost is considered optimal. However, as the number of time points is decreased, the variance of the slope contrast increases and may become unacceptably large. Therefore, DeWoody and Raghavarao suggested evaluating on a product-by-product basis which design may represent the best combination of cost versus the expected degradation rate and variance. Murphy[16] proposed several efficiency measures to show that a typical matrix design where each batch has a different (reduced) time schedule, is inferior to a uniform matrix design where each batch has the same time schedule. The time schedule has been reduced in such a way that the remaining time points are concentrated at the beginning and at the end of the study. If the uniform matrix design is to be considered, it may be prudent to consult with the regulatory agency first to obtain concurrence that there is no concern regarding undue loss of information about stability early on and/or pattern (curvature) of the data. Pong and Raghavarao[17] compared the power for detecting a significant difference between slopes and the mean square error to evaluate the precision of the estimated shelf-life of bracketing and matrixing designs. They found the power of both designs to be similar. Based on the conditions under study, they concluded that bracketing appears to be a better design than matrixing in terms of the precision of the estimated shelf-life.

A different perspective was proposed by Kleijn and Lakeman[11] for postmarketing stability surveillance, i.e., for confirming an approved shelf-life. In this proposal, not only the amount of testing, but also the testing time schedule is challenged. They proposed to put a single batch per year on stability and test all batches on a "selected date" once a year or less often. The use of this approach should be carefully evaluated before applying it. In addition, the applicability of this approach to the estimation of the shelf-life during the marketing application has not been established.

III. METHODS FOR SHELF-LIFE DETERMINATION

A. ANCOVA MODELING OF SIMPLE STABILITY STUDIES

In this section, a drug product that is produced in only one strength and container size is considered. Without loss of generality, one can assume that the drug attribute changes linearly with time, (e.g., potency assay decreases linearly as time increases). Other cases can be treated similarly. Currently, FDA and most pharmaceutical companies use simple linear regression to analyze long-term stability data collected under room temperature conditions. The simple linear regression model for this approach is

$$Y(t) = \alpha + \beta t + \varepsilon_t \tag{22.1}$$

where $Y(t)$ denotes the attribute value of the batch at month t, α and β are the intercept and slope parameters, respectively, and ε_t is the model error term that is iid and follows a $N(0, \sigma^2)$ distribution. α and β are the parameters to be estimated and assumed to be fixed.[5,6,18]

As the data from a single batch cannot capture batch-to-batch variability, a stability study is conducted with a minimum of three batches. To model the linear regressions of multiple batches of the same drug product, the ANCOVA model is often used,

$$Y_i(t) = \alpha_0 + \alpha_i + (\beta_0 + \beta_i)t + \varepsilon_{it} \tag{22.2}$$

where α_0 and β_0 are the common intercept and slope parameters, respectively, shared by all batches, and α_i and β_i are the deviations of the individual intercept and slope of the ith batch from α_0 and β_0, respectively.

One of the most important chemical attributes is the potency assay, whose results represent the contents of the drug substance or active ingredient. It is expressed in percent of label claim or a transformation thereof. If a product has more than one active ingredient, the analysis is performed on each ingredient separately. Degradation products of the active ingredient, whose levels increase with time, are also very important measures of stability and are similarly analyzed. Other attributes, e.g., pH, preservative contents, dissolution, etc., are similarly analyzed, usually in their original units or an appropriate transformation to improve linearity.

In practice, stability data may vary sufficiently between batches so that the individual regression lines may have different intercepts and/or slopes. However, the collected stability data can be fitted with one of the following models:[5]

1. Model 1: different intercepts and different slopes (Figure 22.1a),

$$Y_i(t) = \alpha_0 + \alpha_i + (\beta_0 + \beta_i)t + \varepsilon_{it}$$

2. Model 2: common intercept but different slopes (Figure 22.1b),

$$Y_i(t) = \alpha_0 + (\beta_0 + \beta_i)t + \varepsilon_{it}$$

3. Model 3: common slope but different intercepts (Figure 22.1c),

$$Y_i(t) = \alpha_0 + \alpha_i + \beta_0 t + \varepsilon_{it}$$

4. Model 4: common slope and common intercept (Figure 22.1d),

$$Y_i(t) = \alpha_0 + \beta_0 t + \varepsilon_{it}$$

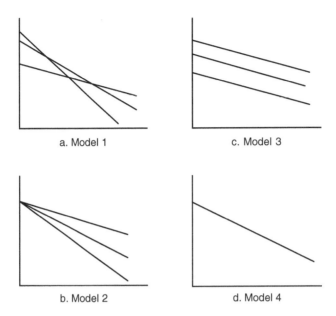

FIGURE 22.1 Four regression models.

Determining which of the above models best fit the data is accomplished by testing the equality of slopes and/or intercepts of the regression lines. If the regression lines are shown to be similar, the data may be pooled to obtain a common slope and/or intercept.

The pooling tests of slope and intercept are conducted in hierarchical order, i.e., the poolability of slopes is tested before the poolability of intercepts. The null and alternative hypotheses of the slope poolability test are,

$$H_0 : \beta_i = 0 \ \forall i, \text{ versus } H_a : \beta_i \neq 0, \text{ for some } i. \qquad (22.3)$$

A common slope is accepted if H_0 is not rejected. Once a common slope is accepted, the poolability of the intercepts is tested by the following hypotheses,

$$H_0 : \alpha_i = 0 \ \forall i, \text{ versus } H_a : \alpha_i \neq 0, \text{ for some } i. \qquad (22.4)$$

A common intercept is accepted if H_0 is not rejected. The determination of the final model is based on the results of the hierarchical testing of hypotheses (22.3) and (22.4).

The hierarchical testing procedure can be carried out in a single ANCOVA modeling step with the hierarchical partitioning of the total sum of squares, i.e., the Type I sums of squares. In fact, with the ANCOVA model and the Type I sums of squares, the following tests are performed.

The total sum of squares, SS_{tot}, is partitioned into the sum of squares because of regression, SS_{reg}, and

$$\sum\sum(Y_{ij} - \bar{Y}_{..})^2 = \underbrace{\sum\sum(\hat{Y}_{ij} - \bar{Y}_{..})^2}_{SS_{reg}} + \underbrace{\sum\sum(Y_{ij} - \hat{Y}_{ij})^2}_{SS_{res}}$$

$$\underbrace{\phantom{\sum\sum(Y_{ij} - \bar{Y}_{..})^2}}_{SS_{tot}}$$

the residual sum of squares, SS_{res} where Y_{ij} is the product characteristic at the jth time point of the ith batch of a drug.

The residual sum of squares is further partitioned into the sum of squares due to the variation about the individual regression equations, SS_{resin}, the sum of squares due to the variation between individual slopes and the average slope, $SS_{slopein}$, the sum of squares due to the variation about the regression of batch means, SS_{regmn}, and the sum of squares due to the variation between the regression of the means and the common slope, $SS_{slopemn}$:

$$\sum\sum(Y_{ij} - a - bX_{ij})^2 = \sum\sum[Y_{ij} - (a_i + b_iX_{ij})]^2 + \sum(b_i - \bar{b})^2\sum(X_{ij} - \bar{X}_{i.})^2$$

$$+ \sum J_i[\bar{Y}_{i.} - (\hat{a} + \hat{b}\bar{X}_{i.})]^2 + \frac{(\bar{b} - b)^2}{\left[\sum J_i(\bar{X}_{i.} - \bar{X}_{..})^2\right]^{-1}\left[\sum\sum(X_{ij} - \bar{X}_{i.})^2\right]^{-1}}$$

The above components are expressed by the following notations:

$$SS_{res} = SS_{resin} + SS_{slopein} + SS_{regmn} + SS_{slopemn}$$

a. *Test for equality of slopes.* With these partitions, the statistic $F_{slope} = MS_{slopein}/MS_{resin}$ follows an $F(I - 1, \Sigma_iJ_i - 2I)$ distribution under H_0 of (22.3). To reject H_0, F_{slope} should have a p-value less than .25.[3,5,6,18,19] The decision of a common slope is made if the F_{slope} test fails to reject H_0 of (22.3).

b. *Test for equality of intercepts given parallel lines.* Similarly, the statistic $F_{intercept} = MS_{regmn}/MS_{resin}$ follows an $F(I - 1, \Sigma_iJ_i - 2I)$ distribution under H_0 of (22.4). To reject H_0, $F_{intercept}$ should have a p-value less than .25. The decision of a common intercept is made if the $F_{intercept}$ test fails to reject H_0 of (22.4).

At the end of the above two hypothesis tests, one of the following models is selected for fitting the stability data of a drug product:

i. Individual slopes and intercepts (i.e., Model 1) if H_0 of (22.3) is rejected. Model 2 is considered as a special case of Model 1,

ii. Individual intercepts but common slope (i.e., Model 3) if H_0 of (22.4) is rejected but H_0 of (22.3) is not,

iii. Common slope and intercept (i.e., Model 4) if H_0 of both (22.3) and (22.4) are not rejected.

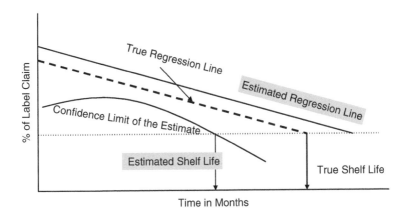

FIGURE 22.2 Shelf-life estimation.

The slopes and intercepts can be estimated using the final ANCOVA model. The standard errors of the estimates and the confidence bands around the regression lines can be obtained according to the selected model. However, even if only individual regression lines can be fitted, the estimated variance of the error term of the full model using data of all batches may be used in the construction of the confidence bands.

In theory, the shelf-life of each batch is the date when the expected value of the regression line intersects the acceptance criteria of the attribute (Figure 22.2). Statistically, the shelf-life is estimated by the time the confidence band intersects with the acceptance criteria of the attribute. When two-sided acceptance criteria are of concern, the proper shelf-life is based on the earliest intersection of the confidence bands with the acceptance criteria. When each batch is represented by an individual regression line, a shelf-life is determined for each batch based on its regression line. The shelf-life estimate for the product is determined by the minimum of all estimated shelf-lives. The same concept applies also when the drug product contains more than one active ingredient or when several product attributes are studied. In these cases, the shelf-life of the drug product is also determined by the minimum of any estimate based on all active ingredients and/or all studied attributes.

When evaluating stability data in support of a proposed shelf-life T_0, which in general may be 3 to 12 months longer than the last observed time point, the (minimum) estimated shelf-life T^* based on all batches will be compared with T_0. T_0 is granted if $T^* > T_0$.

The ANCOVA modeling of shelf-life determination of a single drug product can be illustrated with the following example.

Example 1. The stability data of three batches of a single drug product were collected at 0, 3, 6, 9, 12, and 18 months with the objective to claim 30 months for the shelf-life of the product. The data are shown in Table 22.4.

TABLE 22.4
Stability Data of Three Batches of a Product

Batch	Time Point (month)					
	0	**3**	**6**	**9**	**12**	**18**
Batch 1	103	104	104	103	102	101
Batch 2	102	103	103	102	102	100
Batch 3	103	102	101	101	100	99

The original ANCOVA model is

$$Y_i(t) = \alpha_0 + \alpha_i + (\beta_0 + \beta_i)t + \epsilon_t$$

where $i = 1, 2, 3$ (batch), $t = $ month, $\varepsilon_t \sim N(0, \sigma)$.
The SAS statement of the ANCOVA model used is

$$\text{MODEL } Y = \text{TIME BATCH TIME} \times \text{BATCH/SS1};$$

The three fitted individual lines are

$$Y(t) = 104.07 - 0.1667t$$
$$Y(t) = 103.04 - 0.1310t$$
$$Y(t) = 103.75 - 0.2262t.$$

They intersect the lower acceptance criterion (95% LC) at approximately 39, 39, and 30 months, respectively (Figure 22.3).

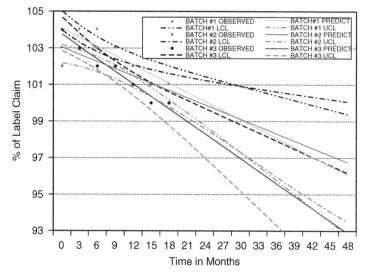

FIGURE 22.3 Individual regression lines of example 1.

TABLE 22.5
ANCOVA Results of Example 1

Source	DF	Sum of Squares	Mean Square	F Value	Pr > F
Model	5	27.167	5.433	14.09	<.0001
Error	15	5.786	0.386		
Corrected Total	20	32.952			
Source	**DF**	**Type I SS**	**Mean Square**	**F Value**	**Pr > F**
Month	1	23.0476	23.0476	59.75	<.0001
batch	2	2.9524	1.4762	3.83	.0454
Month × batch	2	1.1667	0.5833	1.51	.2522

A significance level of .25 is used for both the pooling tests of slope, $H_0 : \beta_i = 0$ and intercept, $H_0 : \alpha_i = 0$. There is no statistically significant difference between the slopes (p-value $= .252$). But the intercepts are considered different (p-value $= .045$) (Table 22.5).

These results lead to three parallel regression lines with different intercepts for the three batches as shown in Figure 22.4. The three fitted regression lines are

$$Y_1(t) = 103.286 - 0.1746t,$$

$$Y_2(t) = 104.144 - 0.1746t,$$

$$Y_3(t) = 103.430 - 0.1746t.$$

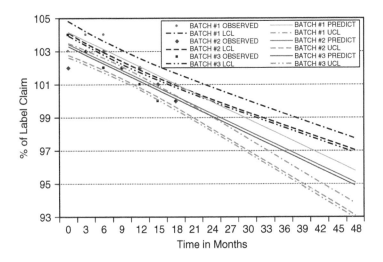

FIGURE 22.4 Parallel regression lines of example 1.

Their 95% confidence bounds intersect with the lower acceptance criterion at approximately 42, 39, and 36 months. Hence a 30-month shelf-life is supported.

B. ANCOVA MODELING OF STABILITY STUDIES DESIGNED WITH MULTIPLE FACTORS

As described in the previous section, the ANCOVA modeling application to the simple three-batch single product study has the feature of hierarchical testing for pooling of slopes and intercepts embedded in the single layout of the ANCOVA results. The equality tests of slopes and intercepts are handled in a hierarchical manner using the type I sum of squares of the ANCOVA model in SAS. Extention of the same ANCOVA application to a complicated multiple factor design requires a prespecified hierarchical ordering of the sums of squares partitions and of the pooling tests. For example, in a stability study designed with multiple levels of strength, container size, and batch, the ANCOVA model with all factors and interactions can be represented by (22.5) below

$$Y_{spbt} = \alpha + \alpha_s + \alpha_p + \alpha_b + \alpha_{sp} + \alpha_{sb} + \alpha_{pb} + \alpha_{spb} + \beta_t + \beta_s t + \beta_p t$$
$$+ \beta_b t + \beta_{sp} t + \beta_{sb} t + \beta_{pb} t + \beta_{spb} t + \epsilon_{spbt} \qquad (22.5)$$

where the subscript $s = 1$ to S represents the level of the strength, $p = 1$ to P represents the level of container size, and $b = 1$ to B represents the level of batch. Moreover, α's represent the intercepts of the regression lines: α_i represents the effect of factor i on the intercept, α_{ij} represents the 2-way interaction effect of factors i and j on the intercept, α_{ijk} represents the 3-way interaction effect of factors i, j, and k on the intercept. Similar to the way of the α's represent the intercept coefficients, the β's represent the slope coefficients of the regression lines. Finally, the random error term follows a standard normal distribution with mean zero and variance σ^2. Here, model (22.5) is known as the preliminarily specified model. Through tests of equality of slopes and intercepts specified in the preliminary model, Model (22.5) may be reduced to a simpler model. Then, the final simpler model reduced from Model (22.5) will be used to estimate the shelf-life for the drug product studied. For example, if through a hierarchical testing procedure, the data support the elimination of $\beta_{spb}, \alpha_{spb}, \beta_{sp}, \alpha_{sp}, \beta_{pb}, \alpha_{pb}, \beta_{sb}, \alpha_{sb}$ in Model (22.5) by not rejecting $H_0 : \beta_{spb} = 0$, $H_0 : \alpha_{spb} = 0$, $H_0 : \beta_{sp} = 0$, $H_0 : \alpha_{sp} = 0$, $H_0 : \beta_{pb} = 0$, $H_0 : \alpha_{pb} = 0$, $H_0 : \beta_{sb} = 0$, $H_0 : \alpha_{sb} = 0$, then the full model is reduced to

$$Y_{spbt} = \alpha + \alpha_s + \alpha_p + \alpha_b + \beta t + \beta_s t + \beta_p t + \beta_b t + \epsilon_{spbt} \qquad (22.6)$$

As a comparison, the linear regression lines fitted with Model (22.6) are more clustered than the regression lines fitted using Model (22.5) and will lead to longer estimated expiration dating periods. Thus, the sponsor may take advantage of choosing a reduced model like (22.6) after testing which terms in Model (22.5) can be dropped to avoid the possibility of getting shorter estimated expiration dating periods for some strength-container size combinations.

To extend the model building process from a single-factor to a multi-factor stability design, the ANCOVA modeling application requires a prespecified hierarchical ordering of the pooling tests. For example, it may be defined as follows,

(a) $H_0 : \beta_{spb} = 0$, strength-by-container size-by-batch interaction for slope
(b) $H_0 : \alpha_{spb} = 0$, strength-by-container size-by-batch interaction for intercept
(c) $H_0 : \beta_{sb} = 0$, strength-by-batch interaction for slope
(d) $H_0 : \alpha_{sb} = 0$, strength-by-batch interaction for intercept
(e) $H_0 : \beta_{pb} = 0$, container size-by-batch interaction for slope
(g) $H_0 : \alpha_{pb} = 0$, container size-by-batch interaction for intercept
(h) $H_0 : \beta_{sp} = 0$, strength-by-container size interaction for slope
(i) $H_0 : \alpha_{sp} = 0$, strength-by-container size interaction for intercept
(j) $H_0 : \beta_b = 0$, batch slope
(k) $H_0 : \alpha_b = 0$, batch intercept
(l) $H_0 : \beta_s = 0$, strength slope
(m) $H_0 : \alpha_s = 0$, strength intercept
(n) $H_0 : \beta_p = 0$, container size slope
(o) $H_0 : \alpha_p = 0$, container size intercept.

Whenever a null hypothesis of the pooling test is rejected, the pooling test of the rest of the interactions or main factors contained in the significant interactions will not be performed. The shelf-life estimate for each strength-container size combination of the product is then determined by the date of the intersection of the one-sided 95% confidence limit based on the reduced model with the specification level for a given attribute. A regulatory shelf-life of each strength-container size combination of the product is determined by comparing the estimate with the shelf-life targeted. If the product has an estimate of shelf-life longer than the proposed shelf-life, the proposed shelf-life will be accepted as the regulatory shelf-life. Otherwise the shorter time estimate will be used as the regulatory shelf-life.

The extension of the single-factor ANCOVA modeling procedure to a multi-factor model causes some serious difficulties in the selection of the final model for expiration dating estimation. First, the hierarchical ordering of pooling tests restricts the possibility of pooling patterns and eliminates many pooling opportunities. Second, using different hierarchical orderings of pooling tests may lead to different final models and result in different estimated shelf-lives for strength-container size combinations of the product. For instance, in the last example, it is also possible to change the ordering of the testing of the interactions of strength with batch, container size with batch, and strength with container size.

With no specific restriction, there are six ordering patterns. Similarly, the ordering of the main factors leads also to six patterns. The 36 distinct orderings may lead to 36 different shelf-life settings for the products.

The heterogeneity test of the slopes across various levels of batch, strength, and container size is carried out by testing the hypotheses,

$$H_0 : \beta_{spb} = 0 \text{ against } H_a : \beta_{spb} \neq 0 \qquad (22.7)$$

Similarly, the heterogeneity test of intercepts across various levels of batch, strength, and container size is carried out by testing

$$H_0 : \alpha_{spb} = 0 \text{ against } H_a : \alpha_{spb} \neq 0 \qquad (22.8)$$

The remaining heterogeneity tests and test for main effects follow the same procedure as in (22.7) and (22.8).

Note that the decision of pooling is made if H_0 of (22.7) or (22.8) is not rejected. Because more degrees of freedom are associated with the estimate of error term variance in the reduced model than in the full fixed model (22.1), the shelf-life estimated by the reduced model is usually longer than that estimated by the full fixed model (22.5). However, with the limited number of observation times, the major concern of the pooling tests is their power to reject the null hypothesis, especially in matrixing and bracketing designs. Hence, in order to reduce the rate of falsely pooling because of lack of testing power, Brancroft[19] and other authors[20–23] proposed the use of a larger significance level such as $\alpha = .25$ for preliminary tests of hypothesis. Controlling the primary and overall type I error rate for the estimation or testing of the proposed shelf-life is of primary concern.

For this reason, the primary objective for the stability study is restated by Chen and Tsong[24,25] and stated as an alternative in ICH Q1E[3] as follows,

$$H_0 : T_{spb} \leq T_0 \text{ for some } s, p, b \text{ versus } H_a : T_{spb} > T_0 \text{ for all } s, p, b \quad (22.9)$$

where T_0 is the manufacturer proposed common shelf-life for all strength-container size combinations of the product within the maximum extension beyond the last time point with observed data, and T_{spb} is the true shelf-life of the specific combination of the product. Clearly, this restated objective of the stability study emphasizes that the stability study is designed to collect data in support of the sponsor's claim of a specific shelf-life T_0 for the product. In order to make the claim, the sponsor is responsible to collect data to demonstrate that batches of each factor level combination tested have shelf-lives longer than the targeted shelf-life T_0. Then, a T_0 shelf-life is statistically supported when H_0 is rejected with data of the available batches (i.e., all batches in each combination of factor level have true shelf-lives longer than T_0). By rejecting H_0, it establishes that all T_{spb}'s are longer than T_0. A good testing procedure is the one that can properly control the type I error rate for testing (22.9).

In addition, for multiple factor stability designs, when the result failed to reject (22.9), the design data are split into subsets for testing different multiple hypotheses to accommodate the different shelf-lives for different strength-container size combinations of the product.

For potency stability, for instance, the hypotheses (22.9) are tested by comparing the lower one-sided 95% confidence limit with the acceptance criterion at T_0. Pooling tests should be considered with properly controlling of the type I error rate in the test of the primary hypotheses (22.9). Chen and Tsong[24] evaluated the simple case of a standard stability study with three batches using various significance levels for the slope pooling test in order to control the type I error rates of the test of the hypotheses (22.9) at .05 and .10 levels under a set of specific conditions, in particular that one of the three batches has an expected shelf-life equal to T_0. In the paper, the simulation algorithm that determined the significance level for testing hypothesis (22.7) so that a type I error rate of .05 or .10 for testing the primary objective null hypothesis (22.9) is preserved, consists of the following two stages: (i) the determination of the detectable parameter value for the slope differences and (ii) the determination of the α significance level for testing hypothesis (22.7). In the first stage, for each specified false positive rate of rejecting the primary objective null hypothesis H_0: $Min_{k=1 \text{ to } 3} (T_k) \leq T_0$, the algorithm determines the slope differences among the three batches such that the rate of falsely rejecting the primary objective null hypothesis H_0, induced by falsely pooling slope differences, is not less than or equal to the prespecified false positive rate. In the second stage, for each specified false positive rate, the algorithm determines the significance level of rejecting the hypothesis of equal slopes under the slope differences determined from the first stage, in order to preserve a prespecified Type I error rate in the test of the hypothesis (22.9). Finally, the significance level for testing the hypothesis of equal slopes is equal to the maximum of the significance levels determined for each false positive rate used in the simulation.

The authors reported that in order to keep the type I error rates at .05 and .1 levels not inflated when testing H_0: $Min_{k=1 \text{ to } 3} (T_k) \leq 18$, significance levels up to .7 and .45, respectively are needed when testing for equality of slopes and using one year data with large standard deviations such as 0.2, 0.4, 0.8, and 1.4% of the labeling claim. Moreover, the simulation study indicated that the curves for the significance levels for the slope pooling tests at the selected false positive rates, which controlled the type I error rates at .05 and .1 levels in the test of hypothesis (22.9), were similar among the four data standard deviations. The curve delineating the relationship between the significance levels for testing the hypothesis (22.7) of slope equality and the false positive rates specified for testing the primary hypothesis of (22.9) using data with standard deviation of 0.2 is presented in Figure 22.5. In this figure, each significance level is determined by the simulation algorithm to bring down the associated false positive rate to the Type I error rate of 5% for testing the primary objective null hypothesis of (22.9).

From Figure 22.5, one notes that the significance level for testing the preliminary hypothesis of equal slopes increases for false positive rates ranging from .05 to .25, and decreases after the false positive rate becomes greater

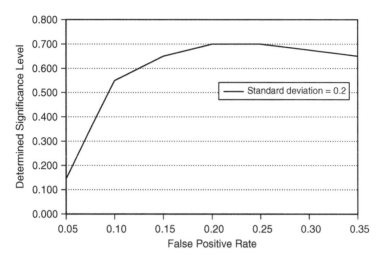

FIGURE 22.5 Significance level required at each false positive rate in keeping Type I error rate of .05 not inflated.

than .25. In order to keep the type I error in the test of the primary objective null hypothesis of (22.9) at .05 not inflated, the maximum significance level could be as high as .7 for controlling a false positive rate of .25.

As mentioned above, this is just a simulation of a simple case of three batches with a requested shelf-life of 18 months. However, the results from this simulation indicate that because of a lack of power for testing slope differences, high significance levels are required to provide higher levels of power. Thus the test procedure is able to detect when the slopes of three batches are different under the most variable condition and brings down the false positive rate to a prespecified Type I error rate in the test of primary objective null hypothesis of (22.9).

A generalization of Bancroft's proposal to the multi-factor stability study was proposed by Fairweather et al.[26] They proposed to use a significance level of .25 for any batch-related pooling test of main factor and interactions and a significance level of .05 for all other pooling tests. These significance levels are currently recommended in ICH Q1E.[3]

Because of the difficulties of directly extending the ANCOVA modeling procedure from a simple single factor three-batch study to a multi-factor study, a more flexible version of ANCOVA modeling is proposed. It is proposed based on a stepwise selection procedure. The basic hierarchical ordering of pooling test is as follows:

1. Testing the slope term before the corresponding intercept term for an interaction or a main effect.
2. Testing a higher level interaction before a lower level interaction.

3. Factors in the interaction test will not be pooled once the interaction is significant. Once an interaction is significant, its members cannot be tested for pooling, whether as lower level interactions or as main effects.

The testing rule for pooling can be described as follow:

1. Fitting the data with the initial ANCOVA model (e.g., full model) and comparing the confidence limit of the attribute with the quality acceptance criterion at T_0. If the confidence limit of the full model, i.e., of each strength-container size combination of the product, is within the acceptance criterion, H_0 of (22.9) is rejected and T_0 is the shelf-life supported for all product combinations with no need of any pooling tests. Otherwise go to step 2.
2. Comparing the p-value of the slope term of the highest order interaction with the properly prespecified significance level for pooling (usually .25 since batch will be one factor). If it is significant (i.e., the p-value is smaller than the significance level), the full model is final. Otherwise the model can be reduced by the highest order interaction term.
3. Refitting the data with the reduced model. Among the next highest level of interactions, if there is more than one term of the same degree, the batch-related terms will be considered for elimination first. Among them, the one with the largest p-value will be considered for elimination first. This is done by comparing the p-value of interaction slope term of the next highest order with the properly prespecified significance level for pooling. If it is significant (i.e., the p-value is smaller than the significance level), this term and all terms of lesser order of the involved factors cannot be eliminated from the model. Otherwise reduce the model by the nonsignificant term.
4. Repeating the procedure for all batch-related interactions of the same order. When all of them could be deleted, repeating the procedure for all nonbatch related interactions of the same order, again starting with the one with the highest p-value. When not all interactions can be deleted, continue with the highest order term having none of the factors that were part of a significant term.
5. Refitting the data with the reduced model and comparing the confidence limit of each strength-container size combination of the product with the quality acceptance criterion at T_0. If all the confidence limits are within the acceptance criteria, H_0 of (22.9) is rejected and T_0 is the shelf-life supported for all strength-container size combinations of the product and no further modeling is needed. Otherwise go to the next step.
6. Repeat the pooling test of Step 2 to 5 for the corresponding intercept of the eliminated slope term until either H_0 of (22.9) is rejected and the associated claim that T_0 is the uniform shelf-life for all

strength-container size combinations of the product, or a final model is identified. When H_0 of (22.9) cannot be rejected for all combinations for a uniform shelf-life, the product shelf-life should be determined individually by comparing the confidence limits of the remaining factors and interactions with the acceptance criterion/criteria at $T \leq T_0$.

For illustrative purpose, the above procedure is applied to single factor with three batches in the example below.

The sample means and the 95% confidence limits of Y_{24} of the three batches calculated from the final model of example 1 are given below:

Estimate and 95% CI using Model (22.2)

Batch	Lower Limit	Mean	Upper Limit
1	99.057	99.952	100.85
2	98.343	99.238	100.13
3	98.200	99.095	99.991

It is clear that the 95% confidence intervals for the assay at 24 months of all three batches are between 95 and 105% of the label claim of the attribute. Hence the null hypothesis of (22.9) is rejected and a 24-month shelf-life is supported.

Example 2 below is used to illustrate the proposed stepwise ANCOVA modeling in a multiple factor stability study.

Example 2. A stability design with two levels of strength (10 mg, 40 mg), four levels of container sizes (3, 30, 100, and 1000 count bottles) and three batches in cross-classification is considered. Measurements were made at 0, 3, 6, 9, 12, and 18 months with the objective of a $T_0 = 30$ months shelf-life. The assay measurements are given in Table 22.6.

For the stability of potency, we consider the two-sided acceptance criteria, $S_L = 95\%$ and $S_U = 105\%$ of label claim. Assume a full linear fixed effects model as the original model,

$$Y_{spbt} = \alpha_0 + \alpha_s + \alpha_p + \alpha_b + \alpha_{sp} + \alpha_{sb} + \alpha_{pb} + \alpha_{spb} + \beta_0 t$$
$$+ \beta_s t + \beta_p t + \beta_b t + \beta_{sp} t + \beta_{sb} t + \beta_{pb} t + \beta_{spb} t + \epsilon_{spbt}$$

where α_0 and β_0 are the general mean intercept and slope, respectively, $\alpha_s >$ and β_s are the strength effect on the intercept and slope, respectively, α_p and β_p are the container size effect on the intercept and slope, respectively, α_{sp} and β_{sp} are the interaction effect between strength and container size effect on the intercept and slope, respectively, α_b and β_b are the batch effect on the intercept and slope, respectively, α_{sb} and β_{sb} are the interaction effect between batch and strength on the intercept and slope, respectively, α_{pb} and β_{pb} are the interaction effect between batch and container size effect on the intercept and slope, respectively, α_{spb} and β_{spb} are the interaction effect among container size, batch,

TABLE 22.6
Stability Data of a Multiple Factor Stability Study

Strength	Container Size	Batch	0	3	6	9	12	18
10	3	1	102	103	103	102	2	100
		2	103	102	103	101	100	101
		3	102	103	102	103	101	101
	30	1	103	102	101	101	100	99
		2	104	103	101	102	101	100
		3	103	103	101	101	101	99
	100	1	104	103	102	101	102	101
		2	104	103	103	101	101	100
		3	103	102	101	102	101	100
	1000	1	103	103	101	102	101	100
		2	102	103	101	102	100	99
		3	103	102	101	101	100	99
40	3	1	104	103	102	103	101	100
		2	103	102	102	101	100	100
		3	103	102	101	101	100	100
	10	1	103	102	102	101	100	100
		2	104	102	103	101	100	100
		3	104	103	101	102	100	99
	100	1	103	103	101	102	100	99
		2	104	103	101	102	100	100
		3	102	103	101	102	100	99
	1000	1	105	104	102	103	101	101
		2	102	103	102	101	100	100
		3	103	103	101	102	100	99

and strength on the intercept and slope, respectively, and ϵ_{spbt} is the data random error term that follows the standard normal distribution with mean zero and variance $\Phi.^2$ In this example, the significance levels of the pooling tests proposed by Fairweather et al. are used.

Results of the ANCOVA using the full model are given in Table 22.7. The first pooling test is $H_0 : \beta_{spb} = 0$ vs. $H_a : \beta_{spb} \neq 0$. Since the p-value of the F test is .9254 > .25, this term can be eliminated from the model.

The reduced model without the β_{spb} term is then used to test the corresponding intercept term α_{spb} by testing $H_0 : \alpha_{spb} = 0$ vs. $H_a : \alpha_{spb} \neq 0$. After removing terms through stepwise modeling and pooling tests, the final model below is obtained.

$$Y_{spbt} = \alpha_0 + \alpha_s + \alpha_p + \alpha_b + \alpha_{sp} + \alpha_{pb} + \beta_0 t + \epsilon_{spbt}$$

TABLE 22.7
Results of ANCOVA of the Original Full Model of Example 2

Source	DF	Sum of Squares	Mean Square	F Value	Pr > F
Model	47	217.417	4.626	10.15	<.0001
Error	96	43.743	0.456		
Corrected Total	143	261.160			

Source	DF	Type III SS	Mean Square	F Value	Pr > F
BATCH	2	1.313	0.656	1.44	.2419
STRENGTH	1	0.591	0.591	1.30	.2576
CONTAINER SIZE	3	0.634	0.211	0.46	.7082
BATCH × CONTAINER SIZE	6	6.224	1.037	2.28	.0425
BATCH × STRENGTH	2	0.931	0.465	1.02	.3640
CONT. SIZE × STRENGTH	3	0.949	0.316	0.69	.5578
BATCH × CONT. × STRENGTH	6	1.363	0.227	0.50	.8080
MONTH	1	185.534	185.534	407.18	<.0001
MONTH × CONTAINER SIZE	3	2.777	0.926	2.03	.1146
MONTH × BATCH	2	0.012	0.006	0.01	.9866
MONTH × STRENGTH	1	1.302	1.302	2.86	.0942
MONTH × BATCH × CONT. SIZE	6	2.237	0.373	0.82	.5585
MONTH × BATCH × STRENGTH	2	0.496	0.248	0.54	.5818
MONTH × CONT. × STRENGTH	3	0.526	0.175	0.38	.7642
MONT × BATCH × CONT. × STREN	6	0.873	0.146	0.32	.9254

TABLE 22.8
ANCOVA Results of the Last Final Model of Example 2

Source	DF	Sum of Squares	Mean Square	F Value	Pr > F
Model	16	205.082	12.818	29.03	<.0001
Error	127	56.078	0.442		
Corrected Total	143	261.160			

Source	DF	Type III SS	Mean Square	F Value	Pr > F
BATCH	2	3.764	1.882	4.26	.0162
STRENGTH	1	0.063	0.063	0.14	.7074
CONTAINER SIZE	3	1.354	0.451	1.02	.3852
BATCH × CONT. S.	6	9.125	1.521	3.44	.0035
CONT. × STRENGTH	3	5.243	1.748	3.96	.0098
MONTH	1	185.534	185.534	420.18	<.0001

TABLE 22.9
Estimates of μ_{spb} at the 30th Month of Each Strength-Container Size-Batch Configuration

Strength	Cont.	Batch	Mean	LCL	UCL	Time of Intersection
10	3	1	97.918	97.319	98.516	36
10	3	2	97.418	96.819	98.016	36
10	3	3	97.501	96.903	98.100	36
10	30	1	96.890	96.292	97.489	36
10	30	2	97.473	96.875	98.072	36
10	30	3	97.140	96.542	97.739	36
10	100	1	97.779	97.181	98.377	36
10	100	2	97.862	97.264	98.461	36
10	100	3	97.362	96.764	97.961	36
10	1000	1	97.696	97.097	98.294	36
10	1000	2	96.779	96.181	97.377	30
10	1000	3	96.696	96.097	97.294	30
40	3	1	97.640	97.042	98.239	36
40	3	2	97.140	96.542	97.739	36
40	3	3	97.223	96.625	97.822	36
40	30	1	97.001	96.403	97.600	36
40	30	2	97.585	96.986	98.183	36
40	30	3	97.251	96.653	97.850	36
40	100	1	97.279	96.681	97.877	36
40	100	2	97.362	96.764	97.961	36
40	100	3	96.862	96.264	97.461	36
40	1000	1	98.196	97.597	98.794	42
40	1000	2	97.279	96.681	97.877	36
40	1000	3	97.196	96.597	97.794	36

Results of ANCOVA using the final model are given in Table 22.8. The p-values of the remaining factors indicate that none of the factors can be eliminated from the model.

The fitted regression lines of all batches of all strength-container size configurations intersect with the S_L at time points no shorter than 30 months (Table 22.9). The results indicate that all observed strength-container size configurations have no less than 30 months of shelf-life. Extrapolating to future batches, one can compare the estimate of Y_{spb} at the 30th month with S_L and S_U to determine if the results support the 30-month shelf-life. In this case, the 95% confidence interval of the mean of Y_{spb} at the 30th month lies between S_L and S_U, which indicates that all batches of all configurations support the proposed 30 months shelf-life (Table 22.9).

The same approach described above can be used for stability studies using incomplete block designs such as the matrix design. When a multi-factor stability design is used, with proper justification based on known chemical properties of the product, some of the factors may be eliminated from the original model to increase the power of the pooling test for the remaining terms in the model.

   Example 3. A matrix stability design with the same two levels of strength (10 mg, 40 mg), four levels of container sizes (3, 30, 100, and 1000 count bottles), and three batches in a cross classification experiment as in Example 2 are considered. Measurements were made incompletely at 0, 3, 6, 9, and 12 months with the objective of a $T_0 = 30$ months shelf-life. The assay measurements are given in Table 22.10.

When planning a matrix stability study, it is assumed that the properties of the chemical used in the product are well known, and that the product has no heterogeneity in degradation changes due to the size of packaging. For example, it may be agreed upon between the manufacturer and the regulatory agency that

TABLE 22.10
Stability Data of a Matrix Design Stability Study

						Time in Months		
Strength	Container Size	Batch	0	3	6	9	12	18
10	3	1	102	X	103	102	101	X
		2	103	102	X	101	100	101
		3	102	103	102	X	101	101
	30	1	103	102	X	101	100	99
		2	104	103	101	X	101	100
		3	103	X	101	101	101	X
	100	1	104	103	102	X	102	101
		2	104	X	103	101	101	X
		3	103	102	X	102	101	100
	1000	1	103	X	101	102	101	X
		2	102	103	X	102	100	99
		3	103	102	101	X	100	99
40	3	1	104	103	X	103	101	100
		2	103	102	102	X	100	100
		3	103	X	101	101	100	X
	10	1	103	102	102	X	100	100
		2	104	X	103	101	100	X
		3	104	103	X	102	100	99
	100	1	103	X	101	102	100	X
		2	104	103	X	102	100	100
		3	102	103	101	X	100	99
	1000	1	105	104	X	103	101	101
		2	102	103	102	X	100	100
		3	103	X	101	102	100	X

TABLE 22.11
ANCOVA Analysis of the Original Model of Example 3

Source	DF	Sum of Squares	Mean Square	F Value	Pr > F
Model	17	157.571	9.269	17.38	<.0001
Error	94	50.143	0.533		
Corrected Total	111	207.714			

Source	DF	Type III SS	Mean Sq.	F Value	Pr > F
PKG	3	1.173	0.391	0.73	.535
BATCH	2	1.320	0.660	1.24	.295
STRENGTH	1	1.283	1.283	2.41	.124
BATCH × STRENGTH	2	0.388	0.194	0.36	.696
MONTH × BATCH	2	0.436	0.218	0.41	.666
MONTH × STRENGTH	1	1.777	1.777	3.33	.071
MONTH × BATCH × STRENGTH	2	0.276	0.138	0.26	.772
MONTH × CONTAINER SIZE	3	2.671	0.890	1.67	.179

all slope interaction terms relating to packaging may be eliminated from linear modeling. In addition, it may also be assumed that there is no expected intercept difference among container sizes. Hence all intercept terms related to packaging may also be eliminated from the initial model. The initial linear fixed effects model to be considered for a product satisfying the above assumptions is as follows:

$$Y_{spbt} = \alpha_0 + \alpha_s + \alpha_p + \alpha_b + \alpha_{sb} + \beta_0 t + \beta_s t + \beta_p t + \beta_b t + \beta_{sb} t + \epsilon_{spbt}$$

The results of the analysis using the model are given in Table 22.11.
Results of the analysis show that the strength-batch slope interaction β_{sb} is first eliminated from the model. The remaining terms that are sequentially eliminated from the ANCOVA model are batch-strength intercept interaction (α_{sb}), batch slope term (β_b), container size slope term (β_p), and container size intercept term (α_p). After removing all the above terms, the reduced ANCOVA model is

$$Y_{spbt} = \alpha_0 + \alpha_s + \alpha_b + \beta_0 t + \beta_s t + \epsilon_{spbt}$$

Results of the analysis using the above-reduced model as the final model are given in Table 22.12.
The 95% confidence intervals of the mean attribute value μ for each of the strength-container size-batch configurations at 30 months based on the final reduced ANCOVA model are given in Table 22.13. Because all the confidence intervals lie between the acceptance limits (i.e., 95% and 105% of label claim), it is clear that the stability data support the 30-month shelf-life for all strength-container size configurations of the product. An alternative way to determine if the requested 30-month shelf-life is supported by the data is by comparing

TABLE 22.12
ANCOVA Results of the Reduced Model of Example 3

Source	DF	Sum of Squares	Mean Square	F Value	Pr > F
Model	8	152.828	19.104	35.85	<.0001
Error	103	54.886	0.533		
Corrected Total	111	207.714			

Source	DF	Type III SS	Mean Square	F Value	Pr > F
PKG	3	0.828	0.276	0.52	.6707
BATCH	2	4.880	2.440	4.58	.0124
STRENGTH	1	1.220	1.220	2.29	.1333
MONTH × STRENGTH	2	147.599	73.799	138.49	<.0001

TABLE 22.13
Estimate of μ Values of Each Configuration at 30th Month and Intersection Time

Strength	Cont. Size	Batch	$\hat{Y}$	LCL	UCL	Time of Size Intersection
10	3	1	98.072	97.301	98.843	36
10	3	2	97.828	97.065	98.592	36
10	3	3	97.565	96.798	98.331	36
10	30	1	98.072	97.301	98.843	36
10	30	2	97.828	97.065	98.592	36
10	30	3	97.565	96.798	98.331	36
10	100	2	97.828	97.065	98.592	36
10	100	3	97.565	96.798	98.331	36
10	1000	1	98.072	97.301	98.843	36
10	1000	2	97.828	97.065	98.592	36
10	1000	3	97.565	96.798	98.331	36
40	3	1	97.190	96.427	97.954	30
40	3	2	96.946	96.180	97.713	30
40	3	3	96.683	95.912	97.454	30
40	30	1	97.190	96.427	97.954	30
40	30	2	96.946	96.180	97.713	30
40	30	3	96.683	95.912	97.454	30
40	100	1	97.190	96.427	97.954	30
40	100	2	96.946	96.180	97.713	30
40	100	3	96.683	95.912	97.454	30
40	1000	1	97.190	96.427	97.954	30
40	1000	2	96.946	96.180	97.713	30
40	1000	3	96.683	95.912	97.454	30

the shortest estimated shelf-life of all configurations with the target shelf-life of 30 months. The estimated shelf-lives are given in Table 22.13. It is clear that a single 30-month shelf-life for all strength-container size configurations is supported.

IV. ALTERNATIVE APPROACHES FOR SHELF-LIFE DETERMINATION

Most of the alternative procedures that have been proposed in the literature are for single-factor designs. However, the generalization to studies using multi-factor designs may be derived. Random or mixed effects ANCOVA models were proposed in the literature for the analysis of the stability study data[27-30] either when batches are nested within some of the main factors or when the number of batches is large. Chow and Shao[27-28] proposed the use of the random or mixed effect model for upscaling or manufacturing stability studies. They also recommended the use of the prediction interval instead of the confidence interval of mean in the estimation of expiration dating periods. Chen, Hwang, and Tsong[31] proposed that when using a mixed effects model in shelf-life determination, a test for zero variance of slope or intercept is needed for pooling data of individual batches.

Ruberg et al.[32-33] proposed an alternative test for pooling data of individual batches. They proposed to test the following hypotheses of slopes and intercepts

$$H_0 : |\beta_j - \beta_{j'}| \geq \delta \text{ for some } j \neq j', \text{ versus } H_a : |\beta_j - \beta_{j'}| < \delta \text{ for all } j,j'$$

and

$$H_0 : |\alpha_j - \alpha_{j'}| \geq \delta' \text{ for some } j,j', \text{ versus } H_a : |\alpha_j - \alpha_{j'}| < \delta' \text{ for } j,j'$$

However, no equivalent limits were proposed in the paper. A simulation study showed comparable results of their slope equality test with the ANCOVA approach with an appropriately chosen equivalent limit Δ. Lin and Tsong[34] discussed the problem of using a fixed equivalence limit in this alternative approach. They showed through simulation that depending on the slope values, but with the same equivalence limit, the test can yield different results and have different impact on the shelf-life estimation of a drug product.

Yoshioka et al.[35,36] revisited the equivalence approach and proposed to pool the batches if the difference in shelf-life between any two batches is within an equivalence limit that is a percentage of the sample mean shelf-life. Yoshioka et al.'s range-based test is proposed to test the hypotheses

$$H_0 : |T_j - T_{j'}| \geq \gamma \text{Max}_j T_j \text{ for some } j \neq j',$$

versus

$$H_a : |T_j - T_{j'}| < \gamma \text{Max}_j T_j \text{ for all } j,j' \qquad (22.10)$$

where γ is a prespecified proportion such that $0 \le \gamma \le 1$. Yoshioka et al.[36] compared the range-based equivalence test with $\gamma = 0.15$ and the ANCOVA approach through a Monte Carlo simulation and found that the proposed method is more powerful in rejecting pooling when the batches have different shelf-lives. However, there is no proper statistical justification for the equivalence approach. Tsong et al.[37] proposed a pooling test based on equivalence testing of the mean value of the characteristic at the proposed shelf-life. Specifically, they proposed the following to test

$$H_0 : |Y_j(T_0) - Y_P(T_0)| \ge \delta_{T_0} \quad \text{for some } j = 1 \text{ to } J$$

versus

$$H_a : |Y_j(T_0) - Y_P(T_0)| < \delta_{T_0} \quad \text{for all } j = 1 \text{ to } J$$

where T_0 is the proposed shelf-life, $Y_j(T_0)$ and $Y_P(T_0)$ are the mean values of the jth batch and the average of all batches at T_0, respectively, and δ_{T_0} is a proposed equivalence limit.

ACKNOWLEDGMENTS

The work has been produced by the authors, Roswitha Kelly, Drs Chi Wen Chen, Wen Jen Chen, Karl K. Lin, Tsae-Yun Daphne Lin, and Yi Tsong in the capacity of federal government employees, as part of their official duty. The work is in the public domain and is not subject to copyright. The views expressed in this chapter are those of the authors and are not necessarily those of the U.S. Food and Drug Administration.

REFERENCES

1. ICH Q1A(R2), Stability Testing of New Drug Substances and Products, Conference on Harmonization, Geneva, Switzerland (http://www.fda.gov/cder/guidance/index.htm), 2003.
2. ICH Q1D, Bracketing and Matrixing Designs for Stability Testing of New Drug Substances and Products, Conference on Harmonization, Geneva, Switzerland (http://www.fda.gov/cder/guidance/index.htm), 2003.
3. ICH Q1E, Stability Data Evaluation, Conference on Harmonization, Geneva, Switzerland (http://www.fda.gov/cder/guidance/index.htm), 2003.
4. FDA. *Guidelines for Submitting Documentation for the Stability of Human Drugs and Biologics*, Rockville MD, Food and Drug Administration, Center for Drugs and Biologics, 1987.
5. Lin, K.K., Lin, T.D., and Kelly, R.E., Stability of drugs, In *Statistics in the Pharmaceutical Industry*, 2nd ed., Buncher, C.R. and Tsay, J.Y., eds., Marcel Dekker, New York, pp. 419–444, 1993.
6. Chow, S.C. and Liu, J.P., *Statistical Design and Analysis in Pharmaceutical Sciences*, Marcel Dekker, New York, 1995.

7. Nakagaki, P., Matrixing and bracketing of solid oral dosage forms for thermal stability studies. AAPS Annual Meeting, Las Vegas, NV, 1990.

8. Helboe, P., New designs for stability testing programs: matrix or factorial designs. Authorities viewpoint on the predictive value of such studies, *Drug Inf. J.*, 26, 629–634, 1992.

9. Helboe, P., New designs for stability testing programs, *Drug Inf. J.*, 26, 629–634, 1992.

10. Nordbrock, E., Statistical comparison of stability study designs, *J. Pharm. Stat.*, 2(1), 91–113, 1992.

11. De Kleijn, J.P. and Lakeman, J., Stability surveillance testing: an effective and efficient approach, *J. Pharm. Sci.*, 82(11), 1130–1133, 1993.

12. Lin, T.-Y.D., Applicability of matrix and bracket approach to stability study design. *Proceedings of the American Statistical Association Biopharmaceutical Section*, pp. 142–147, 1994.

13. Chen, C., U.S. FDA's perspective of matrixing and bracketing, *Proceedings from EFPIA Symposium: Advanced Topics in Pharmaceutical Stability Testing Building on the ICH Stability Guideline*, EFPIA, Brussels, 1996.

14. Ju, H.L. and Chow, S., On stability designs in drug shelf-life estimation, *J. Biopharm. Stat.*, 5(2), 201–214, 1995.

15. DeWoody, K. and Raghavarao, D., Some optimal matrix designs in stability studies, *J. Pharm. Stat.*, 7(2), 205–213, 1997.

16. Murphy, J.R., Uniform matrix stability study designs, *J. Pharm. Stat.*, 6(4), 477–494, 1996.

17. Pong, A. and Raghavarao, D., Comparison of bracketing and matrixing designs for a two-year stability study, *J. Pharm. Stat.*, 10(2), 217–228, 2000.

18. FDA. *Guidelines for submitting documentation for the stability of human drugs and biologics*, Food and Drug Administration, Center for Drugs and Biologics, Rockville, MD, 1987.

19. Bancroft, T.A., On biases in estimation due to the use of preliminary tests of significance, *Ann. Math. Stat.*, 15, 190–204, 1944.

20. Asano, C., Tests due to pooling data through preliminary test on biological direct assay, *Bull. Math. Stat.*, 25–39, 1960.

21. Larson, H.J. and Bancroft, T.A., Sequential model building for prediction in regression analysis, I, *Ann. Math. Stat.*, 34, 231–242, 1963.

22. Bancroft, T.A., Analysis and inference for incompletely specified models involving the use of preliminary tests of significance, *Biometrics*, 20(3), 427–442, 1964.

23. Johnson, J.P., Bancroft, T.A., and Han, C.P., A pooling methodology for regressions in prediction, *Biometrics*, 33, 57–67, 1977.

24. Chen, W.J. and Tsong, Y., Significance level for stability polling test: a simulation study, to appear in *J. Pharm. Stat.*, 13(3), 255–274, 2003.

25. Tsong, Y., Chen, W.J., and Chen, C.W., Statistical analysis of multiple factor design of stability study, to appear in *J. Pharm. Stat.*, 13(3), 375–395, 2003.

26. Fairweather, W., Lin, T.D., and Kelly, R., Regulatory, design, and analysis aspects of complex stability studies, *J. Pharm. Sci.*, 84(11), 1322–1326, 1995.

27. Chow, S.-C. and Shao, J., Test for batch-to-batch variation in stability analysis, *Stat. Med.*, 8, 883–890, 1989.

28. Chow, S.-C. and Shao, J., Estimating drug shelf-life with random batches, *Biometrics*, 47, 1071–1079, 1991.

29. Shao, J. and Chow, S.C., Statistical inference in stability analysis, *Biometrics*, 50, 753–763, 1994.
30. Murphy, J.R. and Weisman, D., Using random slopes for estimating shelf-life, *Proc. Biopharm. Sect. Joint Stat. Meet., Am. Stat. Assoc.*, 196–203, 1990.
31. Chen, J.J., Hwang, J.-S., and Tsong, Y., Estimation of the shelf-life of drugs with mixed effects models, *J. Pharm. Stat.*, 5(1), 131–140, 1995.
32. Ruberg, S.J. and Stegemen, J.W., Pooling data from stability studies: testing the equality of batch degradation slopes, *Biometrics*, 47, 1059–1069, 1991.
33. Ruberg, S.J. and Hsu, J.C., Multiple comparison procedures for pooling batches in stability studies, *Proc. Biopharm. Sect. Joint Stat. Meet., Am. Stat. Assoc.*, 204–209, 1990.
34. Lin, T.-Y.D. and Tsong, Y., Determination of significance level for pooling data in stability studies, *Proc. Biopharm. Sect. Joint Stat. Meet., Am. Stat. Assoc.*, 195–201, 1991.
35. Yoshioka, S., Aso, Y., and Kojima, S., Statistical evaluation of shelf-life of pharmaceutical products estimated by matrixing, *Drug Stab.*, 1, 147–151, 1996.
36. Yoshioka, S., Aso, Y., and Kojima, S., Assessment of shelf-life equivalence of pharmaceutical products, *Chem. Pharm. Bull.*, 45(9), 1482–1484, 1997.
37. Tsong, Y., Chen, W.J., Lin, T.-Y.D., and Chen, C.W., Pooling batch based on equivalence test, *J. Pharm. Stat.*, 13(3), 431–449, 2003.

23 When and How to Do Multiple Comparisons

Charles W. Dunnett and Charles H. Goldsmith

CONTENTS

I. INTRODUCTION

In many of the drug experiments performed in the pharmaceutical industry, at least two drugs or at least two levels of one drug are considered. As a consequence of these experiments, questions related to picking out drugs or dose levels which are different from others are often generated. However, it is rare that some overall test of a null hypothesis provides researchers with specific details to answer the questions of interest. Because overall tests tend to average out real effects with negligible effects, they may fail to detect important features. Even if an overall test is significant, further analyses may be necessary to determine which specific differences among the treatments are clinically important. These "further analyses" constitute performing multiple comparisons among the treatments to detect those effects which are of prime interest to the researchers.

II. DESCRIPTION AND TAXONOMY OF MULTIPLE COMPARISON PROCEDURES

A. TERMS

Suppose we have a drug trial with k distinct treatments (different dosage levels, for example) that are randomly allocated to distinct experimental units (rats, patients, baboons, etc.). Suppose y_{ij} is the response of the jth experimental unit in the ith treatment group. If the responses are quantitative (interval or ratio scale), it is common to summarize the responses of the n_i experimental units to the ith treatment by their *arithmetic mean*, $\bar{y}_i$.

A **linear combination** of treatment means is defined as

$$L_1 = c_1\bar{y}_1 + c_2\bar{y}_2 + \cdots + c_k\bar{y}_k \quad \left(= \sum_{i=1}^{k} c_i\bar{y}_i \right) \quad (23.1)$$

where the c_i are given constants. If $(c_1 + c_2 + \cdots + c_k)$ equals zero

$$\left[\sum_{i=1}^{k} c_i = 0 \right]$$

this linear combination is known as a *contrast*. A contrast is said to be *pairwise* if exactly two of the coefficients c_i are nonzero (one being the negative of the other in value and the other $k - 2$ being zero).

If there is a second contrast

$$L_2 = d_1 \bar{y}_1 + d_2 \bar{y}_2 + \cdots + d_k \bar{y}_k \quad \left(= \sum_{i=1}^{k} d_i \bar{y}_i \right) \qquad (23.2)$$

where $(d_1 + d_2 + \cdots + d_k)$ equals zero

$$\left[\sum_{i=1}^{k} d_i = 0 \right]$$

the two contrasts L_1 and L_2 are said to be orthogonal if those are uncorrelated, i.e., provided

$$\frac{c_1 d_1}{n_1} + \frac{c_2 d_2}{n_2} + \cdots + \frac{c_k d_k}{n_k} = 0 \qquad \left[\sum_{i=1}^{k} \frac{c_i d_i}{n_i} = 0 \right]$$

A set of $k - 1$ (or fewer) contrasts is said to be an *orthogonal set of contrasts* provided all possible pairs of contrasts in the set are orthogonal.

A contrast is said to be an *a priori* contrast if its coefficients were determined before the results of the experiment were analyzed, whereas a contrast is an *a posteriori* contrast if the coefficients were only formulated after the results of the experiment had been looked at (implying that the coefficients were chosen after seeing patterns in the results).

A treatment is said to be a *control* if it is the standard of comparison in the experiment. A control may be a *placebo* if it contains no pharmacologically active agent, or it may be some active treatment that has become the *standard* comparison in that clinical, experimental, research, or therapeutic area.

Numbers assigned to objects in the process of measurement, can have various properties, which determine the kinds of things that can be done with the measurements in their analysis. The four measurement scales are: nominal, ordinal, interval, and ratio. A measurement is said to be *nominal* when it serves only to distinguish the objects being measured into mutually exclusive and exhaustive groups. The most common examples of nominal scales in pharmaceutical trial are the presence or absence of various outcomes, viz., side effects, deaths, strokes, tumors, etc., where presence of the outcome is indicated by 1 and its absence by 0. The measurements are said to possess the ordering property in addition to distinguishability when the measurements taken on the objects can be ordered (oriented) in some sensible way, and under such circumstances the scale of measurement is said to be *ordinal*. Severity scales and quality-of-outcome judgments are common ordinal scales used in drug trial. Measurements made on nominal or ordinal scales are commonly called *qualitative* measurements because these tend to reflect qualitative aspects of the things measured. In addition to the distinguishability and ordering properties, intervals of the same length chosen from various locations on the scale have equal meaning in case of measurements made on an *interval* scale. Measurements of time at a location and temperature on a Fahrenheit or Celsius scale in a drug study are interval measurements. In addition to these three previously mentioned properties (distinguishability, ordering, and equality of intervals), if the measurements are such that the ratio of the two observations gives the sense of their relative magnitude, the scale of measurements is said to be *ratio*. This latter property also generally means that the zero point on the scale corresponds to absence of the item or count being measured. Heights, weights, volumes, concentrations and time intervals are common examples of ratio scales in pharmaceutical studies.

If the responses y_{ij} are at least ordinal (ordinal, interval, or ratio), they can be ranked from smallest to largest and these *ranks* are denoted by r_{ij}. For each of $i = 1, 2, ..., k$, the *rank sums* are

$$R_i = r_{i1} + r_{i2} + \cdots + r_{in_i}. \qquad \left(= \sum_{i=1}^{n_i} r_{ij} \right)$$

and the *mean ranks* are

$$\bar{R}_i = \frac{R_i}{n_i}$$

The *overall mean rank* is $\bar{R} = (N + 1)/2$, where

$$N = \sum_{i=1}^{k} n_i$$

Multiple comparisons with ordinal scales generally use contrasts of rank means instead of the response means, or contrasts of rank sums if the sample sizes are equal.

If the observations are made on a nominal scale (with one denoting the presence and zero the absence of the trait being studied) then the mean response $\bar{y}_i$ is the proportion of the sample possessing the trait. With these nominal scales, multiple comparisons are based on contrasts of proportions. Although it is clear that multiple comparisons can be used with all kind of measurements, the type of procedure and its properties and the critical value tables used will somewhat vary.

As a test of the significance of a contrast, its computed value is compared with that of a certain *allowance* and if the absolute value of the contrast exceeds its allowance, it is significant at a chosen level of probability (statistical significance). Two-sided confidence limits may also be obtained by adding the allowance to and subtracting it from the value of the contrast. The differences between the various multiple comparison procedures lie in the way in which the respective allowances are determined.

Before we indicate how the allowances are calculated, it is essential to understand the concept of *error rates*. *Error* means the error of rejecting a null hypothesis when it is true (the so-called Type I error).

Tukey[1] distinguished among three error rates. For the present purposes, however, only two of those can be focused on, viz., the comparison error rate and the family (or, more correctly, "familywise") error rate. Tamhane[2] defined a family as a set of contextually related inferences (comparisons) from which some common conclusions are drawn or decisions are made. The determination of what constitutes a family is difficult and is a controversial issue among statisticians. For further elaboration of this point, see Miller[3] (pp. 31–35) and Westfall et al.[4] (p. 5). We also include another error rate, called the false discovery rate, which was introduced by Benjamini and Hochberg.[5]

The following definitions are based on a long series of such comparisons made over many experiments:

Comparison error rate

$$= \frac{\text{Number of comparisons leading to rejecting a true null hypothesis}}{\text{Total number of comparisons}}$$

Family (familywise) error rate

$$= \frac{\text{Number of families in which one or more true null hypotheses are rejected}}{\text{Total number of families}}$$

False discovery rate (FDR)

$$= \frac{\text{Number of comparisons leading to rejecting a true null hypothesis}}{\text{Total number of rejected null hypotheses}}$$

First a standard t test is considered for comparing two treatment means. This consists of determining the difference between the two means and dividing by its standard error. The null hypothesis that the two groups have same population mean is rejected, if the absolute value of the result exceeds the appropriate critical value tabulated for the Student's t distribution at the probability level α. Thus, the allowance for the difference between the two means is the critical value of Student's t multiplied by the standard error of the difference between the two means. Such a test controls the comparison error rate at level α.

Now the effect of performing multiple t tests in the same experiment is considered, each one at the probability level α. Provided that the contrasts are selected in advance (that is, these are not determined on the basis of the results of the experiment), it will still be true that, among many such tests in a large number of experiments, a proportion α of those for which the null hypothesis is actually true, will be falsely labeled significant. This outcome is not altered by the fact that the tests performed within the same experiment are correlated to some extent. Thus, for multiple t tests carried out at a fixed level of significance, α, the comparison error rate is controlled at the level α.

With family being the unit, the *family error rate* takes into account the entire set of comparisons. It measures the relative frequency with which families containing one or more comparisons falsely labeled significant occur among all families. This is appropriate in situations where conclusions are based on the whole set of comparisons in the family. Under such situations the existence of a single error within a family might jeopardize the conclusions. For example, suppose an experiment is performed to compare several new treatments with a standard with the object of selecting one of them for future use. The family of comparisons of interest might consist of each new treatment vs. the standard. The experiment would be totally baseless if the comparison in error happened to be the one involving the selected treatment because it could result in the replacement of the standard by a treatment that was not really superior to it.

When the family error rate is controlled, the allowance depends upon the number of treatment groups but not upon the actual number of comparisons within the family. Thus, without affecting the nominal value of error rate, some of the methods can be extended to a wider class of contrasts, so that additional comparisons can be added after observing how the data have turned out.

When the family contains a large number of inferences, controlling the family error rate may be too stringent a requirement, resulting in the test procedure with low power. Under such situation, the FDR may be useful as it provides control of the family error rate only when all the null hypotheses in the family are true. This is called "weak control" of the family error rate.

In a family of multiple comparisons, we can make correct or incorrect decisions. For a family F, the error rate is $P(F)$, the probability of making an incorrect decision, hence $1 - P(F)$ is the probability of making a correct decision when the null hypothesis is true. Suppose there are s individual statements in the family which may be correct or incorrect. If $P(S_j)$ is the probability that the jth statement is incorrect, then the Bonferroni inequality

$$1 - P(F) \geq 1 - P(S_1) - P(S_2) - \cdots - P(S_k) = 1 - \sum_{j=1}^{s} P(S_j) \qquad (23.3)$$

can be used to place a lower bound on the probability of making a correct decision for the family. For example, if $s = 5$

$$P(S_j) = 0.05, \qquad 1 - P(F) \geq 1 - 5\alpha = 0.75$$

It is noticed that this inequality does not rely on the knowledge of joint relationships among the decisions. Games[6] gives a table based on Šidák's[7] inequality, which produces a better lower bound. Šidák's inequality is

$$1 - P(F) \geq [1 - P(S_1)][1 - P(S_2)]\cdots[1 - P(S_s)] = \prod_{j=1}^{s}[1 - P(S_j)] \quad (23.4)$$

and with the same values used in the evaluation of the Bonferroni inequality, the Šidák bound is

$$1 - P(F) \geq (1 - \alpha)^5 = (0.95)^5 = 0.77$$

In drug studies, some or all of k treatments are sometimes related to each other in a quantitative way. If certain treatments are related as if these were measured on either an interval or a ratio scale of measurement, the functional relationship among these treatments can be exploited to determine functional relationships among the responses to these treatments. Quite often this occurs when the experimenter is interested in a dose–response relationship and may use functions such as orthogonal polynomials to determine the degree of the polynomial that best fits the dose–response curve.

B. DESCRIPTIONS OF MULTIPLE COMPARISON PROCEDURES

In what follows, $\bar{y}_1, \bar{y}_2, \ldots, \bar{y}_k$ refer to the observed treatment means and s^2 to an estimate of variance (from an analysis of variance table) that is based on, say, f degrees-of-freedom (df). Also, s is the positive square root of s^2 and is known as the standard deviation. These means and the standard deviation summarize the experimental results of interest for making treatment comparisons, regardless of what experimental design was used to generate the data. It will be assumed that the variances within each treatment group are homogeneous. Where this is not true, the formulas quoted will require modification, as described in some of the references given.

1. The Least Significant Difference and Multiple t Test Procedures

The least significant difference (LSD) procedure and the multiple t test use the well known Student's t test but the LSD procedure is a two-step method, starting with an F-test at level α and followed by multiple t-tests only if the value of F is significant, see Hochberg and Tamhane[8] (p. 3). Use of the LSD procedure without the preliminary F test is sometimes called the "unprotected" LSD procedure. For any contrast, say L_1, which is defined in Equation 23.1, the allowance is

$$\text{LSD} = t_{\alpha,f} s_c = t_{\alpha,f} s \sqrt{c_1^2/n_1 + \cdots + c_k^2/n_k} \qquad (23.5)$$

where s_c is the standard error of the contrast, and $t_{\alpha,f}$ is the appropriate two-tailed upper α point of Student's t distribution with f df. If the intention is to compare two treatments in a pairwise comparison, such as treatment 1 and treatment 2 as the difference between their means

$$\bar{y}_1 - \bar{y}_2 \ (c_1 = +1; \ c_2 = -1; \ c_j = 0 \ \text{for } j = 3, 4, \ldots, k).$$

the allowance becomes

$$\text{LSD} = t_{\alpha,f} s_d = t_{\alpha,f} s \sqrt{n_1^{-1} + n_2^{-1}} \qquad (23.6)$$

where s_d is the standard error of the difference between the two means. Use of the unprotected LSD procedure or multiple t tests for *a priori* comparisons with quantitative data will lead to the occurrence of results falsely labeled significant in a proportion α of the comparisons; that is, the procedure controls the comparison error rate at the level α. If the absolute value of the computed contrast exceeds the allowance, the contrast is said to be statistically significant and an appropriate interpretation can be made.

2. S Method

The S method, otherwise known as Scheffé's[9] fully-significant-difference (FSD) method, controls the familywise error rate at any desired level α. This is achieved by replacing $t_{\alpha,f}$ in the formula for the LSD allowance by

$$\sqrt{(m-1)F_{\alpha,m-1,f}}$$

where $F_{\alpha,m-1,f}$ is the upper α point of the F distribution with $m-1$ numerator df and f denominator df.

$$[\text{Note}:\ \text{when}\ m=2,\ \sqrt{(m-1)F_{\alpha,m-1,f}}=\sqrt{F_{\alpha,1,f}}=t_{\alpha,f}.]$$

Here m is the number of means involved in the family of comparisons ($m \leq k$), while the allowance for any contrast, say L_1, is given by

$$\begin{aligned}\text{FSD} &= s_c\sqrt{(m-1)F_{\alpha,m-1,f}}\\ &= s\sqrt{(m-1)F_{\alpha,m-1,f}(c_1^2/n_1+\cdots+c_m^2/n_m)}\end{aligned}\tag{23.7}$$

Since the S method controls the familywise error rate at the level α for all possible contrasts which can be formed from the treatment means, it is not necessary to specify *a priori* the particular contrasts of interest. *A posteriori* contrasts suggested by the data can be added and tested without affecting the nominal value of the error rate.

3. T Method

Like the S method, the T method, otherwise known as Tukey's[1] wholly-significant-difference (WSD) method, controls the family error rate. It is particularly well suited, when the main interest is in testing all the differences between $m \leq k$ treatment means when these are taken in pairs, because the allowances for these contrasts are considerably smaller than those for the S method. The allowance for any contrast, say L_1, is given by

$$\text{WSD} = q_{\alpha,m,f}s\,\frac{\displaystyle\sum_{i=1}^{m}\sum_{j=1}^{m}c_i^+c_j^-\sqrt{n_i^{-1}+n_j^{-1}}}{\dfrac{1}{2}\displaystyle\sum_{i=1}^{m}|c_i|}\tag{23.8}$$

where $|c|$ represents the absolute value of the constant c, $c_i^+ = \max(c_i, 0)$, $c_j^- = \min(c_j, 0)$ and $q_{\alpha, m, f}$ is the upper α point of the distribution of the Studentized range for m means and f df. For a difference such as $\bar{y}_1 - \bar{y}_2$, the allowance simplifies to

$$\text{WSD} = q_{\alpha, m, f} s \sqrt{1/2(n_1^{-1} + n_2^{-1})} \qquad (23.9)$$

4. Orthogonal Contrasts

Another method, also from Tukey,[1] controls the family error rate when the family consists of a set of orthogonal contrasts (TOC: Tukey orthogonal contrasts). To obtain the required allowance, $t_{\alpha, f}$ in Equation 23.5 for the LSD is replaced with $t'_{\alpha, p, f}$, the upper α point of the distribution of the Studentized maximum modulus, where p is the number of contrasts in the orthogonal set with f df. The Studentized maximum modulus is the maximum of p independent normal variates with mean zero, divided by an estimate of the standard error. This distribution coincides with Student's t for a single comparison ($p = 1$) but its percentage points exceed those of Student's t for two or more orthogonal contrasts in the set. With this method, the allowance for any contrast L_1 in a set of p mutually orthogonal contrasts is

$$\text{TOC} = t'_{\alpha, p, f} s_c = t'_{\alpha, p, f} s \sqrt{c_1^2/n_1 + \cdots + c_k^2/n_k} \qquad (23.10)$$

This concept can be extended to test other contrasts that can be expressed as linear combinations of the p contrasts in the orthogonal set without modifying the error rate.

Orthogonal contrasts arise in analysis of variance when a treatment sum of squares is partitioned into single-degree-of-freedom components. In a clinical trial with four distinct treatments, for example, the treatment sum of squares can be partitioned into three mutually orthogonal contrasts of interest. One way to obtain a single overall test is to add together these three orthogonal sums of squares and apply an F test with 3 and f df. Another way is to test the $p = 3$ contrasts separately by using this multiple comparison procedure based on the Studentized maximum modulus distribution. The latter tests will have the same type I error probability as the F test, but with greater power to detect a failure in validity which has affected one or more of the specified orthogonal contrasts.

5. Comparisons with a Control or Standard

Many times in clinical trials and dose–response studies, one of the groups has a special status and the comparisons of interest are those between the other treatment means and the specified mean. Examples of such comparisons are between several test treatments and a control or standard treatment and between a new drug and several reference standard drugs. Let $\bar{y}_1$ be the mean for the specified group; then the contrasts of primary interest are $\bar{y}_2 - \bar{y}_1, \bar{y}_3 - \bar{y}_1, ..., \bar{y}_k - \bar{y}_1$.

For control of the family error rate, the upper α point of a multivariate Student's t distribution is required in place of $t_{\alpha,f}$ in the LSD allowance (Equation 23.5). This procedure is frequently called Dunnett's test; the allowance for these contrasts (MCC: Multiple Comparisons with a Control) is

$$\text{MCC} = t''_{\alpha,k-1,f}s_d = t''_{\alpha,k-1,f}s\sqrt{n_i^{-1} + n_1^{-1}} \qquad (23.11)$$

where $t''_{\alpha,k-1,f}$ is the upper α point of a $(k-1)$-variate Student's t distribution with correlations $\rho_{ij} = \lambda_i\lambda_j$, $\lambda_i = 1/\sqrt{1 + n_1/n_i}$, and f df. The allowance can be extended to test any weighted mean of the treatment means vs. the control mean.

6. Stepwise (Step-down and Step-up) Tests

In testing a set of k contrasts, such as a set of orthogonal contrasts or a set of contrasts representing differences between several treatments and a specified treatment, the power for detecting true differences can be increased by performing the tests in "stepwise" fashion. Denoted by t_i the statistic for testing the ith contrast, ranked in ascending order so that $|t_1| \le \cdots \le |t_k|$, where $|t_i|$ denotes the absolute value (the value with any negative sign deleted) of t_i. (For one-sided tests, the actual t's instead of their absolute values should be ordered.) Denote by $c_1, \ldots, c_k$ a set of critical values to be used in the tests, c_i being the critical value to be used with $|t_i|$. In stepwise testing, the tests are carried out sequentially. Step-down tests start with the largest one, $|t_k|$, and continue downwards towards $|t_1|$ until an insignificant result is obtained. At this point testing stops (and all remaining tests are automatically insignificant). In other words, the ith contrast is declared significant provided that $|t_k| \ge c_k, |t_{k-1}| \ge c_{k-1}, \ldots, |t_i| \ge c_i$. The reason for the increase in power is that the c's become smaller as i decreases, making it easier to find significance. In fact, the smallest one, c_1, is the same as used in the LSD test.

Step-up tests, on the other hand, start with $|t_1|$ and continue upwards towards $|t_k|$. As long as an insignificant result occurs, testing continues to the next t_i. As soon as a significant result is obtained, the testing stops (and all remaining tests are automatically significant). In other words, the ith contrast is declared significant if at least one of $|t_1|, |t_2|, \ldots, |t_i|$ exceeds its critical value.

The critical constants needed for the tests depend upon the particular contrasts being tested. The set of c's required for step-up tests will ordinarily be slightly larger than the c's required for step-down tests, except for c_1, which is the same for both. Depending on how many of the k contrasts are expected to correspond to real effects it can be concluded whether a step-down or a step-up procedure is better in terms of power. If there are only one or a few in this category, step-down is better; if all or most of them are in this category, step-up is better (see Dunnett and Tamhane,[10] who considered the case of testing a set of equally-correlated contrasts). In Section III.B, a practical example is described.

7. Multiple Range Tests

The multiple range tests, known as the Student–Newman–Keuls (SNK) and Duncan (DCN) procedures, after Newman,[11] Keuls[12] and Duncan,[13] may be considered as modifications of the T method although these were developed independently. These are stepwise tests and are used when pairwise comparisons of the treatment means are of interest.

These procedures are illustrated for the case where the means are based on equal sample sizes. The k treatment means are ranked from the lowest to the highest:

$$\bar{y}_{(1)} \leq \bar{y}_{(2)} \leq \cdots \leq \bar{y}_{(k)}$$

To test the difference between any two means, say

$$\bar{y}_{(i)} - \bar{y}_{(i')} \qquad (i > i')$$

the WSD allowance is $q_{\alpha,k',f} s_{\bar{y}}$ no matter which pair is being compared, where $s_{\bar{y}} = s/\sqrt{n}$ is the standard error of a mean. The SNK procedure, on the other hand, uses the allowance

$$\text{SNK} = q_{\alpha,k',f} s_{\bar{y}} \tag{23.12}$$

where k' is the number of means lying between and including the two being compared (i.e., $k' = |i - i'| + 1$, where i and i' represent the rank order of the two means being compared). Thus the SNK allowance is smaller than the WSD allowance except for comparisons of two extreme means, in which case these are equal. Once a pair of ordered means $(\bar{y}_{(i')}, \bar{y}_{(i)})$ is tested and is found to be insignificant, no other pair of treatments whose means fall between $\bar{y}_{(i')}$ and $\bar{y}_{(i)}$ can be declared to be significant.

In Duncan's multiple range test, the allowance is

$$\text{DCN} = q_{\alpha',k',f} s_{\bar{y}} \tag{23.13}$$

where k', as in the SNK allowance (Equation 23.12), is the number of means between and including the two being tested, while α' is equal to $1 - (1 - \alpha)^{k'-1}$. This choice of the percentage point of the Studentized range statistic is based on the concept of *error rate per degree-of-freedom*.[13] The DCN (Equation 23.13) allowances are smaller than the WSD (Equation 23.8) and the SNK allowances (Equation 23.12) but larger than those of the LSD (Equation 23.5) method.

The SNK method does not control the family error rate to be $\leq \alpha$ in all cases. Several authors have proposed modifications to correct this deficiency. The Tukey–Welsch modification[8] (p. 69), which proceeds as in the SNK procedure except that α in Equation 23.6 is replaced by $\alpha_{k'} = 1 - (1 - \alpha)^{k'/k}$ for $k' \leq k - 2$ and is a good method to be used. Regarding DCN, the error rate per degree-of-freedom concept on which it is based has been criticized by Miller[3] (pp. 87–89), Hsu[14] (pp. 129–130) and others; most statisticians no longer recommend it.

Duncan has also developed another method,[15] called an *adaptive k-ratio t test* for comparing all treatments in pairs, in which the size of the allowance is a function of the value of the F-statistic for testing treatment homogeneity. However, multiple range tests continue to be popular among practitioners, particularly in the agricultural areas, although considerable criticism exists about their indiscriminant use.[16]

8. Confidence Intervals

In most of the discussion above, it has been assumed that the interest is in significance testing. The estimate of the value of each contrast is simply the observed value of the contrast; two-sided confidence limits are easily obtained by adding and subtracting the value of the appropriate allowance. There is the same choice between methods of determining the allowance in confidence interval estimation as in significance testing: the confidence coefficient, $1 - \alpha$, may apply to each confidence interval separately or jointly to all the confidence intervals in a family. Thus, corresponding to the comparison and family error rates of multiple hypotheses testing, separate and joint (or simultaneous) confidence coefficients for confidence interval estimation are available. There is no confidence interval procedure corresponding to the SNK and DCN tests.

9. Comparisons with the Best

A method called *multiple comparisons with the best* (MCB) was developed by Hsu[14] (chapter 4, pp. 81–118). It is related to the MCC method above, although it is quite different from it. Instead of comparing the treatments with a specified treatment as in the MCC method, each treatment is compared with whichever one of the remaining treatments appears to be the best one. Thus we compare $\bar{y}_i$ with $\max_{j\neq i}\bar{y}_j$ (assuming a larger treatment effect is better). The resulting contrasts, $\bar{y}_i - \max_{j\neq i}\bar{y}_j$, are not linear contrasts like the others we have discussed, but are a particular kind of nonlinear function of the means. However, these can be used to form a set of simultaneous confidence intervals for the corresponding parameters $\mu_i - \max_{j\neq i}\mu_j$ where μ_i denotes the true mean for the ith treatment. The MCB method uses the MCC allowance $t''_{\alpha,k-1,f}s_d$, but with the following difference from the customary confidence intervals: if a one-sided value of $t''_{\alpha,k-1,f}$ is specified, the confidence intervals are constrained to contain the value zero. The effect of above leads to a confidence interval for the ith treatment whose lower limit is zero meaning the treatment to be the best. Similarly, a confidence interval with upper limit as zero means that the treatment is not the best, but it does not provide a lower bound on how much worse it is than the true best. If a two-sided value $t''_{\alpha,k-1,f}$ is specified, the confidence intervals are not constrained in this way and these have the same form as the usual two-sided confidence intervals. For an illustrative numerical example, see Hsu[14] (pp. 86–87 and 108).

10. Nonparametric Procedures

The multiple comparison procedures discussed so far have dealt exclusively with quantitative data. However, many times in clinical trial or dose-response animal studies, the data which need to be analyzed are only qualitative.

Using the ranks, r_{ij}, of the observations and the mean ranks $\bar{R}_i$, the family error rate is controlled and the allowance for a one-way design is approximately (KWA: after Kruskal and Wallis)

$$\text{KWA} = q_{\alpha,k,\infty}\sqrt{\frac{k(kn+1)}{12}} \tag{23.14}$$

where $q_{\alpha,k,\infty}$ is the upper α percentile point of the range of k independent standard normal random variables. Here two treatments are said to be significantly different if the absolute value of the difference of their mean ranks is larger than the allowance KWA. The procedure does not apply to general contrasts.

If one wishes to compare the $k-1$ treatments with a control when the data are ranks, controlling the family error rate yields an allowance that is approximately (KWC: after Kruskal–Wallis control)

$$\text{KWC} = |m|_{\alpha,k-1,1/2}\sqrt{\frac{k(kn+1)}{6}} \tag{23.15}$$

where $|m|_{\alpha,k-1,1/2}$ is the upper α point of the maximum absolute value of $k-1$ standard normal random variables with correlation $\frac{1}{2}$. Both of these are based on the Kruskal–Wallis[17] test.

If the ranks came from a two-way design where the k treatments are ranked within each of n blocks, control of the family error rate for all pairwise comparisons yields an approximate allowance of

$$\text{FRI} = q_{\alpha,k,\infty}\sqrt{\frac{k(k+1)}{12n}} \tag{23.16}$$

where $q_{\alpha,k,\infty}$ is, as before, the upper α point of the range of k independent standard normal random variables (FRI: Friedman).

When treatment 1 is the control or standard and the paired comparisons of interest all involve treatment 1, the ranks derived from a two-way design provide an experimentwise control of the error rate with the approximate allowance

$$\text{FRC} = |m|_{\alpha,k-1,1/2}\sqrt{\frac{k(k+1)}{6n}} \tag{23.17}$$

where $|m|_{\alpha,k-1,1/2}$ is the upper α point of the maximum absolute value of $k-1$ standard normal random variables with the correlation $\frac{1}{2}$ (FRC: Friedman control). Both of these allowances are based on the Friedman[18] test statistic. When ties are present in the ranks, these procedures need to be modified.[19]

11. Multiple Comparisons between Dose Levels and a Zero Dose

The procedures proposed by Williams[20,21] are found to be appropriate in the special multiple comparisons case, where the object is to establish the minimum dose at which some undesirable response is first observed when compared with a zero dose. Where the usual normality assumption is not justified in data, Shirley[22] outlined a similar procedure based on the means of ranks of responses rather than the responses themselves. These procedures assume that the dose–response curve is monotonic even though the observed data may not be.

If the first treatment 1 is the zero dose control and the other $k - 1$ treatments are a series of increasing doses of the same therapeutic agent, then for the Williams test, the response to the ith dose is determined by

$$\hat{M}_i = \max_{2 \le u \le i} \min_{i \le v \le k} \sum_{j=u}^{v} \frac{\bar{y}_j}{v - u + 1} \qquad (23.18)$$

for $i = 2, 3, ..., k$. This estimate guarantees that $\hat{M}_2 \le \hat{M}_3 \le \cdots \le \hat{M}_{k-1} \le \hat{M}_k$. Once these estimates are obtained, the differences $\hat{M}_i - \bar{y}_1, i = k, k - 1, ..., 3, 2$ are successively compared to the allowances (WIL: Williams)

$$\text{WIL} = \bar{t}_{\alpha,k-1,f} s_{\bar{y}} \sqrt{2} \qquad (23.19)$$

where $\bar{t}_{\alpha,k-1,f}$ is the upper α percentage point of the averaged Student's t distribution for $k - 1$ dosage levels (apart from the control) and f residual df.

12. Multiple Comparisons of Proportions (0–1 Data)

If the k experimental groups contain binary responses so that the means $\bar{y}_i$ are proportions of experimental units in that group with the characteristics of interest, Knoke[23] showed that multiple comparisons based on the F distribution such as Scheffé's procedure (Equation 23.7) are suitable provided $n \ge 10$ and the true proportions lie between .2 and .8.

When a two-way design has been used to obtain the proportions of interest, Bhapkar and Somes[24] showed how the procedures of weighted least squares and suitably chosen χ^2 values can be used to construct allowances based on the Scheffé-type multiple comparison.

It is recommend that readers refer to the book on resampling-based multiple testing methods by Westfall and Young[25] for a different approach to these applications which is also applicable to a wide range of other problems where assumptions of normality and homogeneous variances may not be justified.

13. Other Methods

The commonly used multiple comparison tests have been described, but there are several others that have been proposed in the literature. A method has been described by Gabriel[26] that tests groups of means on the basis of their sums of squares values, as in an analysis of variance, rather than dealing with contrasts. Krishnaiah[27] describes what he calls a *finite intersection* method for testing a set of contrasts chosen *a priori*; the critical region for these contrasts is the intersection of the usual critical regions for testing the individual contrasts with its size equated to $1 - \alpha$. His method coincides with the standard methods if the set of contrasts coincides with that of one of the standard methods, such as all differences from a control, or all pairs of treatment differences. If it is not possible to determine the critical region exactly, he uses Bonferroni or Sidák bounds as an approximation. Hochberg and Rodriguez[28] have devised a class of "intermediate" procedures for testing contrasts which are, in a sense, midway between the Tukey T method and the Scheffé S method. These are based on enlarging the set of contrasts of primary interest to the investigator from the set of all pairwise comparisons, on which the T method is based, to include additional contrasts of a specific type, such as all differences between single treatment means and means of two treatments, or all differences between means of pairs of treatments. The method produces shorter allowances than either the T method or the S method for contrasts of the particular type specified. Several authors, such as Bradu and Gabriel[29] and Johnson,[30] have advocated multiple comparison procedures for testing contrasts of the interaction effects in two-way experimental designs, but the examples used to illustrate the methods raise questions concerning their actual utility in practice.

14. Allocation of Observations among the Treatment Groups

For most of the methods, the contrasts of interest are symmetric in the treatment groups and there is no reason for having certain means estimated more precisely than others by allocating unequal numbers of observations to the treatment groups. An exception occurs when the investigator has special interest in one of the treatment means, such as the mean for control or standard. Intuitively, one should allocate a higher proportion of the observations to the control or standard, if the investigator is interested mainly in the treatment vs. control contrasts. The problem of optimum allocation in this situation has been investigated by Bechhofer[31] and Bechhofer and Nocturne.[32] They showed that, when the variances are equal in the various treatment groups, the optimum allocation approaches the familiar "square root" rule asymptotically, namely, the ratio of the number of observations assigned to the control to the number assigned to any treatment should be $\sqrt{k}$, where k is the number of noncontrol treatments. This is optimum as the size of the experiment approaches infinity; the optimum can be quite different than this, when the sample sizes are small and error rates larger than the customary 1% or 5% are adopted.

TABLE 23.1
Summary Taxonomy of Multiple Comparison Procedures

Allowance	Error rate	Type of contrast	Design	Parametric/ Nonparametric	Distribution
LSD	Comparison	General	Any	Parametric	t
FSD	Family	General	Any	Parametric	F
WSD	Family	General	Any	Parametric	Studentized range
TOC	Family	Orthogonal	Any	Parametric	Studentized maximum modulus
MCC	Family	Control	Any	Parametric	Multivariate t
SNK	Family	Pairwise	Any	Parametric	Studentized range
DCN	df	Pairwise	One-way	Nonparametric	Normalized range
KWC	Experiment	Control (pairwise)	One-way	Nonparametric	Correlated multivariate normal
FRI	Experiment	Pairwise	Two-way	Nonparametric	Normalized range
FRC	Experiment	Control (pairwise)	Two-way	Nonparametric	Correlated multivariate normal
WIL	Experiment	Control	Any	Parametric	Averaged t

C. SUMMARY TAXONOMY

The purpose of Table 23.1 is to summarize all the techniques discussed in Section II.B of this chapter by considering the allowance short-form name, the error rate, whether it is pairwise oriented or general-contrast-oriented and the key distribution that is needed to compute the allowance.

D. COMMON SOURCES OF TABLES

When it comes to applying multiple comparison procedures, one needs to refer to tabulations of percentage points of the needed distributions. Student's t and F distributions can be found in many statistics books, so none will be recommended here. Table 23.2 outlines the common sources of tables.

TABLE 23.2
Multiple Comparison Critical Table Sources

Distribution	Symbol	f	k	%	Reference
Studentized range	$q_{\alpha,k}$	ν	r	5,1	3 (pp. 234–238)
Studentized range, for $\alpha' = 1 - (1 - \alpha)^{k-1}$	$q_{\alpha',k}$	ν	p	5,1	3 (pp. 243–246)
Studentized maximum modulus	$t'_{\alpha,p}$	ν	k	10,5,1	3 (p. 278)
Multivariate t	$t''_{\alpha,k}$	ν	p	20,10,5,1	33 (pp. 70–343)
Normalized range	$q_{\alpha,k,\infty}$	∞	k	20,10,5,...,0.01	19 (p. 330)
Correlated multivariate normal	$\|m\|_{\alpha,k-1,\frac{1}{2}}$	∞	ℓ	5,1	19 (p. 365)
Averaged t	$\bar{t}_{\alpha,k-1}$	ν	k	5,1	20 (pp. 107–108)

III. MULTIPLE COMPARISON TESTS IN PRACTICE

It may be recalled that the experiment has been performed to study the effects of k different treatments. The experimenter will be interested in making inferences about the "true" values of the treatment effects, which may take the form of either tests of hypotheses concerning certain contrasts or the estimation of confidence limits on their population values. There may be several contrasts which are of interest to the experimenter, but this does not necessarily mean that one of the multiple comparisons procedures must be used to make the inferences. The choice between using a multiple comparison test or an ordinary t test (or some equivalent method) depends on whether it is more appropriate to control the family error rate or the comparison error rate. If the user cannot decide which error rate is more appropriate, some statisticians would advise the user to use a multiple comparison procedure on the grounds that it is the conservative course of action to take, since setting the family error rate at some value α ensures that the comparison error rate will be less than α.

These error rates refer to Type I error (rejecting null hypotheses which are true). But there are other types of error to be concerned about as well, namely, failing to reject null hypotheses which are false (Type II errors) and the use of a multiple comparison procedure in place of a standard test, such as a t test will result in an increase in the probability of making a Type II error. In other words, the power of the test decreases.

A. IS A MULTIPLE COMPARISON PROCEDURE NEEDED?

Here, some typical examples arising in pharmaceutical research to illustrate some of the reasons for using (or not using) multiple comparison procedures will be considered. In general, the use of an appropriate multiple comparison test to make inferences concerning treatment contrasts is indicated in the following situations:

1. To make an inference concerning a particular contrast which has been selected on the basis of how the data have turned out.
2. To make an inference which requires the simultaneous examination of several treatment contrasts.
3. In "data dredging," viz., assembling the data in various ways to determine whether some interesting differences will emerge.

On the other hand, multiple comparison procedures are usually not appropriate when particular contrasts to be tested are selected in advance and are reported individually rather than as a group. In such situations, the comparison error rate is usually of primary concern and the standard tests of significance can be used, rather than a multiple comparison test.

For simplicity, it will be assumed in the examples considered in the rest of this section that the responses observed in an experiment, give rise to quantitative data, that the latter satisfy standard assumptions of model I (treatments fixed) analysis of variance and that there is equal replication of each of the k treatments. Thus (as in Section II.B), the data from the experiment can be summarized in the form of a set of values: $\bar{y}_1, \bar{y}_2, ..., \bar{y}_k$ and s^2 where $\bar{y}_i$ is the mean response for the ith treatment ($i = 1, 2, ..., k$) and s^2 is a variance estimate based on f df. The standard error of any treatment difference $\bar{y}_i - \bar{y}_j$ is represented by s_d. For a one-way design with n observations on each treatment, for example, $f = k(n - 1)$ and $s_d = s\sqrt{2/n}$.

1. Testing a Selected Contrast

When a set of experimental data is examined, it often happens that some particular feature of the configuration of treatment means raises questions as to whether or not it is significant. Consider, for example, the data shown in Table 23.1 of Dunnett[35] which represent measurements of the percentage fat content of breast muscle in cockerels on four different treatments: 1, 2, 3, and 4. The following mean values were obtained:

$$\bar{y}_1 = 2.493, \qquad \bar{y}_2 = 2.398, \qquad \bar{y}_3 = 2.240, \qquad \bar{y}_4 = 2.494$$

The birds that received treatment 1 were untreated controls while treatments 2, 3 and 4 were particular drugs. Each treatment mean shown was based on 20 independent values. The error mean square was $s^2 = 0.1086$ with $f = 64$ df, calculated from the analysis of variance, from which the standard error of the difference between any two treatments is $s_d = \sqrt{0.1086 \times 2/20} = 0.104$. The analysis of variance F test for testing the between-treatments mean square was significant, although it is not necessary to do a preliminary F test before proceeding with multiple comparisons (as some texts recommend). Performing a preliminary F test may miss important single effects which become diluted (averaged out) with other effects.

On examining these results, the experimenter was somewhat surprised at the low value for treatment group 3 and raised a question whether it is significantly different from the control. Thus, he is asking whether the contrast $\bar{y}_1 - \bar{y}_3 = 0.253$ is significantly different from zero.

To test the significance of a contrast, its observed value is compared with an allowance which is calculated by one of the methods described in Section II. Using the LSD, we have $LSD = t_{\alpha,f} s_d$, where $t_{\alpha,f}$ is the upper α point of Student's t distribution with $f = 64$ df. From tables of Student's t percentage points, we find that $t_{.05,64} = 2.00$ and the LSD allowance becomes .208, so the contrast $\bar{y}_1 - \bar{y}_3 = 0.253$ would be judged significant. However, the LSD is inappropriate as an allowance in this case, because it does not take into account the fact that $\bar{y}_1 - \bar{y}_3$ is a selected contrast: it was chosen specifically because the value of $\bar{y}_3$ was observed to be low.

To decide on the appropriate allowance to use in this case, it is necessary to determine the family of contrasts from which this one was selected. In the present case, if it can be assumed that only contrasts which involve differences from the control would be considered for statistical testing, then the family consists of $\bar{y}_1 - \bar{y}_2$, $\bar{y}_1 - \bar{y}_3$ and $\bar{y}_1 - \bar{y}_4$. The appropriate allowance for the selected contrast is MCC $= t''_{\alpha,k,f} s_d$; taking $t''_{0.05,4,64} = 2.41$ from Dunnett,[35] (Table 2) in we obtain MCC $= 0.251$. Thus, the contrast of interest is still significant although barely so.

On the other hand, if other contrasts might also have caught the experimenter's eye and the configuration of observed treatment means turned out differently, then the family would have to be enlarged and a different multiple comparison test used. For instance, if all differences between two means are included, the T method of Tukey should be used and the allowance becomes WSD $= q_{\alpha,k,f} s_{\bar{y}} = 3.74 \times 0.0737 = 0.276$, where $q_{0.05,4,64} = 3.74$ was obtained from tables of the Studentized range.

The need to test selected contrasts arises frequently in pharmaceutical research. Suppose a new drug is under development and many chemicals of related structure to a known active compound can be synthesized. It may happen that several potential candidates become available, and a choice has to be made to decide which one should be carried through to the clinical trial stage.

Let k be the number of candidates, where $k \geq 2$, and suppose an experiment is to be performed to measure a particular response, with the one producing the highest mean response to be selected. It may be noted that it is not a question of determining one which is significantly better than the others but simply of picking the one which produces the highest observed mean. There are interesting statistical problems involved in the design of the experiment so that the best candidate will have sufficiently high probability of producing a higher mean than any of the others. We will not consider these here, but we refer the interested reader to Gibbons et al.[36]

In such an experiment, a control or placebo treatment is often included for the purpose of estimating the "no-effect" response level. Let the no-effect treatment mean be $\bar{y}_0$ and let the observed treatment means be $\bar{y}_1, \bar{y}_2, ..., \bar{y}_k$. Then the experimenter chooses $\bar{y}_{max} = \max\{\bar{y}_1, \bar{y}_2, ..., \bar{y}_k\}$ and the drug corresponding to $\bar{y}_{max}$ is the one chosen to undergo further development in preparation for clinical trials. Having chosen it, however, the company management might wish to be assured that $\bar{y}_{max}$ is significantly different from $\bar{y}_0$. What p-value can we associate with $\bar{y}_{max} - \bar{y}_0$? Clearly, this is a selected contrast and the family consists of all $\bar{y}_i - \bar{y}_0$, $i = 1, 2, ..., k$. Thus the appropriate p-value is determined from the MCC test previously discussed. Calculation of $t'' = (\bar{y}_{max} - \bar{y}_0)/s_d$ and reference to the percentage points of the multivariate t distribution, with the degrees-of-freedom associated with s_d, tabulated in Bechhofer and Dunnett[33] gives the required p-value by interpolation. Or it can be computed using software based on the algorithm in Ref. 34, which can be downloaded from http://lib.stat.cmu.edu/apstat/251. Note that if a different number n_0 of observations had been obtained on the control than the number n on each treatment, then $s_d = s\sqrt{n^{-1} + n_1^{-1}}$ and the correlation coefficient $\rho = 1/(1 + n_0/n)$ would be used instead of $\rho = \frac{1}{2}$ in using either the tables or the computing software.

2. Comparisons between a New Drug and Active and Placebo Controls

This example illustrates that there are situations where the set of contrasts of interest in an experiment forms more than one family. Suppose a pharmaceutical company has developed a new drug that it wishes to market. To obtain permission from the regulatory authorities to do this, detailed information about the new drug must be submitted, including evidence about its compliance with the claimed activity and superiority over the existing drugs already in the market. Such evidence is obtained from clinical trials, in which the efficacy of the new drug is compared with one or more reference drugs and a placebo. In addition to providing a baseline for measuring the efficacy of the new drug, the purpose of the placebo is to verify that the trial is able to distinguish between the placebo and the known active drugs (referred to as the sensitivity of the trial). For ethical reasons it may not always be possible to include a placebo.

One way to design the efficacy trials would be to set up a number of trials, in each of which there are two treatment groups, one receiving the new drug and the other one of the reference drugs, and perhaps a third group receiving the placebo. However, a more efficient experimental design is to include all the treatments of interest together in each clinical trial. Suppose there are $k(\geq 1)$ reference drugs. Then each trial provides a set of $k + 2$ observed treatment means: $\bar{y}_1, \bar{y}_2, ..., \bar{y}_k$ the means for the k reference drugs, $\bar{y}_T$ the mean for the test drug and $\bar{y}_0$ the mean for the placebo. Comparisons can be made either between the observed means within each trial or between appropriate mean values over the entire set of trials. In either case, multiple comparisons are involved and the statistician is faced with the problem of deciding which is the proper test to use.

It is necessary to consider first which treatment comparisons are of interest to the pharmaceutical company and to the regulatory agency. Although any contrast among the $k + 2$ treatment means is potentially of some interest, it must be remembered that the main purpose of the trial is to: (1) demonstrate that the new drug is active relative to the placebo, (2) verify the sensitivity of the trial by comparing the known actives with the placebo and (3) compare the efficacy of the new drug with that of the reference drugs. Other comparisons, such as comparisons among the known actives, are superfluous to the main purpose of the trial. Thus, the comparisons of primary interest are limited to the particular set of $2k + 1$ contrasts and form three families: (1) $\bar{y}_T - \bar{y}_0$ representing the difference between the test drug and placebo, (2) $\bar{y}_1 - \bar{y}_0, ..., \bar{y}_k - \bar{y}_0$ representing the differences between the reference drugs and placebo and (3) $\bar{y}_T - \bar{y}_1, ..., \bar{y}_T - \bar{y}_k$ representing the differences between the test drug and the reference drugs.

Inferences concerning this set of contrasts can be made either by performing significance tests or by calculating confidence limits. For significance testing, appropriate null hypotheses have to be specified. Since the pharmaceutical firm must establish that the new drug is active, the first step is to compare it with the placebo by testing the null hypothesis that the difference of the true mean of the new drug and the true mean of the placebo is zero, vs. the alternative hypothesis that the true difference is nonzero (or perhaps positive). The contrast for testing the null hypothesis is $\bar{y}_T - \bar{y}_0$ and because this contrast is chosen because it is pertinent for this particular null hypothesis, not because it is selected on the basis of the observed data as in the previous example (even though it may indeed be the largest contrast in the set), the appropriate allowance for determining its significance is the LSD (Equation 23.5). Use of the LSD test at a particular significance level α guarantees that the probability of finding a significant difference between its new drug and the placebo when the new drug is really not different from the placebo, does not exceed α. This error rate is not affected by the fact that there are other treatments in the experiment.

Unless this particular treatment contrast $\bar{y}_T - \bar{y}_0$ is sufficiently significant, i.e., has a sufficiently small p-value associated with it to establish that the response to the new drug is indeed different from the placebo response, the testing of the remaining contrasts involving $\bar{y}_T$ is rather academic. Thus the testing of the remaining contrasts is conditional on a significant difference having been obtained for $\bar{y}_T - \bar{y}_0$.

The next set of contrasts to test, namely $\bar{y}_1 - \bar{y}_0, ..., \bar{y}_k - \bar{y}_0$, pertains to the sensitivity of the trial. Because these are differences between known actives and a placebo, we expect all of them to test significant. If any of them fail to show significance, then we have failed to establish the sensitivity of the trial, at least with respect to the particular reference drugs which do not differ significantly from the placebo. Berger[37] had the insight to realize that the type of test where all null hypotheses are to be rejected, to establish that a particular state of affairs pertains, requires a different type of multiple comparisons test. The null hypothesis to be tested is that at least one of the differences between the true mean of a reference standard and the true mean of the placebo is zero, vs. the alternative hypothesis that all the differences are positive (for a 1-sided test), or nonzero (for a 2-sided test). As Berger showed, the correct test for each is an ordinary comparisonwise test at level α (i.e., a t-test). This was considered in detail by Laska and Meisner[38] and was the basis of their "min" test. Thus, each of the contrasts $\bar{y}_i - \bar{y}_0$ is tested for significance by a t-test and sensitivity is established if all of the $\bar{y}_i - \bar{y}_0$ exceed their allowances.

Dunnett and Tamhane[39] proposed the use of a step-up test (see Section AII.B.7), with the critical value c_1 identical with that of a t-test so that the step-up test also establishes sensitivity when the min test does. The advantage of the step-up test is that if one or more of the $\bar{y}_i - \bar{y}_0$ fail to exceed the allowance based on c_1, it might still be possible to establish "partial sensitivity" with respect to some of the reference drugs. For example, if $\bar{y}_1 - \bar{y}_0$ does not reach significance with respect to its allowance based on c_1 but $\bar{y}_2 - \bar{y}_0$ is significant with respect to c_2, then it can be concluded that, although the first reference standard fails to satisfy the sensitivity criterion, all the remaining standards do (we assume we have ordered the reference drugs according to their t-values as described for stepwise testing).

While ordinarily it is not necessary for the pharmaceutical company to establish a significant difference between a new drug and any of the reference drugs to justify it being allowed to go on the market, it would clearly be to the company's advantage to be able to do so if it can. The null hypothesis to be tested is that the new drug is not superior to any of the reference drugs, vs. the alternative that the new drug is superior to at least one of the reference drugs. Rejection of the null hypothesis indicates that the new drug is superior to at least one of the reference drugs and thus strengthens the case of the pharmaceutical company to have it allowed on the market.

To test the null hypothesis with a specified upper bound on the probability of rejecting the null hypothesis when it is true, an extension of the step-down procedure described for equal sample sizes in Miller[3] (p. 86) can be used; see Dunnett and Tamhane.[40] The t-statistics for the set of contrasts $\bar{y}_T - \bar{y}_1, ..., \bar{y}_T - \bar{y}_k$ are ordered as described in Section II.B.7 and compared with critical values $c_1, c_2, ..., c_k$. These critical values are the same as those used in the MCC allowance (Equation 23.11). The largest t statistic t_k is thus compared with the MCC allowance for k comparisons; if it is significant, the next largest t_{k-1} is compared with the MCC allowance for $k - 1$ comparisons; and so on. This step-down procedure is analogous to the step-down of the Studentized range in the SNK procedure in Section II.B.8 of this chapter.

Thus the three families of contrasts for comparing first the test drug with the placebo, then the known active drugs with the placebo and finally the test drug with the known active drugs, can each be tested separately using an appropriate α-level test for each family. Because each family is tested conditionally on significance having been found for any previous families, the use of level α for each family ensures that the overall error rate is also less than α. So there is no need to consider the entire set of $2k + 1$ contrasts as a single family, which would result in a decrease in the power. This is discussed in more detail in Ref. 39.

For example, suppose $k = 2$ and the following treatment means are obtained: $\bar{y}_0 = 6.9$, $\bar{y}_T = 10.2$, $\bar{y}_1 = 7.6$ and $\bar{y}_2 = 9.0$ with $s_d = 1.22$ and $f = 20$ degrees-of-freedom. Then the new drug would be declared significantly different from the placebo since $(\bar{y}_T - \bar{y}_0)/s_d = 2.70$, which exceeds the $\alpha = 0.01$ point (two-tail) of Student's t with 20 df ($t_{.01,20} = 2.086$). Next, it would be declared superior to drug 1, since $\bar{y}_T - \bar{y}_1 = 2.6$ exceeds the allowance MCC $= t''_{0.05,2,20}$ $s_d = (2.03)(1.22) = 2.5$, but not to drug 2, since $\bar{y}_T - \bar{y}_2 = 1.2$ does not exceed the allowance MCC $= t''_{.05,1,20}$ $s_d = (1.72)(1.22) = 2.1$ (using one-tail values for these tests, due to the fact that the alternative hypothesis is one-sided).

3. Combination Drugs

The use of combination drugs has been a problem of special concern to pharmaceutical companies and the regulatory authorities. There are many possible reasons for combining more than one drug together in the same tablet or capsule. Sometimes, a second drug is added to counteract a possible side effect of the main drug. Sometimes the range of action can be increased by including more than one drug, such as, in controlling an infection where it is not known which drug would be the best one to use against the particular microorganism causing the infection. Whatever may be the reason for combining two or more drugs together, the regulatory agency would require evidence from the sponsor of the product that of the combination is more useful medically than each of its components (see Gibson and Overall[41]).

The whole question of demonstrating the efficacy of a combination drug product is very complex, and only one aspect of it will be considered here to illustrate the use of simultaneous inference. Suppose there is just one response to the drug to be considered, such as a fall in systolic blood pressure. If a combination drug is proposed to bring about this response, it would be necessary to establish that the combination is significantly better than each of the others. This would involve simultaneous inferences concerning the differences between the mean for the combination drug (e.g., drug 1) and the means for each of the components (drugs $2, 3, ..., k$) assumed to be $k - 1$ in number. It will be required to test the null hypothesis, that the true mean of the combination drug is less than or equal to the true mean of at least one component vs. the alternative that it exceeds all the components. The similarity between the null hypothesis being tested here and the one for testing for sensitivity in the previous example may be noted. Here, rejection of the null hypothesis requires each of the differences $\bar{y}_1 - \bar{y}_i$, $i = 2, 3, ..., k$, to fall in the rejection region rather than merely the largest one. The critical value needed to test these differences, chosen to achieve a test of size α for all true differences consistent with the null hypothesis, is based on the α-point of univariate (not multivariate) Student's t.

4. Data Dredging

In most experiments, the main treatment comparisons of interest are determined prior to doing the experiment. The purpose of doing the experiment is usually to estimate certain prespecified treatment effects, not to look for new leads to follow up. Nevertheless, having tested the main treatment effects of interest, it can be tempting to look at the data in other ways just in case "something might show up." This may be particularly the case in medical experiments involving human patients, since a large amount of subsidiary information is usually available about the patients, and it may be worthwhile to examine other effects too. In a trial to compare two or more treatments, for example, in addition to comparing the mean responses of the treatment groups, the experimenter may wish to make additional comparisons between subgroups of patients. For instance, the experimenter may wish to determine whether male patients respond more than females, whether the age of the patient is a factor, and so on. This process can generate quite a large number of comparisons to be made in addition to the primary comparisons which were the main reasons for doing the experiment.

The best way to treat such comparisons is in an ad hoc manner, without trying to attach any p-value to them or doing any formal test of significance. Any effect which looks interesting (by virtue of it being large compared to its standard error) should be looked upon as something to be studied further in another trial. However, if the experimenter must calculate a p-value, it would be necessary to take account of the actual number of comparisons those have been attempted, and use the Bonferroni method to arrive at a p-value, which would be an upper bound on the actual value of p. Shafer and Olkin[42] have considered this problem and obtained a mathematical justification for the use of the Bonferroni method in this way.

For example, suppose a clinical trial is done to compare two drugs, denoted by A and B, with $n = 100$ subjects assigned to each of the treatments. The main comparison in the trial would be the mean response $\bar{y}_A$ on drug A vs. the mean response $\bar{y}_B$ on drug B and the standard error of $\bar{y}_A - \bar{y}_B$ could be determined. Now suppose the subjects are split according to their sex, and measures of the treatment differences obtained separately for the males and females, giving $\bar{y}_{A,m} - \bar{y}_{B,m}$ for the males and $\bar{y}_{A,f} - \bar{y}_{B,f}$ for the females. Similar splits could be obtained on the basis of age, disease severity, and a number of other factors, each one providing a measure of the treatment difference and a standard error depending on the number of subjects. Selecting a particular treatment difference because it is large compared to its standard error would have to be assessed by referring the value of its $(\bar{y}_A - \bar{y}_B)/s_d$ to Student's t distribution with the appropriate degrees-of-freedom, and multiplying the p obtained from the t distribution by the total number of such comparisons made, according to the Bonferroni method. Thus, if the .005 point of Student's t were reached and 30 such tests had been made, an upper bound on the p-value associated with the comparison would be $(0.005)(30) = 0.15$.

5. Drug Screening

The purpose of drug screening is to test chemical compounds for a desired type of activity separating the active compounds from inactive ones. Over the years, many improvements have been developed in the laboratory testing procedures, particularly from the *in vivo* testing (i.e., in animals) as originally used to *in vitro* and in silicon testing methods which are common today: see Ruben and Neubauer[43] and Lam et al.[44] These changes have greatly increased the numbers of compounds which can be screened, leading to so-called "high throughput screening" methods.

Let k be the number of compounds tested in a screening experiment and denote by $\bar{y}_i$ the observed response for the ith compound ($i = 1, 2, ..., k$). Usually there is a control group producing a response $\bar{y}_0$ to estimate the inactive response level, although sometimes the mean response of all the compounds in the experiment is used instead, on the assumption that most of the compounds are inactive. Then a decision to accept a compound as active (which is called a "lead" or a "positive"), to reject it or to repeat the test is based on the magnitude of the difference $\bar{y}_i - \bar{y}_0$ ($i = 1, 2, ..., k$), or on its cumulative mean value if a multistage testing procedure is used and the compound has been tested previously. In terms of hypothesis testing, let θ_i denote the increase in activity between the ith compound and the control. We test the hypothesis H_i: $\theta_i \leq 0$ vs. the alternative that $\theta_i > 0$; rejection of H_i means that the ith compound has been classified as "positive." For a particular drug screening procedure, among its important properties are the proportions of compounds which are correctly classified as active or inactive in the long run. Similar issues arise in the analysis of DNA microarray data (see Lee and Whitmore[45]).

Because the main interest is usually to make separate inferences for each compound tested in the experiment, screening methods traditionally have been designed to control the comparison error rate to be $\leq \alpha$. A false positive will be detected by subsequent testing but valuable resources are used in the process. On the other hand, a false negative may mean that an effective treatment has been lost. For specified sample sizes, the value of α is chosen to achieve a balance between these two errors by discarding most of the inactives while selecting most of the actives (see Davies[46]). Some approaches choose α indirectly by seeking to optimize a measure of the efficiency of the screening procedure, such as the expected number of active compounds detected for a given amount of screening (see Davies[46] and also King[47]). However α is determined, the critical constant(s) for determining which compounds to select depend directly on the value of α. Examples of screening procedures for detecting anticancer compounds are given in Armitage and Schneiderman[48] and Vogel and Haynes.[49]

The FDR offers a different approach. Developed by Benjamini and Hochberg[5] as an alternative to controlling the family error rate, they also recommended its use in screening applications. Their procedure can be applied to the p-values corresponding to the test statistics arising from a screening experiment. Denote the ordered p-values by $p_{(1)} \leq p_{(2)} \leq \cdots \leq p_{(k)}$. These are compared in a stepwise manner to a set of critical bounds $c_1, \ldots, c_k$ which are certain fractions of α. In their method, these bounds are defined as $c_i = i\alpha/k \ (i = 1, \ldots, k)$, which vary from α/k for $i = 1$ to α for $i = k$ in a linear manner. The aim is to determine a number m, denoting the number of compounds to be selected, where m is defined as the largest i for which $p_{(i)} \leq c_i$. Then we classify the m compounds with p-values $\leq c_m$ as positives. This method is step-up, which means that it starts with the least significant p-value, $p_{(k)}$. Thus, we first try $m = k$: if $p_{(k)} \leq c_k = \alpha$, then $m = k$ and we stop. If not, we try $m = k - 1$: if $p_{(k-1)} \leq c_{k-1} = (k-1)\alpha/k$, then $m = k - 1$ and we stop; etc. The final step, if we go this far, is to try $m = 1$: if $p_{(1)} \leq c_1 = \alpha/k$, then $m = 1$, otherwise $m = 0$ and no compound is selected as positive.

For example, suppose there are $k = 100$ compounds in the screening experiment and we wish to control the FDR to be $\leq \alpha = .10$. Then the critical bounds for the ordered p-values are $.001, .002, \ldots, .100$ and we apply the rule given above to find the value of m. Say we obtain $m = 5$: then $c_m = .005$ and we select the five compounds with p-values $\leq .005$ as positive.

Which of these two approaches, controlling the comparison error rate or the FDR, is more suitable depends on the needs of the particular application. If the main interest is to make inferences about each compound separately, without regard to the decisions made about other compounds tested in the same experiment, a method for which the comparison error rate is $\leq \alpha$ is a reasonable choice, using an appropriate value of α. It enables the investigator, by the choice of α, to have direct control over the criterion which determines whether a compound is selected for further investigation.

Control of the FDR may be more appropriate in a situation where the experimenter has insufficient information about the population of compounds under test to make an appropriate choice of the value of α for controlling the comparison error rate: for example, if a new category or class of compounds is being tested and no information is available about the proportion of true actives it contains. With FDR control, which provides weak control of the family error rate, the probability of finding a false lead when no true actives are present is equal to the value chosen for α. On the other hand, if the new class turns out to be a rich source of true actives, FDR control adapts to this by increasing the probability of finding leads.

B. ANALYSIS OF A RANDOMIZED TRIAL

The following fictitious randomized trial was constructed to illustrate a variety of different multiple comparison procedures with the same set of data.

This trial was mounted by Canpharm Pharmaceutical Company to test out a new nonsteroidal anti-inflammatory drug (NSAID) called Arthritol. Animal studies had shown that the relative potency of Arthritol was estimated to be 0.90 when compared with plain aspirin. Consequently, a one-way randomized trial was designed with a placebo, a standard of 20 mg aspirin, and four dose levels of Arthritol: 10, 15, 20, and 25 mg. Sample size calculations dictated that $n = 11$ patients were to be randomly allocated to each of the six treatment groups.

The outcome measure chosen was the pooled index developed by Smythe et al.,[50] which was measured by an independent assessor (IA) in these Rheumatoid Arthritis (RA) patients before and after a 2-week treatment period. The IA was unaware of the treatment group to which any patient belonged.

The results of this trial are displayed in Table 23.3. Preliminary analyses showed there was no difference in the measures of variation[51] [$F_{max} = 3.36$, critical $F_{max}(\alpha = .05., k = 6, v = 10) = 6.92$]. For purposes of estimating the variance to be used in the multiple comparison procedures, a one-way analysis of variance was calculated and is displayed in Table 23.4.

Although this ANOVA showed that the treatments were quite different ($P \leq .001$), this was anticipated. Before the study was conducted, however, the following questions were of interest:

1. Is any dose of Arthritol different from placebo?
2. What is the lowest dose of Arthritol that is better than placebo?
3. Is any dose of Arthritol different from aspirin at 20 mg?
4. What is the nature of the dose-response of Arthritol? Is it linear, or does it need a higher degree polynomial?

It was also agreed that once a specific multiple comparison procedure was chosen to answer a question, the testing would be done at $\alpha = .05$.

TABLE 23.3
Results of Arthritol Randomized Trial

Patient Number (j)	Placebo	Aspirin (20 mg)	Arthritol dose (mg)				Total
			10	15	20	25	
	$i = 1$	2	3	4	5	6	
1	1.0	1.3	2.1	1.9	2.5	6.5	
2	−0.6	2.7	1.1	1.0	2.0	3.0	
3	0.7	2.1	2.4	0.9	4.0	2.4	
4	1.4	0.7	0.1	1.7	4.0	3.5	
5	1.0	3.6	0.1	1.9	1.9	4.3	
6	1.8	1.9	−0.1	1.5	3.3	3.3	
7	0.2	3.9	−0.3	2.2	4.3	2.3	
8	1.7	−0.8	0.8	3.7	2.1	2.7	
9	0.4	2.2	−0.6	0.1	2.8	2.6	
10	1.0	1.9	0.6	−0.1	2.4	4.7	
11	0.2	2.8	0.3	0.6	2.7	4.7	
n	11	11	11	11	11	11	66
$\sum_{j=1}^{11} y_{ij}$	8.8	22.3	6.5	15.4	32.0	40.0	125.0
$\sum_{j=1}^{11} y_{ij}^2$	12.18	62.59	12.95	33.08	100.54	162.16	383.50
$\bar{y}_i$	0.80	2.03	0.59	1.40	2.91	3.64	1.89
s_i	0.72	1.32	0.95	1.07	0.86	1.29	1.50

Observations were generated by adding $N(0,1)$ random variables to the six treatment effects 0.5, 2.0, 0.6, 1.3, 3.0 and 4.1, respectively.

TABLE 23.4
ANOVA of Arthritol Trial

Source	df	SS	MS	F	P
Mean	1	236.742			
Treatments (cfm)[a]	5	79.4521	15.89	14.17	0.001
Residual	60	67.3054	1.12		
Total	66	383.5			
Mean	1	236.742			
Total (cfm)	65	146.75			

[a] cfm, corrected for the mean.

To answer question 1, the MCC allowance (Equation 23.11) is employed where $s = \sqrt{1.121} = 1.059$, $f = 60$, $k = 4 + 1 = 5$, the four doses of Arthritol plus the placebo. Then $t''_{.05,4,60} = 2.51$:

$$\text{MCC} = \frac{(2.51)(1.059)(\sqrt{2})}{\sqrt{11}} = 1.133$$

The paired comparisons of interest are

$$\bar{y}_3 - \bar{y}_1 = -0.21, \ \bar{y}_4 - \bar{y}_1 = 0.60, \ \bar{y}_5 - \bar{y}_1 = 2.11, \ \bar{y}_6 - \bar{y}_1 = 2.84$$

Doses 20 and 25 mg of Arthritol are significantly different from placebo, but doses 10 and 15 are not significantly different from placebo.

To answer question 3, the same allowance MCC is used. This time, the paired comparisons of interest are

$$\bar{y}_3 - \bar{y}_2 = -1.44, \ \bar{y}_4 - \bar{y}_2 = -0.63, \ \bar{y}_5 - \bar{y}_2 = 0.88, \ \bar{y}_6 - \bar{y}_2 = 1.61$$

Consequently, 10 mg of Arthritol is significantly lower than the 20 mg of aspirin and the 25 mg of Arthritol is significantly higher than the aspirin dose. Also, both the 15 and 20 mg doses of Arthritol are not significantly different from the aspirin dose.

Question 2 can be dealt with by using the WIL (Equation 23.19) allowance. Here $\alpha = .05$, $k - 1 = 4$, $f = 60$ so $\bar{t}_{.05,4,60} = 1.78$. Now

$$\text{WIL} = \frac{(1.78)(1.059)(\sqrt{2})}{\sqrt{11}} = 0.804$$

Then

$$\hat{M}_3 = \frac{\bar{y}_1 + \bar{y}_3}{2} = 0.695, \ \hat{M}_4 = \bar{y}_4 = 1.40, \ \hat{M}_5 = \bar{y}_5 = 2.91, \ \hat{M}_6 = \bar{y}_6 = 3.64$$

Hence

$$\hat{M}_6 - \bar{y}_1 = 2.84, \ \hat{M}_5 - \bar{y}_1 = 2.11, \ \hat{M}_4 - \bar{y}_1 = 0.60, \ \hat{M}_3 - \bar{y}_1 = -0.105$$

By comparing these differences to the allowance WIL = .804, a dose of 20 mg of Arthritol or more gives a significantly higher response than the placebo.

To answer question 4, a set of orthogonal contrasts is applied to the four treatment means $\bar{y}_3$, $\bar{y}_4$, $\bar{y}_5$ and $\bar{y}_6$. Since the linear, quadratic and cubic polynomial terms can be fitted to four means, $p = 3$. Also $\alpha = .05$, $f = 60$ and the critical value used is

$$t'_{.05,3,50} = 2.46 \text{ for TOC} = \frac{(2.46)(1.059)}{\sqrt{11}} \sqrt{c_1^2 + \cdots + c_6^2}$$

where, for these contrasts, $c_1 = c_2 = 0$. Table 23.5 displays the actual computations.

Since only the linear contrast exceeds its critical value given by TOC, the evidence indicates that response of Arthritol can be described as linear in the dose range given. Strictly speaking, this conclusion should cause the experimenter

TABLE 23.5
Orthogonal Polynomials of Arthritol Doses

Contrast Name	Arthritol (mg)				$\sqrt{c_3^2 + c_4^2 + c_5^2 + c_6^2}$	TOC	Contrast Value
	$\bar{y}_3 = 0.59$	$\bar{y}_4 = 1.40$	$\bar{y}_5 = 2.91$	$\bar{y}_6 = 3.64$			
	c_3	c_4	c_5	c_6			
Linear	-3	-1	1	3	$\sqrt{20} = 4.47$	3.513	10.66
Quadratic	1	-1	-1	1	$\sqrt{4} = 2$	1.571	-0.08
Cubic	-1	3	-3	1	$\sqrt{20} = 4.47$	3.513	-1.48

to revise the answers to questions 1 and 3. If the response function is linear down to zero, *any* dose is different from the placebo; and bioassay methods could be used to estimate the dose which gives the same response as aspirin. These could also be used to estimate the dose which is equivalent to placebo.

REFERENCES

1. Tukey, J.W., The problem of multiple comparisons, 1953, In *The Collected Works of John W Tukey, Vol. VIII, Multiple Comparisons: 1948–1983*, Braun, H.I., ed., Chapman & Hall, New York and London, pp. 1–300, 1994.
2. Tamhane, A.C., Multiple comparisons, *Handbook of Statistics*, Vol. 13, Ghosh, S. and Rao, C.R., eds., pp. 587–630, 1996.
3. Miller, R.G. Jr., *Simultaneous Statistical Inference*, 2nd ed., Springer, New York, 1981.
4. Westfall, P.H., Tobias, R.D., Rom, R.D., Wolfinger, R.D., and Hochberg, Y., *Multiple Comparisons and Multiple Tests Using the SAS System*, SAS Institute Inc., Cary, NC, 1999.
5. Benjamini, Y. and Hochberg, Y., Controlling the false discovery rate: a practical and powerful approach to multiple testing, *J. Roy. Stat. Soc. B*, 57, 1289–1300, 1995.
6. Games, P.A., An improved t table for simultaneous control on g contrasts, *J. Am. Stat. Assoc.*, 72, 531–534, 1977.
7. Šidák, Z., Rectangular confidence regions for the means of multivariate normal distributions, *J. Am. Stat. Assoc.*, 62, 626–633, 1967.
8. Hochberg, Y. and Tamhane, A.C., *Multiple Comparison Procedures*, Wiley, New York, 1987.
9. Scheffé, H., A method for judging all contrasts in the analysis of variance, *Biometrika*, 40, 87–104, 1953.
10. Dunnett, C.W. and Tamhane, A.C., A step-up multiple test procedure, *J. Am. Stat. Assoc.*, 87, 162–170, 1992.
11. Newman, D., The distribution of the range in samples from a normal population, expressed in terms of an independent estimate of standard deviation, *Biometrika*, 31, 20–30, 1939.
12. Keuls, M., The use of the Studentized range in connection with an analysis of variance, *Euphytica*, 1, 112–122, 1952.

13. Duncan, D.B., Multiple range and multiple F-tests, *Biometrics*, 11, 1–42, 1955.

14. Hsu, J.C., *Multiple Comparisons: Theory and Methods*, Chapman & Hall, London, 1996.

15. Duncan, D.B. and Brant, L.J., Adaptive *t* tests for multiple comparisons, *Biometrics*, 39, 790–794, 1983.

16. Bryan-Jones, J. and Finney, D.J., On an error in "Instructions to Authors", *Hortic. Sci.*, 18, 279–282, 1988.

17. Kruskal, W.H. and Wallis, W.A., Errata to "Use of ranks in one-criterion variance analysis", *J. Am. Stat. Assoc.*, 48, 907–911, 1953.

18. Friedman, M., The use of ranks to avoid the assumption of normality implicit in the analysis of variance, *J. Am. Stat. Assoc.*, 32, 675–701, 1937.

19. Hollander, M. and Wolfe, D.A., *Nonparametric Statistical Methods*, Wiley, New York, 1973.

20. Williams, D.A., A test for differences between treatment means when several dose levels are compared with a zero dose control, *Biometrics*, 27, 103–117, 1971.

21. Williams, D.A., The comparison of several dose levels with a zero dose control, *Biometrics*, 28, 519–531, 1972.

22. Shirley, E., A nonparametric equivalent of Williams' test for contrasting increasing dose levels of a treatment, *Biometrics*, 33, 386–389, 1977.

23. Knoke, J.D., Multiple comparisons with dichotomous data, *J. Am. Stat. Assoc.*, 71, 849–853, 1976.

24. Bhapkar, V.P. and Somes, G.W., Multiple comparisons of matched proportions, *Commun. Stat. Theor. Methods A*, 5, 17–25, 1976.

25. Westfall, P.H. and Young, S.S., *Resampling-Based Multiple Testing*, Wiley, New York, 1993, chap. 5, pp. 146–183.

26. Gabriel, K.R., A procedure for testing the homogeneity of all sets of means in analysis of variance, *Biometrics*, 20, 459–477, 1964.

27. Krishnaiah, P.R., Some developments on simultaneous test procedures, *Developments in Statistics*, Vol. 2, Krishnaiah, P.R., ed., New York, Academic Press, pp. 157–201, 1979.

28. Hochberg, Y. and Rodriguez, G., Intermediate simultaneous inference procedures, *J. Am. Stat. Assoc.*, 72, 220–225, 1977.

29. Bradu, D. and Gabriel, K.R., Simultaneous statistical inference on interactions in two-way analysis of variance, *J. Am. Stat. Assoc.*, 69, 428–436, 1974.

30. Johnson, E.E., Some new multiple comparison procedures for the two-way AOV model with interaction, *Biometrics*, 32, 929–934, 1976.

31. Bechhofer, R.E., Optimal allocation of observations when comparing several treatments with a control: multivariate analysis, II, *Proceedings of the Second International Symposium on Multivariate Analysis*, Academic Press, New York, pp. 463–473, 1969.

32. Bechhofer, R.E. and Nocturne, D.J.-M., Optimal allocation of observations when comparing several treatments with a control, II: 2 sided comparisons, *Technometrics*, 14, 423–436, 1972.

33. Bechhofer, R.E. and Dunnett, C.W., Tables of percentage points of multivariate Student *t* distributions, *Sel. Tables Math. Stat.*, 11, 1–371, 1988.

34. Dunnett, C.W., Multivariate normal probability integrals with product correlation structure. Algorithm AS251, *Appl. Stat.*, 38, 564–579, 1989, To download software, go to http://lib.stat.cmu.edu/apstat/251

35. Dunnett, C.W., New tables for multiple comparisons with a control, *Biometrics*, 20, 482–491, 1964.

36. Gibbons, J.D., Olkin, I., and Sobel, M., *Selection and Ordering Populations: A New Statistical Methodology*, Wiley, New York, 1977.

37. Berger, R.L., Multiparameter hypothesis testing and acceptance sampling, *Technometrics*, 24, 295–300, 1982.

38. Laska, E.M. and Meisner, M.J., Testing whether an identified treatment is best, *Biometrics*, 45, 1139–1151, 1989.

39. Dunnett, C.W. and Tamhane, A.C., Comparisons between a new drug and active and placebo controls in an efficacy clinical trial, *Stat. Med.*, 11, 1057–1063, 1992.

40. Dunnett, C.W. and Tamhane, A.C., Step-down multiple tests for comparing treatments with a control in unbalanced one-way layouts, *Stat. Med.*, 10, 939–947, 1991.

41. Gibson, J.M. and Overall, J.E., The superiority of a drug combination over each of its components, *Stat. Med.* 8 1479–1484, 1989.

42. Shafer, G. and Olkin, I., Adjusting p-values to account for selection over dichotomies, *J. Am. Stat. Assoc.*, 78, 674–678, 1983.

43. Ruben, R.L. and Neubauer, R.H., Semiautomated colorimetric assay for in vitro screening of anticancer compounds, *Cancer Treat. Rep.*, 71, 1141–1149, 1987.

44. Lam, R.L.H., Welch, W.J., and Young, S.S., Uniform coverage designs for molecule selection, *Technometrics*, 44, 99–109, 2002.

45. Lee, M.-L.T. and Whitmore, G.A., Power and sample size for DNA microarray studies, *Stat. Med.*, 21, 3543–3570, 2002.

46. Davies, O.L., The design of screening tests in the pharmaceutical industry, *Bull. Int. Stat. Inst.*, 36, 226–241, 1958.

47. King, E.P., A statistical design for drug screening, *Biometrics*, 19, 429–440, 1963.

48. Armitage, P. and Schneiderman, M., Statistical problems in a mass screening program, *Ann. N. Y. Acad. Sci.*, 76, 896–908, 1958.

49. Vogel, A. and Haynes, J., Experiences with sequential screening for anticancer agents, *Cancer Chemother. Rep.*, 22, 23–30, 1962.

50. Smythe, H.A., Helewa, A., and Goldsmith, C.H., "Independent assessor" and "pooled index" as techniques for measuring treatment effects in rheumatoid arthritis, *J. Rheumatol.*, 3, 144–152, 1977 (Reprinted in: *Physiother. Can.* 30, 175–180, 1978.).

51. Hartley, H.O., The maximum F-ratio as a short-cut test for heterogeneity of variances, *Biometrics*, 37, 308–312, 1950.

24 Reference Intervals (Ranges): Distribution-Free Methods vs. Normal Theory

Paul S. Horn and Amadeo J. Pesce

CONTENTS

I. INTRODUCTION

The reference interval, also known as the reference range or normal range, includes the central 95% of an analyte (where an analyte is "any substance or chemical constituent of blood, urine, or other body fluid that is analyzed") measured in a presumed healthy population. The reference interval is used when there is no clear definition of disease. By this definition, unhealthy, or abnormal patient analyte values, would lie in the lower and upper 2.5%. In cases where the disease is defined, for example,[1] glucose concentration levels above 110 mg/dL are associated with diabetes,[2] the reference interval derived for the central 95% of the population is not used. It should be noted that the reference interval is by its nature a guideline and when combined with other clinical data helps define the clinical status of a patient. However, often in clinical practice the reference interval is misused as an absolute definition of health status. For this reason, the traditional term "normal range" has been mostly replaced by "reference range," or more correctly, "reference interval," in current practice.

For reasons of simplicity the reference intervals derived by hospitals are often all-inclusive. This means that the population of interest may contain many diverse subgroups, e.g., age groups, genders, ethnic groups, etc., and they may be combined. Therefore, the published reference intervals may be inaccurate for the individual subgroups. In clinical trials one may have a well-defined cohort for which the published reference intervals do not apply. In this chapter we discuss strategies for obtaining reference intervals for these cohorts.

The derivation of the reference intervals are based on results from nonparametric statistics as well as classical Normal theory.[10] Examples of the use of the reference interval for serum chemistry analytes include creatinine, albumin, and total protein. High creatinine values are indicative of poor kidney function. Low value of albumin occurs with poor nutrition and/or leakage through the glomerular membrane, while high value occurs in dehydration. Low values of total protein are often due to low values of albumin, while high values may be due to overproduction of immunoglobulins.[3] Two professional organizations have provided guidelines for the determination of reference intervals. The National Committee for Clinical Laboratory Sciences (NCCLS)[1] and the International Federation of Clinical Chemistry (IFCC)[4-9] are in general agreement.

II. REFERENCE INTERVALS AND PERCENTILE ESTIMATORS

Consider a sample of n independent and identically distributed random variables from a population with cumulative distribution function (cdf) $F(\cdot)$, and continuous probability density function (pdf), $f(\cdot)$. In other words, $\tilde{X} = (X_1, X_2, ..., X_n) \sim F(\cdot)$, and the reference interval based on this sample is defined as $(L(\tilde{X}), U(\tilde{X}))$ where $L(\tilde{X})$ and $U(\tilde{X})$ are the lower and upper endpoints of the reference interval. The $100(1-\alpha)\%$ reference interval is the same as a prediction interval, i.e., if X_{n+1} is another (independent) random variable from the same population then,

$$P(L(\tilde{X}) \leq X_{n+1} \leq U(\tilde{X})) = 1 - \alpha \qquad (24.1)$$

Here X_{n+1} is the patient's analyte value and the purpose is to see whether or not this value lies within the limits set by the reference interval. Further, it is customary for the reference interval to be symmetric in the sense that the central $100(1 - \alpha)\%$ of the population will lie within its limit. Hence, $L(\tilde{X})$ and $U(\tilde{X})$ are estimators of the lower and upper $(\alpha/2)$ percentiles, respectively. For the traditional 95% reference interval, $\alpha = 0.05$, and the reference interval consists of estimates of the lower and upper 2.5 percentiles.

III. TRADITIONAL NORMAL-THEORY APPROACH

Consider the classical situation where $X_1, X_2, ..., X_n$ form a random sample from a Gaussian (Normal) distribution with unknown mean, μ, and variance, σ^2, i.e., $X_i \sim N(\mu, \sigma^2)$, for $i = 1, ..., n$. Further, the "future" observation, X_{n+1}, is also from this population and independent from the random sample. Thus, we have the following results based on Normal theory:

$$\frac{\bar{X} - \mu}{\sigma} \sim N\left(0, \frac{1}{n}\right),$$

$$\frac{X_{n+1} - \mu}{\sigma} \sim N(0, 1),$$

yielding,

$$\frac{X_{n+1} - \bar{X}}{\sigma} \sim N\left(0, 1 + \frac{1}{n}\right),$$

$$\frac{X_{n+1} - \bar{X}}{\sigma\sqrt{1 + 1/n}} \sim N(0, 1),$$

and

$$\frac{X_{n+1} - \bar{X}}{S\sqrt{1 + 1/n}} \sim t_{n-1}, \tag{24.2}$$

where S is the sample standard deviation, $S = \left((1/(n-1)) \sum_{i=1}^{n} (X_i - \bar{X})^2\right)^{1/2}$, and t_{n-1} is a Student's t-distribution with $(n-1)$ degrees of freedom.[11] Thus, the 95% prediction interval for X_{n+1}, or, in other words, the reference interval is:

$$\bar{x} \pm t_{\alpha/2}^{(n-1)} s \sqrt{1 + \frac{1}{\sqrt{n}}} \tag{24.3}$$

where $\bar{x}$ is the observed sample mean, s is the observed sample standard deviation, $t_{\alpha/2}^{(n-1)}$ is the upper $\alpha/2$ percentile from a Student's t-distribution with $(n-1)$ degrees of freedom, and n is the sample size. In a formula,

$$L(\tilde{x}) = \bar{x} - t_{\alpha/2}^{(n-1)} s \sqrt{1 + \frac{1}{n}},$$

and

$$U(\tilde{x}) = \bar{x} + t_{\alpha/2}^{(n-1)} s \sqrt{1 + \frac{1}{n}}, \tag{24.4}$$

where $\tilde{x} = (x_1, x_2, ..., x_n)$ are the observed values.

For example, consider the data in Table 24.1 that represent a sample of 120 determinations of lactate dehydrogenase (LDH) in young females. The data are from an unscreened population and is representative of what is most easily

TABLE 24.1
Serum Lactate Dehydrogenase for Young Females: Observations and Order Statistics

i	$X_{(i)}$	i	$X_{(i)}$	i	$X_{(i)}$
1	321	41	537	81	717
2	324	42	538	82	720
3	357	43	544	83	723
4	377	44	547	84	729
5	387	45	549	85	739
6	403	46	550	86	762
7	423	47	552	87	766
8	428	48	553	88	792
9	431	49	555	89	797
10	434	50	564	90	814
11	436	51	569	91	814
12	442	52	572	92	819
13	447	53	573	93	825
14	448	54	575	94	828
15	448	55	576	95	830
16	452	56	576	96	838
17	457	57	581	97	838
18	466	58	590	98	845
19	467	59	603	99	853
20	469	60	608	100	864
21	469	61	609	101	900
22	472	62	622	102	934
23	472	63	635	103	939
24	478	64	642	104	958
25	480	65	644	105	983
26	481	66	650	106	1023
27	483	67	651	107	1077
28	490	68	653	108	1082
29	492	69	663	109	1130
30	493	70	672	110	1144
31	500	71	673	111	1168
32	509	72	674	112	1333
33	512	73	684	113	1368
34	513	74	687	114	1383
35	519	75	691	115	1385
36	531	76	694	116	1404
37	532	77	698	117	2327
38	533	78	713	118	2614
39	534	79	716	119	4537
40	536	80	717	120	66592

collected from a pediatric population. The sample mean and standard deviation are equal to 1277.8 and 6031.7 IU. Using Equation 24.4 above, the limits of the 95% reference interval are derived as follows:

$$L(\tilde{x}) = 1277.8 - t_{0.025}^{(119)} \times 6031.7 \times \sqrt{1 + \frac{1}{120}} = -10,715$$

$$U(\tilde{x}) = 1277.8 + t_{0.025}^{(119)} \times 6031.7 \times \sqrt{1 + \frac{1}{120}} = 13,271$$

Note the effect that the large outliers have on these traditional estimates of the mean and standard deviation, and thus on the derived reference interval. While this example is extreme, it is illustrative of the problem of outliers that will be discussed later. Also note that the lower limit of the reference interval is less than zero (which is physiologically impossible). As a general practice, when the lower limit is less than zero, it should be reported as equal to zero.

Note that the reference interval represented by Equation 24.4 is valid only in the case where the population of analytical values has a Gaussian distribution. This is true regardless of the number of observations because even when the Central Limit Theorem holds (i.e., the distribution of the sample mean is approximately Gaussian), the distribution of X_{n+1} is the same as the parent population; thus Equation 24.2 does not hold in general. This is in contrast to the problem of deriving a confidence interval for the population mean, μ, where use of the Central Limit Theorem is (generally) valid.[11]

IV. DATA TRANSFORMATION TO ACHIEVE NORMALITY

It is often the case that real data are skewed and therefore not Gaussian. However, it is often possible to transform the data, so that the transformed sample appears to have come from a Gaussian population. A popular family of transformations is the power transformations from Box and Cox:

$$y = \begin{cases} \dfrac{x^\lambda - 1}{\lambda} & \lambda \neq 0 \\ \ln(x + c) & \lambda = 0 \end{cases} \qquad (24.5)$$

where x is the original, untransformed data point. The constants, λ and c are derived using maximum likelihood methodology.[12]

For example, consider the data from Table 24.1. The value for λ for the 120 observations was 0.7. The histogram for the transformed data is given in Figure 24.1. Clearly, these transformed data appears closer to a Gaussian distribution than the original data in Figure 24.2. Applying the estimators in Equation 24.4, and then backtransforming to get the original scale, yields the following 95% reference interval: (351, 1730).

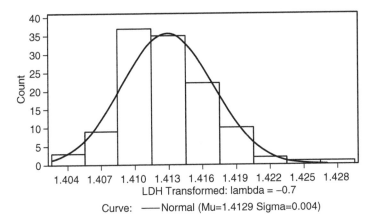

FIGURE 24.1 Histogram of transformed LDH values for female children with fitted Gaussian curve. The value of the λ-parameter is approximately $= -0.7$. The p-value for the Anderson-Darling test is approximately 0.06.

V. NONPARAMETRIC APPROACH USING ORDER STATISTICS

For the reason stated above, it is desirable to use quantile or percentile estimators that do not depend on the underlying distribution of analytical values. Such distribution-free estimators are based on the order statistics from the sample. Consider the random sample $X_1, X_2, ..., X_n$, from the distribution, $F(\cdot)$, and the associated order statistics $X_{(1)} \leq X_{(2)} \leq ... \leq X_{(n)}$. An estimator of the pth

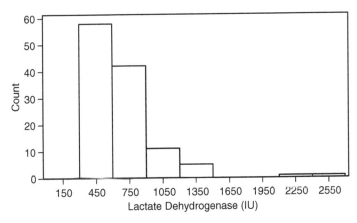

FIGURE 24.2 Histogram of LDH values for female children. 118 out of the 120 values are included in the figure. The two largest values were omitted to prevent the scale from being distorted. The p-value for the Anderson-Darling test is less than 0.005 (small p-values indicate a nonGaussian distribution).

quantile, $F^{-1}(p)$, is $X_{(\xi_n)}$ where ξ_n is approximately equal to $n \times p$. For example, if the sample size is 100, then an estimator of the 95th percentile is $X_{(95)}$. It can be shown that the quantile estimator based on order statistics are consistent for $F^{-1}(p)$ and do not depend on $F(\cdot)$ so long as $\xi_n/n \to p$ when $n \to \infty$.[13] Such estimators are referred to as nonparametric estimators.

It should be noted that there is no generally accepted exact form for the sample quantile estimator, except for the sample median. For example, if the sample size is 100, then two reasonable estimators of $F^{-1}(.95)$, $\hat{F}^{-1}(.95)$, are $X_{(95)}$ and $(X_{(95)} + X_{(96)})/2$. Further, the statistical software package (SAS®) allows for the choice of five different definitions of the estimator of the pth quantile, or percentile:

Definition 1.

$$\hat{F}^{-1}(p) = (1 - r)X_{(j)} + rX_{(j+1)}$$

where $j = [np]$ and $r = np - j$;

Definition 2.

$$\hat{F}^{-1}(p) = \begin{cases} X_{(i)} & r \neq 0.5; \\ X_{(j)} & r = 0.5 \quad \text{and } j \text{ is even}; \\ X_{(j+1)} & r = 0.5 \quad \text{and } j \text{ is odd}; \end{cases}$$

where $i = [np + 0.5]$

Definition 3.

$$\hat{F}^{-1}(p) = \begin{cases} X_{(j)} & r = 0; \\ X_{(j+1)} & r > 0; \end{cases}$$

Definition 4.

$$\hat{F}^{-1}(p) = \begin{cases} (X_{(j)} + X_{(j+1)})/2 & r = 0; \\ X_{(j+1)} & r > 0; \end{cases}$$

Definition 5.

$$\hat{F}^{-1}(p) = (1 - r)X_{(j)} + rX_{(j+1)}$$

where $j = [(n + 1)p]$, $r = (n + 1)p - j$, and $X_{(n+1)} \equiv X_{(n)}$;

where $[x]$ is the integer part of x. For our purposes we use the percentile estimator corresponding to Definition 4.[14] (Note that this is the same as PCTLDEF number 5 in SAS®, which is the default.) In contrast, both the NCCLS[1] and Harris and Boyd (1995)[10] use the percentile estimator corresponding to Definition 5.

For example, consider the data from Table 24.1. The standard 95% reference interval consists of estimates of the 2.5 and 97.5 percentiles. Thus, to compute the 97.5 percentile, $p = 0.975$ and $n = 120$ in this case. Using Definition 4 above, the 2.5 percentile is computed as follows:

$$j = [120 \times 0.025] = 3 \qquad \text{and} \qquad r = 120 \times 0.025 - j = 0.$$

Thus, the 2.5 percentile is estimated by $(X_{(3)} + X_{(4)})/2 = (357 + 377)/2 = 367$. Similarly, the 97.5 percentile is computed as follows:

$$j = [120 \times 0.975] = 117 \qquad \text{and} \qquad r = 120 \times 0.975 - j = 0.$$

Thus, the 97.5 percentile is estimated by $(X_{(117)} + X_{(118)})/2 = (2327 + 2614)/2 = 2470.5$. The resulting 95% reference interval, based on Definition 4 is approximately $(367, 2471)$.

Using Definition 5 above, the 2.5 percentile is computed as follows:

$$j = [(120 + 1) \times 0.025] = 3 \qquad \text{and} \qquad r = (120 + 1) \times 0.025 - 3 = 0.025,$$

so the 2.5 percentile is estimated by $(1 - 0.025)X_{(3)} + 0.025X_{(4)} = 0.975 \times 357 + 0.025 \times 377 = 357.5$. Similarly, the 97.5 percentile is computed as follows:

$$j = [(120 + 1) \times 0.975] = 117 \qquad \text{and}$$

$$r = (120 + 1) \times 0.975 - 117 = 0.975,$$

so the 97.5 percentile is estimated by $(1 - 0.975)X_{(117)} + 0.975X_{(118)} = 0.025 \times 2327 + 0.975 \times 2614 = 2606.825$. The resulting 95% reference interval, based on Definition 5 is approximately $(358, 2607)$.

It is not unusual for extreme percentiles to differ depending upon the definition used. In the example above, the nonparametric reference interval based on Definition 5 is approximately 7% wider than that based on Definition 4.

Another nonparametric quantile estimator is described by Harrel and Davis (1982)[15] and is a smoother estimator being a weighted average of all of the order statistics in the sample:

$$\hat{F}^{-1}(p) = \sum_{i=1}^{n} W_{n,i} X_{(i)}, \qquad (24.6)$$

where

$$W_{n,i} = I_{i/n}\{p(n+1), (1-p)(n+1)\} - I_{(i-1)/n}\{p(n+1), (1-p)(n+1)\} \qquad (24.7)$$

and $I_x(a,b)$ is the incomplete beta function, i.e.,

$$I_x(a,b) = \frac{\Gamma(a+b)}{\Gamma(a)\Gamma(b)} \int_0^x t^{a-1}(1-t)^{b-1}dt \qquad (24.8)$$

and $\Gamma(y)$ is the gamma function, i.e.,

$$\Gamma(y) = \int_0^\infty t^{y-1}e^{-t}dt \qquad (24.9)$$

(see Davis[16]). Equation 24.6 represents a bootstrap calculation of the quantile estimator represented by Definition 5. Consider a pseudo-sample consisting of n observations that are sampled, with replacement, from the original data set (consisting of n values). From this pseudo-sample the quantile estimator is computed according to Definition 5. The bootstrapped estimator (Equation 24.6) is then the average of all such possible estimators.[17]

Using the data in Table 24.1, the 95% reference interval based on the Harrel and Davis percentile estimators is approximately (361, 7651). Note that because these estimators are smoother than the traditional nonparametric estimators, all data values get nonzero weight. As a result, the gross outlier, 66592, has an adverse effect on the upper limit. Here is another case where there is a clear need to identify and eliminate outliers from the calculations of the reference intervals.

The derivation of extreme quantiles poses a delicate balancing act. Information must be extracted from that portion of the sample where the data may exhibit extreme behavior. The robust method of deriving reference intervals was proposed by Horn et al.[18] Recall the reference interval based on the Gaussian distribution (Equation 24.3): $\bar{x} \pm t_{\alpha/2}^{(n-1)}s\sqrt{(1+(1/n))}$. This can be rewritten as:

$$\bar{x} \pm t_{\alpha/2}^{(n-1)}\sqrt{s^2 + \frac{s^2}{n}}.$$

The sample mean, $\bar{x}$, is the estimate of the center of the distribution, s^2/n is an estimate of the variability of $\bar{x}$, and s^2 is an estimate of the variability of the next value drawn from the distribution, X_{n+1}. These estimators give equal weight to all observations and are therefore susceptible to outliers (see below). The robust method uses estimators that give different weights (between zero and one) to each observation depending on how far away the observation is from the bulk of the data. See Horn et al.[18] for details. Since the robust estimators are not formally functions of the order statistics they are amenable to transformation, like the Gaussian estimator in Equation 24.3.

We end this section by noting the effect of the sample size, n, on the nonparametric estimator. Using the percentile estimator in Definition 5, it is clear that,

$$(n+1)p \geq 1 \quad \text{or} \quad n \geq \frac{1}{p} - 1, \qquad (24.10)$$

where p is the lower percentile $(p < 0.5)$. For example, to calculate a 95% reference interval, the lower percentile corresponds to $p = 0.025$, and thus, at least 39 observations are required. In this case, the 95% reference interval is defined by $x_{(1)}$ and $x_{(n)}$, the observed minimum and maximum values. If fewer than 39 observations are available and a 95% reference interval is required, then the nonparametric approach may not be valid.

VI. PRECISION OF REFERENCE INTERVAL ENDPOINTS

The reference interval is defined by the two estimators, $L(\tilde{X})$ and $U(\tilde{X})$ defined in Equation 24.1. These statistics are point estimators of the parameters $F^{-1}(\alpha/2)$ and $F^{-1}(1 - \alpha/2)$, respectively. It is often desirable to derive confidence intervals for these parameters. The NCCLS recommends that 90% confidence intervals be used for the endpoints of 95% reference intervals.[1,19] Calculations of the confidence intervals for the reference interval endpoints will be described for the classical Normal-based case and the nonparametric case.

The $(1 - \alpha)100\%$ reference interval based on the assumption that the data come from a Gaussian distribution (Equation 24.4) is as follows:

$$L(\tilde{x}) = \hat{F}^{-1}(\alpha/2) = \bar{x} - t^{(n-1)}_{\alpha/2} s\sqrt{1 + \frac{1}{n}} \quad \text{and}$$

$$\hspace{8cm} (24.11)$$

$$U(\tilde{x}) = \hat{F}^{-1}(1 - \alpha/2) = \bar{x} + t^{(n-1)}_{\alpha/2} s\sqrt{1 + \frac{1}{n}}$$

Using mathematical theory, it is can be shown that the $(1 - \gamma)100\%$ confidence intervals for $F^{-1}(\alpha/2)$ and $F^{-1}(1 - \alpha/2)$ are as follows,

$$\hat{F}^{-1}(\alpha/2) \pm z_{\gamma/2} \cdot s_{\alpha/2} \quad \text{and} \quad \hat{F}^{-1}(1 - \alpha/2) \pm z_{\gamma/2} \cdot s_{\alpha/2}$$

where

$$s_{\alpha/2} = \sqrt{(2 + z^2_{\alpha/2}) \cdot \frac{s^2}{2n}} \hspace{3cm} (24.12)$$

and $z_{\alpha/2}$ is the upper $(\alpha/2)$ percentile from a standard Gaussian distribution.[8] For example, the 90% confidence intervals $(\gamma = 0.10)$ for the lower and upper endpoints of the 95% reference interval are as follows:

$$\hat{F}^{-1}(.025) \pm 2.81 \cdot \frac{s}{\sqrt{n}} \quad \text{and} \quad \hat{F}^{-1}(.975) \pm 2.81 \cdot \frac{s}{\sqrt{n}}, \hspace{1.5cm} (24.13)$$

where $\hat{F}^{-1}(.025)$ and $\hat{F}^{-1}(.975)$ are computed using Equation 24.11 above. Using the data from Table 24.1 and the reference interval computed using Equation 24.4, the 90% confidence interval for the lower limit $(-10,715)$ of the 95% reference interval is as follows:

$$-10,715 \pm 2.81 \times \frac{6031.7}{\sqrt{120}} = (-12{,}262, -9{,}168).$$

However, if the lower limit was set equal to zero, then the confidence interval would be $(-1547, 1547)$. As before, if negative limits are set equal to zero, the reported 90% confidence interval for the lower limit would be $(0, 1547)$.

Similarly, the 90% confidence interval for the upper limit $(13{,}271)$ of the 95% reference interval is as follows:

$$13,271 \pm 2.81 \times \frac{6031.7}{\sqrt{120}} = (11{,}724, 14{,}818).$$

As shown in Figure 24.2, the raw data do not follow a Gaussian distribution. Recall that applying the Box-Cox transformation in Equation 24.5 to these data resulted in a value of $\lambda = -0.7$ and after back-transforming resulted in the 95% reference interval: $(351, 1730)$. In order to compute confidence intervals for each of these two endpoints, confidence intervals for each must first be derived on the transformed data, and then back-transformed. This process yields the 90% confidence interval for the lower limit as $(330, 374)$. Similarly, that for the upper limit is $(1448, 2120)$. Note that as a result of the transformation, the point estimates of the reference interval limits are not exactly in the center of their respective confidence intervals.

The nonparametric reference interval endpoints are based on sample order statistics. In this case

$$L(\tilde{x}) = \hat{F}^{-1}(\alpha/2) = x_{(r)} \qquad \text{and} \qquad U(\tilde{x}) = \hat{F}^{-1}(1 - \alpha/2) = x_{(n-r+1)}$$

where $x_{(r)}$ is the rth order statistic or a linear (convex) combination of adjacent order statistics, depending on which of the five definitions of the sample percentile is used. The upper endpoint, $x_{(n-r+1)}$, is the symmetric counterpart to $x_{(r)}$, in other words, if $x_{(r)} = g \cdot x_{(i)} + (1 - g) \cdot x_{(i+1)}$, where i is an integer and $0 \le g \le 1$, then $x_{(n-r+1)} = g \cdot x_{(n-i+1)} + (1 - g) \cdot x_{(n-i)}$. Again, using mathematical theory, it is easily shown that the $(1 - \gamma)100\%$ confidence interval for $F^{-1}(\alpha/2)$ consists of the interval defined by the two order statistics $(x_{(l)}, x_{(r)})$ where,

$$\sum_{i=l}^{r-1} \binom{n}{i} (\alpha/2)^i (1 - \alpha/2)^{n-i} \ge \gamma. \tag{24.14}$$

Since the indices of the order statistics are not unique it is reasonable to chose l and r so that $r - l$ is as small as possible. By symmetry, the $(1 - \gamma)100\%$ confidence interval for $F^{-1}(1 - \alpha/2)$ consists of the interval defined by the two order statistics $(x_{(n-r+1)}, x_{(n-l+1)})$ where l and r are defined by Equation 24.14 above.[20]

For the Harrel and Davis and robust methods (transformed and not transformed) there are no formulas for the confidence intervals of the reference interval endpoints. For these methods bootstrap simulations are used to derive 90% confidence intervals for the estimators of the reference interval limits.

Recall that there is a minimum required sample size for the $(1 - \alpha)100\%$ reference interval that depends on α. For example, a 95% reference interval requires at least 39 observations (this interval would consist of the minimum and maximum values). There is also a minimum required sample size to determine the $(1 - \gamma)100\%$ confidence interval for the nonparametric reference interval endpoints. This minimum sample size increases as the desired level of confidence increases. The NCCLS recommends a minimum of 120 observations be used to determine reference intervals. Note that this is the minimum sample size required to derive 90% confidence intervals for the nonparametric 95% reference interval endpoints. Thus, if $n = 120$ then the 90% confidence intervals for the lower and upper endpoints of the 95% reference interval are as follows[1]:

$$(x_{(1)}, x_{(7)}) \qquad \text{and} \qquad (x_{(114)}, x_{(120)})$$

Using the data from Table 24.1, the 90% confidence interval for the lower limit of the nonparametric 95% reference interval is (321, 423), and that of the upper limit is (1383, 66592).

VII. OUTLIERS

In an ideal situation all of the data would be from a clearly defined healthy test population and contain no outliers. However, as can be seen from the real data in Table 24.1 this is often not the case. Thus, it is desirable to minimize the effect that the outliers have on the estimation of the reference interval. Many methods of outlier detection have been described in the literature.[21] The NCCLS recommends Dixon's method if outlier detection is desired.[1] In this method, $x_{(n)}$ is identified as an outlier if $x_{(n)} - x_{(n-1)} > (x_{(n)} - x_{(1)})/3$. If $x_{(n)}$ is identified as an outlier then $x_{(n-1)}$ is examined similarly. The process is repeated until no other outliers are found. Using the data from Table 24.1, with $n = 120$, it can be seen that $(66592 - 4537) = 62055 > (66592 - 321)/3 = 66271/3$, or, 22090.33. Next the value of 4537 is tested in the same manner and found to be an outlier as well. Lastly, the value of 2614 is tested and found not to be an outlier. Thus, Dixon's method would identify the two largest values, $x_{(119)}$ and $x_{(120)}$, as outliers.

Another method of identifying outliers is due to Tukey.[22] This method identifies outside values as those that are less than $Q_1 - 1.5 \times IQR$ or greater than $Q_3 + 1.5 \times IQR$, where Q_1 and Q_3 are the lower and upper quartiles and $IQR = Q_1 - Q_3$, the inter-quartile range. It should be noted that for a Gaussian population, only 0.7% of the values lies outside these (population) limits. Using Definition 4 for the quartile estimates, Q_1 is $(x_{(30)} + x_{(31)})/2$, or

496.5, Q_3 is $(x_{(90)} + x_{(91)})/2$, or 814, and the IQR = 814 − 496.5 = 317.5. Thus, this method would identify as outliers those values less than $496.5 − 1.5 \times 317.5 = 20.25$ or greater than $814 + 1.5 \times 317.5 = 1290.25$, i.e., the nine largest values, $x_{(112)}$ through $x_{(120)}$.

Lastly, a method for outlier detection is presented, which was developed for the reference interval problem. This method first transforms the data using the Box-Cox approach (Equation 24.5) and then identifies outliers using the Tukey method on the transformed data.[23] Using this approach on the data from Table 24.1, the two largest values, $x_{(119)}$ and $x_{(120)}$, are identified as outliers.

Dixon's method can fail to identify all of the outliers if they occur in a cluster. This is often referred to as the "masking effect." In other words, if $x_{(n-1)}$ is itself a gross outlier, it can mask the fact that $x_{(n)}$ is a gross outlier. Tukey's method may identify too many observations as outliers if the data are skewed. The last method may identify too few outliers if the outliers cause a transformation that masks their effect. There are no welldefined rules unless strict assumptions are made as to the nature of the underlying population.

For example, consider the data from Table 24.1 with the two largest values deleted as outliers. We will refer to this as the truncated sample. The distribution of the truncated sample can be seen in Figure 24.2 (note that the two largest values were omitted from the histogram so as not to distort the scale). Note, however, Figure 24.3 gives a histogram of the transformed truncated sample. In this case, the Anderson-Darling test[24] of Normality does not reject.

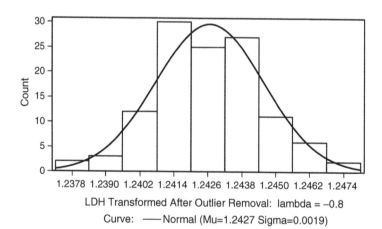

FIGURE 24.3 Histogram of transformed LDH values for female children with fitted Gaussian curve. The two largest values were identified as outliers and removed. The subsequent value of the λ-parameter is approximately = −0.8. The p-value for the Anderson-Darling test is greater than 0.25.

VIII. SUMMARY OF METHODS TO DERIVE REFERENCE INTERVALS

There are a number of choices that can be made to derive reference intervals. These include the nonparametric estimators (as recommended by the NCCLS[1]), traditional Normal theory estimators as well as robust estimators, which may require transformation of the data. Outliers pose a potential problem, and in general, may make the reference interval too wide, thus misclassifying nonhealthy individuals as healthy. Table 24.2 summarizes the results using the data from Table 24.1. We observe that outliers drastically affect the reference interval calculation. As demonstrated in this example outlier detection is necessary. With outliers removed the recommended nonparametric procedure provides reasonably medically conservative limits, i.e., erring on the side of false positives as opposed to false negatives. However, removal of outliers in this case reduces the number of usable observations to the extent that the recommended

TABLE 24.2
Comparison of Reference Interval Estimators for Serum LDH in 120 Young Females

	95% Reference Interval	90% Confidence Intervals	
		Lower Limit	Upper Limit
Results Based on 120 Observations from Table 24.1			
Method			
Nonparametric	(367, 2471)	(321, 423)	(1383, 66592)
Harrel-Davis	(361, 7651)	(332, 409)	(1463, 39498)
Gaussian			
Not Transformed	(0, 13271)	(0, 1547)	(11724, 14818)
Transformed	(351, 1730)	(330, 374)	(1448, 2120)
Robust			
Not Transformed	(361, 1991)	(321, 423)	(1310, 2691)
Transformed	(341, 1668)	(322, 377)	(1372, 2192)
Results Based on 118 Observations from Table 24.1			
Method			
Nonparametric	(357, 1404)	a	a
Harrel-Davis	(352, 1829)	(328, 402)	(1342, 2370)
Gaussian			
Not Transformed	(36, 1357)	(0, 112)	(1271, 1443)
Transformed	(362, 1567)	(343, 383)	(1329, 1894)
Robust			
Not Transformed	(352, 1567)	(337, 383)	(1246, 1859)
Transformed	(359, 1578)	(337, 383)	(1305, 1922)

a Sample size, 118, is too small to compute 90% Confidence Intervals.

90% confidence intervals for the nonparametric limits are not attained. The Gaussian and robust methods are not as adversely affected in terms of confidence interval computation.

We observed that, transforming the data is necessary if Gaussian methods are used, but transformation is not as critical for the robust methods. All of the methods, except for the Gaussian using untransformed data, give reasonable results when the outliers are removed.

In conclusion, if the sample has no outliers removed, or has them removed and is reasonably large (at least 120), then any of these methods should give reasonable reference intervals. (The exception is the Gaussian method on nonNormal data.) However, if the sample size is smaller, then the robust methods should be considered.

REFERENCES

1. National Committee for Clinical Laboratory Standards, How to define and determine reference intervals in the clinical laboratory: approved guideline. NCCLS document C28-A and C28-A2, 1995, 2001.
2. Association, A.D., Type 2 diabetes: diagnosis and lab tests, 2003.
3. Kaplan, L.A., Pesce, A.J., and Kazmierczak, S.C., eds., *Clinical Chemistry: Theory, Analysis, and Correlation*, 4th ed., Mosby, St. Louis, 2003.
4. Solberg, H.E., Approved recommendation (1986) on the theory of reference values. Part 1. The concept of reference values, *Clin. Chim. Acta*, 167, 111–118, 1987.
5. PetitClerc, C. and Solberg, H.E., Approved recommendation (1987) on the theory of reference values. Part 2. Selection of individuals for the production of reference values, *Clin. Chim. Acta*, 170, S1–S12, 1987.
6. Solberg, H.E. and PetitClerc, C., Approved recommendation (1988) on the theory of reference values. Part 3. Preparation of individuals and collection of specimens for the production of reference values, *Clin. Chim. Acta*, 177, S1–S12, 1988.
7. Solberg, H.E. and Stamm, D., Approved recommendation (1988) on the theory of reference values. Part 4. Control of analytical variation in the production, transfer and application of reference values, *Eur. J. Clin. Chem. Clin. Biochem.*, 29, 531–535, 1991.
8. Solberg, H.E., Approved recommendation (1987) on the theory of reference values. Part 5. Statistical treatment of collected reference values: determination of reference limits, *Clin. Chim. Acta*, 170, S33–S42, 1987.
9. Dybkaer, R. and Solberg, H.E., Approved recommendation (1987) on the theory of reference values. Part 6. Presentation of observed values related to reference values, *Clin. Chim. Acta*, 170, S33–S42, 1987.
10. Harris, E.K. and Boyd, J.C., *Statistical Bases of Reference Values in Laboratory Medicine*, Marcel Dekker, New York, 1995.
11. Hogg, R. and Craig, A., *Introduction to Mathematical Statistics*, 5th ed., Prentice Hall, Upper Saddle River, 1995.
12. Box, G. and Cox, D., An analysis of transformations, *J. Roy. Stat. Soc.*, B26, 211–252, 1964.

13. Mosteller, F., On some useful inefficient statistics, *Ann. Math. Stat.*, 17, 377–407, 1946.
14. SAS Institute Inc., SAS OnlineDoc®, Version 8, SAS Institute Inc., Cary, NC, USA, 1999.
15. Harrell, F. and Davis, C., A new distribution-free quantile estimator, *Biometrika*, 69, 635–640, 1982.
16. Davis, P., Gamma function and related functions, In *Handbook of Mathematical Functions with Formulas, Graphs, and Mathematical Tables*, Abramowitz, M. and Stegun, I., eds., Dover Publications, New York, pp. 253–294, 1972.
17. Efron, B., *The jackknife, the bootstrap, and other resampling plans, CBMS-NSF regional conference series in applied mathematics*, Society of Industrial and Applied Mathematics, Philadelphia, p. 92, 1982.
18. Horn, P., Pesce, A., and Copeland, B., A robust approach to reference interval estimation and evaluation, *Clin. Chem.*, 44, 622–631, 1998.
19. Reed, A., Henry, R., and Mason, W., Influence of statistical method used on the resulting estimate of normal range, *Clin. Chem.*, 17, 275–284, 1971.
20. Arnold, B., Balakrishnan, N., and Nagaraja, H., *A First Course in Order Statistics, wiley series in probability and mathematical statistics*, Wiley, New York, p. 279, 1992.
21. Barnett, V. and Lewis, T., *Outliers in Statistical Data*, 3rd ed., Wiley, New York, p. 604, 1994.
22. Tukey, J., *Exploratory Data Analysis*, Addison-Wesley, Reading, p. 688, 1977.
23. Horn, P., Feng, L., Li, Y., and Pesce, A., Effect of outliers and nonhealthy individuals on reference interval estimation, *Clin. Chem.*, 47, 2137–2145, 2001.
24. Stephens, M., Anderson-Darling tests for goodness of fit, In *Encyclopedia of Statistical Sciences,* Volume 1, Kotz, S. and Johnson, N., eds., Wiley, New York, pp. 81–85, 1982.

Index